# The HEART
# & SOUL of
# CHANGE
## Second Edition

# The HEART & SOUL of CHANGE

## Second Edition

### Delivering What Works in Therapy

*Edited by*

Barry L. Duncan, Scott D. Miller,
Bruce E. Wampold, and Mark A. Hubble

American Psychological Association • Washington, DC

Published by
American Psychological Association
750 First Street, NE
Washington, DC 20002
www.apa.org

To order
APA Order Department
P.O. Box 92984
Washington, DC 20090-2984
Tel: (800) 374-2721; Direct: (202) 336-5510
Fax: (202) 336-5502; TDD/TTY: (202) 336-6123
Online: www.apa.org/books/
E-mail: order@apa.org

In the U.K., Europe, Africa, and the Middle East, copies may be ordered from
American Psychological Association
3 Henrietta Street
Covent Garden, London
WC2E 8LU England

Typeset in Goudy by Circle Graphics, Inc., Columbia, MD

Printer: Sheridan Books, Ann Arbor, MI
Cover Designer: Mercury Publishing Services, Rockville, MD
Technical/Production Editor: Harriet Kaplan

The opinions and statements published are the responsibility of the authors, and such opinions and statements do not necessarily represent the policies of the American Psychological Association.

**Library of Congress Cataloging-in-Publication Data**

The heart and soul of change : delivering what works in therapy / edited by Barry L. Duncan . . . [et al.]. — 2nd ed.
    p. ; cm.
    Rev. ed. of: The heart & soul of change / [edited by] Mark A. Hubble, Barry L. Duncan, and Scott D. Miller. c1999.
    Includes bibliographical references and index.
    ISBN-13: 978-1-4338-0709-1
    ISBN-10: 1-4338-0709-2
    1. Psychiatry—Differential therapeutics. 2. Psychotherapy. 3. Strategic therapy.
I. Duncan, Barry L. II. American Psychological Association.
III. Heart & soul of change.
    [DNLM: 1. Psychiatry—methods. 2. Psychotherapy. 3. Decision Making.
4. Mental Disorders—therapy. 5. Treatment Outcome. WM 420 H4365 2010]

    RC480.52.H43 2010
    616.89'14—dc22
                                    2009021158

**British Library Cataloguing-in-Publication Data**

A CIP record is available from the British Library.

*Printed in the United States of America*
*Second Edition*

Dedicated to the memory of Saul Rosenzweig

When, in 1936, I published my first paper on psychotherapy, it was to me just a statement of the obvious which, as we know, is for that very reason, often overlooked. That in the meantime the paper has gained special recognition is, of course, a matter of personal satisfaction. But more important is the fact that others, like Lester Luborsky and now Barry Duncan and Scott Miller[1] have substantiated the statement and have developed the message.

It is thus a privilege to usher in this new edition of *The Heart and Soul of Change*, and this timely event demonstrates that seminal ideas often do mellow with age.

—Saul Rosenzweig (1907–2004)

---

[1]Bruce Wampold and Mark Hubble were not yet a part of the second edition project.

# CONTENTS

Contributors ................................................................ *xiii*

Foreword .................................................................. *xix*
*David E. Orlinsky*

Preface .................................................................. *xxvii*

Prologue: Saul Rosenzweig: The Founder of Common Factors ................. 3
*Barry L. Duncan*

Chapter 1.     Introduction ............................................... 23
               *Mark A. Hubble, Barry L. Duncan, Scott D. Miller,*
               *and Bruce E. Wampold*

**I. What Works and What Does Not:**
**The Empirical Foundations for the Common Factors** ...................... 47

Chapter 2.     The Research Evidence for Common Factors
               Models: A Historically Situated Perspective ............... 49
               *Bruce E. Wampold*

Chapter 3.    Clients: The Neglected Common Factor
              in Psychotherapy ............................................... 83
              *Arthur C. Bohart and Karen Tallman*

Chapter 4.    The Therapeutic Relationship .................................. 113
              *John C. Norcross*

Chapter 5.    Putting Models and Techniques in Context ............... 143
              *Timothy Anderson, Kirk M. Lunnen,
              and Benjamin M. Ogles*

Chapter 6.    Evidence-Based Practice: Evidence or Orthodoxy? .... 167
              *Julia H. Littell*

Chapter 7.    Psychiatric Drugs and Common Factors:
              An Evaluation of Risks and Benefits for
              Clinical Practice ............................................. 199
              *Jacqueline A. Sparks, Barry L. Duncan,
              David Cohen, and David O. Antonuccio*

**II.  Delivering What Works: Practice-Based Evidence** ....................... 237

Chapter 8.    "Yes, It Is Time for Clinicians to Routinely
              Monitor Treatment Outcome" ................................. 239
              *Michael J. Lambert*

Chapter 9.    Outcomes Management, Reimbursement,
              and the Future of Psychotherapy ........................... 267
              *G. S. (Jeb) Brown and Takuya Minami*

Chapter 10.   Transforming Public Behavioral Health Care:
              A Case Example of Consumer-Directed
              Services, Recovery, and the Common Factors ........... 299
              *Robert T. Bohanske and Michael Franczak*

**III.  Special Populations**.................................................. 323

Chapter 11.   Evidence-Based Treatments and
              Common Factors in Youth Psychotherapy ................ 325
              *Susan Douglas Kelley, Leonard Bickman,
              and Earta Norwood*

Chapter 12.   Common Factors in Couple and Family Therapy:
              Must All Have Prizes? .................................... 357
              *Jacqueline A. Sparks and Barry L. Duncan*

Chapter 13.   What Works in Substance Abuse
              and Dependence Treatment ........................ 393
              *David Mee-Lee, A. Thomas McLellan,
              and Scott D. Miller*

**IV. Conclusions** ................................................. **419**

Chapter 14.   Delivering What Works ............................. 421
              *Scott D. Miller, Mark A. Hubble,
              Barry L. Duncan, and Bruce E. Wampold*

Index ...................................................................... 431

About the Editors ............................................... 453

# CONTRIBUTORS

**Timothy Anderson, PhD,** is an associate professor of psychology at Ohio University. His research focuses on a variety of psychotherapy processes, including therapist effects, alliance, in-session emotional experience, and therapist training. He is the 2004 recipient of the Early Career Award from the Society for Psychotherapy Research.

**David O. Antonuccio, PhD,** is a professor in the Department of Psychiatry and Behavioral Sciences at the University of Nevada School of Medicine. A fellow of the American Psychological Association and an American Board of Professional Psychology diplomate in clinical psychology, he is internationally known for his work in depression and smoking cessation. His articles on the comparative effects of psychotherapy and pharmacotherapy have received extensive coverage by the national media. He was named Outstanding Psychologist by the Nevada Psychological Association in 1993, received an award of achievement in 1999 from the Nevada Psychological Association, was awarded the 2000 McReynolds Foundation Psychological Services Award for "outstanding contributions to clinical science," and received the Association for Psychologists in Academic Health Settings Bud Ogel Award for Distinguished Achievement in Research in 2006.

**Leonard Bickman, PhD,** holds the Betts Chair and is professor of psychology, psychiatry, and public policy at Vanderbilt University, where he also directs the Center for Evaluation and Program Involvement. He is the coeditor of two major methods handbooks and the Applied Social Research Methods Series, and he is the editor of the journal *Administration and Policy in Mental Health and Mental Health Services Research.* He has received several national awards, including the Secretary of Health and Human Services Award for Distinguished Service and the education and the research in public services awards from the American Psychological Association. He is a past president of the American Evaluation Association and the Society for the Psychological Study of Social Issues.

**Robert T. Bohanske, PhD,** is the chief of clinical services and clinical training at Southwest Behavioral Health Services in Phoenix, Arizona, where he supervises postdoctoral fellows and psychology residents. He received his doctorate in rehabilitation psychology from the University of Arizona. He holds adjunct faculty positions at Arizona State University, Tempe, and Argosy University, Washington, DC, in clinical psychology and Ottawa University, Ottawa, Ontario, Canada, in professional counseling. He consults with the Arizona Department of Health Services—Division of Behavioral Health as a member of the Best Practices Committee and chair of the Clinical Supervision Committee.

**Arthur C. Bohart, PhD,** is currently affiliated with Saybrook Graduate School and Research Center, San Francisco, California, and is also professor emeritus of California State University, Dominguez Hills. He is a fellow of the American Psychological Association, the author of a number of professional articles and chapters, and the coauthor of *How Clients Make Therapy Work: The Process of Active Self-Healing* (1999).

**G. S. (Jeb) Brown, PhD,** a graduate of Duke University, Durham, North Carolina, is a licensed psychologist residing in Salt Lake City, Utah, where he maintains a part-time psychotherapy practice. For the past 2 decades he has worked to promote outcomes measurement. In 1998, he formed the Center for Clinical Informatics, a consulting group devoted to helping large health care organizations implement outcome-informed care. In 2006, with the encouragement of interested researchers in various academic settings, the Center for Clinical Informatics provided funding and technical assistance for the creation of A Collaborative Outcomes Resource Network (the ACORN Organization, Inc.), a nonprofit organization devoted to fostering collaboration between practitioners and researchers interested in furthering the science and practice of outcome-informed care.

**David Cohen, PhD,** is a professor of social work at the Stempel School of Public Health of Florida International University, Miami, and has also taught in Canada and France. He is the author of more than 120 publications on psychiatric drugs, medicalization, and law and psychiatry. In 2003, he received the Eliot Freidson Award for outstanding publication in medical sociology. Recently, he designed CriticalThinkRx, a publicly funded critical curriculum on psychotropic medications.

**Michael Franczak, PhD,** is the vice president of behavioral health services for the Marc Center in Mesa, Arizona. He received his doctorate in psychology in 1976, and for the past 30 years he has been involved in mental health, substance abuse, and development disability services in Pennsylvania, North Carolina, and Arizona. He was the chief of clinical services for the Arizona Department of Health—Division of Behavioral Health. He has been the primary investigator on numerous grants from the Substance Abuse Mental Health Service Administration, including Housing Approaches for Persons with a Serious Mental Illness, Jail Diversion for Persons with a Serious Mental Illness, Integrated Substance Abuse Mental Health Treatment Models, and System of Care Practices for Children and Adolescents.

**Susan Douglas Kelley, PhD,** is a research associate at the Center for Evaluation and Program Improvement at Vanderbilt University, Nashville, Tennessee. She is also a licensed clinical psychologist and adjunct lecturer for Simmons College, Boston, Massachusetts. She received her doctorate in clinical psychology from Vanderbilt University and completed pre- and postdoctoral training at Children's Hospital Boston; Harvard Medical School, Boston; and Harvard University, Cambridge, Massachusetts. She is a section editor for the journal *Administration and Policy in Mental Health and Mental Health Services Research*.

**Michael J. Lambert, PhD,** is a professor in the Department of Psychology at Brigham Young University, Provo, Utah, where he teaches in the clinical psychology doctoral training program. He is an associate editor of the *Journal of Consulting and Clinical Psychology* and is on the editorial board of numerous scientific journals. He has also served as a consultant to the National Institute of Mental Health and other funding agencies that evaluate the effects of psychotherapy. He is coauthor of the Outcome Questionnaire and Youth Outcome Questionnaire (measures of patient change used in private practice, public mental health, and managed care settings) and editor of the fifth edition of *Bergin and Garfield's Handbook of Psychotherapy and Behavior Change* (2004).

**Julia H. Littell, PhD,** is a professor at the Graduate School of Social Work and Social Research at Bryn Mawr College, Bryn Mawr, Pennsylvania, where she teaches doctoral courses in research methodology and master's courses in human behavior and child welfare. She received her master's and doctorate from the University of Chicago's School of Social Service Administration, Chicago, Illinois. She is editor and cochair of the international Campbell Collaboration's Social Welfare group. She has written numerous articles on psychosocial interventions for families and children and is coauthor of the book *Systematic Reviews and Meta-Analysis* (2008).

**Kirk M. Lunnen, PhD,** received his doctoral degree in psychology from Ohio University, Athens, Ohio. He is currently an associate professor in the Department of Psychology at Westminster College in New Wilmington, Pennsylvania, and the clinical director of People In Need, Inc., a nonprofit community mental health center in New Castle, Pennsylvania. His research interests include psychotherapy process and outcome, instrument development, and the assessment and treatment of depression.

**A. Thomas McLellan, PhD,** is a psychologist, professor of psychiatry at the University of Pennsylvania, Philadelphia, and the CEO of the Treatment Research Institute in Philadelphia. He was educated at Colgate University, Hamilton, New York; Bryn Mawr College, Bryn Mawr, Pennsylvania; and Oxford University, Oxford, England. He has published more than 400 articles and chapters in addiction research and serves as the editor in chief of the *Journal of Substance Abuse Treatment.* He and his colleagues have explored questions such as "What are the active and inactive ingredients of treatment?" and "How do we transfer findings from treatment research into practical applications for the practitioner and provider?"

**David Mee-Lee, MD,** received his medical degree from the University of Queensland, Queensland, Australia, and his psychiatric training affiliated with Ohio State University, Columbus, and Harvard Medical School, Boston, Massachusetts. He is currently involved in full-time training and consulting both nationally and internationally. He has more than 25 years of experience in treatment and program development for people with co-occurring mental and substance use disorders. He is chief editor of the American Society of Addiction Medicine's Patient Placement Criteria, which includes criteria for co-occurring mental and substance-related disorders.

**Takuya Minami, PhD,** is an assistant professor in the Department of Educational Psychology at the University of Utah, Salt Lake City. His research areas are psychotherapy process and outcome, therapist effects, and psychotherapy modeling, particularly within the context of natural clinical settings.

**John C. Norcross, PhD,** is professor of psychology and Distinguished University Fellow at the University of Scranton, Scranton, Pennsylvania; a clinical psychologist in part-time practice; and editor of the *Journal of Clinical Psychology: In Session*. The author of more than 300 publications, he has cowritten or edited 17 books, including *Leaving It at the Office: Psychotherapist Self-Care; Clinician's Guide to Evidence-Based Practice in Mental Health and Addictions; Psychotherapy Relationships That Work;* and *Systems of Psychotherapy: A Transtheoretical Analysis,* now in its seventh edition. Among his awards are the American Psychological Association's Distinguished Career Contributions to Education and Training, Pennsylvania Professor of the Year from the Carnegie Foundation, the Rosalee Weiss Award from the American Psychological Foundation, and election to the National Academies of Practice.

**Earta Norwood, MS,** obtained her bachelor's and master's degrees in psychology from Brigham Young University, Provo, Utah, and is currently pursuing her doctoral degree in clinical psychology at the University of Maryland at College Park.

**Benjamin M. Ogles, PhD,** is currently serving as dean of the College of Arts and Sciences at Ohio University, Athens. He is a clinical psychologist with a long-standing interest in the practical application of therapy research and outcome assessment to practice. He has published a number of articles and chapters regarding various aspects of therapy research, including two books with coauthors about applying outcome assessment methods in practice: *Essentials of Outcome Assessment* (2002) and *Assessing Outcome in Clinical Practice* (1996). With his students and support from the Southern Consortium for Children and the Ohio Department of Mental Health, he developed the Ohio Scales for Youth, which are brief, practical measures of outcome for children receiving mental health services.

**David E. Orlinsky, PhD,** is a professor in the Department of Comparative Human Development, Social Sciences Division, and College at the University of Chicago, Chicago, Illinois; a clinical psychologist in part-time practice; and principal coordinator for the international study of the development of psychotherapists conducted by the Collaborative Research Network of the Society for Psychotherapy Research. The author of many articles and chapters on psychotherapy research, he has cowritten or coedited three books, including *Varieties of Psychotherapeutic Experience, How Psychotherapists Develop,* and *The Psychotherapist's Own Psychotherapy,* as well as the definitive chapter analyzing research on therapeutic process and outcome in four successive editions of *Bergin and Garfield's Handbook of Psychotherapy and Behavior Change.* His awards include those for distinguished career contributions granted by the American Psychological Association Division of Psychotherapy, the Society for Psychotherapy Research, and the Illinois Psychological Society; and the University of Chicago's Quantrell Award for Excellence in Undergraduate Teaching.

**Jacqueline A. Sparks, PhD,** is an associate professor of family therapy at the University of Rhode Island, Kingston. She is a clinical member and approved supervisor of the American Association of Marriage and Family Therapy and is a coauthor of *The Heroic Client* (2004) and *Heroic Clients, Heroic Agencies: Partners for Change* (2002). She has published and presented widely on the overprescription of psychotropic medication for children and the application of client-directed, outcome-informed work with children and families. She is coauthor and research investigator of the Child Outcome Rating Scale and Child Session Rating Scale, and she consults with agencies to transform practices from theory to client-driven services.

**Karen Tallman, PhD,** conducts quantitative and qualitative research to identify successful service practices for Kaiser Permanente in Oakland, California. She has published or presented research in the areas of physician–patient communication, physician job satisfaction, transfer of successful operational practices, cultural interactions, panel management, successful team functioning, physician leadership, drivers of patient satisfaction within ancillary services, and patient responses to various care delivery innovations. She coauthored, with Arthur Bohart, *How Clients Make Therapy Work: The Process of Active Self-Healing* (1999).

# FOREWORD

DAVID E. ORLINSKY

A joke circulated among insiders some years ago about psychotherapy being a field of applied science for which the science that was applied had not yet been developed. The humorous bite of this old joke hit home when it was made in the middle of the last century because it reflected a situation that was largely true at the time. Systematic scientific research on psychotherapy was in its infancy, and there was little beyond traditional clinical theories and illustrative case histories to serve as bases for training and practice. Now, 6 decades later, a substantial body of knowledge does exist, thanks to the efforts of a large and growing number of psychotherapy researchers in many countries. This body of knowledge is based on well-replicated findings about therapeutic processes, outcomes, and clients' characteristics, and thus the situation in which psychotherapists work today is very different. By the end of the 20th century, the real joke (now sad rather than funny) was that too few therapists knew there was a sound scientific foundation for their practice. The great contribution of *The Heart and Soul of Change: What Works in Therapy* when it appeared in 1999 was to systematically digest and present this research to psychotherapists. Research has continued to accumulate rapidly over the past decade. Moreover, to those (like the editors of this volume) who have thought about it, the implications of this research-based knowledge for therapeutic practice have become ever clearer. These are the reasons for a new edition of this volume.

A brief historical sketch of the relationship between psychotherapy research and practice may be in order to help readers appreciate the accomplishment that this volume represents. Systematic empirical research on psychotherapies began as long ago as the late 1940s (e.g., Muench, 1947; Raimy, 1948; Raskin, 1949) and commenced in earnest during the early 1950s (e.g., Eysenck, 1952; Powdermaker & Frank, 1953; Rogers & Dymond, 1954; Snyder, 1953; Wolff & Precker, 1952). Although the field continued to flourish during the 1950s and 1960s, it is probably fair to say that for the first 25 or 30 years of this field's history, studies of psychotherapy taught us more about how to improve our research techniques than they did about how to improve clinical practice. As late as 1969, a leading therapy researcher who contributed as much or more than anyone to this field could publish an article titled "Research Cannot Yet Influence Clinical Practice" (Luborsky, 1969). Clinicians and clinical theorists who had turned expectantly to these early studies for validation or guidance were inevitably disappointed. Many turned away, and for a long time practitioners could afford to disregard research as largely irrelevant to questions of clinical practice.

The tide began to turn in the 1980s with the introduction of meta-analysis (e.g., Smith, Glass, & Miller, 1980) and the publication of the second and third editions of the *Handbook of Psychotherapy and Behavior Change* (Garfield & Bergin, 1978, 1986), which provided comprehensive synopses and syntheses of research results from the preceding decades. Viewed cumulatively, it became apparent that an already massive body of data had established the general effectiveness of psychotherapeutic treatment and had begun to indicate the features of therapy that contributed to its effectiveness (e.g., Orlinsky & Howard, 1986). By the early 1990s, there was compelling reason to reconsider the rift between research and practice, which researchers began to do in the mid-1990s (Aveline & Shapiro, 1995; Talley, Strupp, & Butler, 1994). In the volume titled *Psychotherapy Research and Practice: Bridging the Gap* (Talley et al., 1994), Luborsky's pessimistic outlook of prior years was replaced by a chapter that he now titled "The Benefits to the Clinician of Psychotherapy Research: A Clinician– Researcher's View" (Luborsky, 1994). My own contribution to the same volume was a chapter titled "Research-Based Knowledge as the Emergent Foundation for Clinical Practice" (Orlinsky, 1994). Within 5 years, the first edition of *The Heart and Soul of Change* provided clinicians with an extensive and systematic account of how therapeutic practice should and can be informed by research results (Hubble, Duncan, & Miller, 1999).

From its uncertain beginnings in the mid-20th century, the field of psychotherapy research had truly come of age by the century's end. Indeed, certain findings had been so well replicated that they could be viewed as established facts; for example, findings regarding the therapeutic value of the patient–therapist relationship (Norcross, 2002; chap. 4, this volume). Although research by its nature is open-ended, not given to declaring certainties or making broad generalizations, the accumulated evidence had grown sufficiently to serve as a guide to clinical practice. In the 1st decade of this 21st century, the pace of research on therapy has only increased. Interested clinicians could keep up with some of this new work through occasional articles appearing in newsletters like the *Psychotherapy Networker* (e.g., those collected in Lebow, 2006), but enough has been done since the 1990s to justify this new and enriched second edition of *The Heart and Soul of Change*.

However, this new edition is more than a survey of research findings that have been translated for practitioners. It presents a research-based paradigm of psychotherapy that has emerged as a more accurate alternative to the established but overly narrow, ill-fitting one based on an analogy between psychotherapy and pharmacology (e.g., Orlinsky, 2006; Wampold, 2001; see also chap. 2, this volume). Briefly, the old (and largely still accepted) paradigm assumes that treatment is basically a process of applying psychological techniques to emotional or behavioral disorders, that therapeutic efficacy inheres in the procedures used, that there is a set of optimal procedures for use in treating each disorder, that patients are "carriers" of diagnosable disorders and are more or less cooperative recipients of treatment, and that therapists are more or less discerning diagnosticians and are more or less skillful at administering the optimal procedures for each diagnosed disorder. This view fits well with the individualistic and mechanistic suppositions of modern culture (e.g., Berger, Berger, & Kellner, 1974), which probably accounts for its persistence. Unfortunately, it does not fit very well with 6 decades of accumulated research findings and therefore does not serve very well as a paradigm for psychotherapy.

The alternative paradigm, articulately presented and expertly documented in this volume, holds that therapeutic efficacy inheres primarily in the patient's experience and in the use of a remoralizing, resource-enhancing, and motivating relationship with a therapist who is supportive and challenging (in proportions and at times that suit the patient's needs and abilities). The therapist's procedures are important but become effective largely by contributing to the formation and development of this relationship in the patient's experience.

This view provides a better fit with the cumulative findings of psychotherapy research than does the pharmacological paradigm, as various chapters in this book show. Moreover, this view is grounded implicitly in the following facts of species biology: individuals are born into environments primarily comprising human relationships; for many formative years, individual survival depends on the nurture, discipline, and education provided by relationships;

lives take form and persons grow by participating in relationships that are more or less satisfying and more or less stressful, occurring in social and cultural communities that are more or less cohesive and coherent. From this perspective, it is not surprising to find that relationships that are experienced as discerningly perceptive, genuinely caring, and practically encouraging should be effectively therapeutic.

Implicit recognition of this new paradigm is reflected in the fact that the architects of this new edition have abandoned the traditional distinction between *common factors* and *specific factors* as an organizing framework (in which *specific factors* refers primarily to differences in therapists' procedures or techniques) and have replaced that with a simpler, more inclusive emphasis on *therapeutic factors*. They insist, correctly, that they are not proposing another new theoretical orientation or school of therapy. Rather, they present a comprehensive view of all psychotherapy based on research that demonstrates the factors that contribute to effective change for clients. When described in terms of effectiveness rather than outward forms and arrangements, there is really only one psychotherapy—defined by "what works"—and what works derives from elements that are combined more or less effectively in all forms of therapy.

The idea that there is basically one psychotherapy emphatically does not mean that all forms of psychotherapy are equivalent, nor does it mean that any particular form of therapy is just as well suited (or effective) for all clients and all types of problems. It does not mean that any form of therapy is as well suited as any other to the diverse talents and limitations of particular therapists or can be learned as readily and practiced as effectively by all therapists. There are individual differences among clients in relationship skills and in their ability to be moved by cognitive, affective, imaginal, or enactive aspects of experience. There are also individual differences among therapists in these respects. Some clients are more receptive and ready, with some therapists, using some procedures to engage in and benefit from an effectively therapeutic relationship. Some therapists are more proficient, with some clients, and with some types of problems in creating and cultivating an effective therapeutic relationship. Some procedures are more efficient with some clients, in some circumstances, and in the hands of some therapists in producing and maintaining an effective therapeutic relationship. These are all variables in the therapeutic equation, but the constant in psychotherapy is a relationship, cocreated and sustained by client and therapist, that is applied by clients effectively as a source of corrective influence in their lives.

The findings on which this paradigm is based have implications for practice as well as research. One of the most interesting (and underrated) results of process–outcome research concerns differences between observational perspectives (e.g., Orlinsky, Rønnestad, & Willutzki, 2004, p. 312). There is typically only partial convergence in ratings of therapeutic processes and outcomes by clients, therapists, and external observers—even when focused on what is nominally a fairly specific concept such as empathy—and the same has been found to be true with regard to the evaluation of outcomes. This differs strikingly from epistemological expectations based on the physical sciences, in which high levels of agreement between observers can be achieved and residual disagreements can be statistically discounted as error. Yet lawful relations between process and outcome are found within and between perspectives, indicating that not just measurement unreliability or random errors of observation are at issue. The epistemological situation in the human sciences is simply more complex than in the physical sciences because participant–observers (and external observers, in a different way) are inherently more extensively involved in constructing the reality they observe. In a most basic sense, observations are relative to the perspective from which they are made. Findings validated from one perspective cannot be assumed valid for other perspectives until it has been empirically demonstrated that they are.

Therapists and supervisors cannot assume that impressions and assessments of events in therapy constitute privileged data (i.e., the "expert knows best") or that they know what has really happened because they have participated in a session or witnessed it themselves. They must assume instead that they have access only to part of that reality (their part of it); that there are certainly other legitimate viewpoints in any shared event; and that learning what was experienced by other parties, on the basis of their participation in the event, contributes to a better understanding of what is really happening. This point is made forcefully in the second edition's emphasis on "delivering what works," linked to the practice of routinely monitoring clients' experiences to provide feedback for therapists from the client's perspective (see chap. 8, this volume). This is how therapists can know that the relationships in which they engage with clients are progressing effectively toward therapeutic ends. Integration of perspectives is integral to the new paradigm both in research and in practice.

If these ideas make sense, then read on—for they are lucidly expounded, critically examined, and pragmatically explored in this new edition of *The Heart and Soul of Change*. The evidence supporting these ideas is reviewed and synthesized with practice in mind, and readers will likely find that *The Heart and Soul of Change* will improve their understanding of what is truly therapeutic in the diverse forms of psychotherapy practiced today. Therapists and supervisors will also find an integrative conceptual framework through which to connect what they currently know and do as a therapist or supervisor to a broader range of research and practice that will enable them to know more and do more, without negating the essentials of what they currently know and do.

# REFERENCES

Aveline, M., & Shapiro, D. A. (1995). *Research foundations for psychotherapy practice*. Chichester, England: Wiley.

Berger, P., Berger, B., & Kellner, H. (1974). *The homeless mind: Modernization and consciousness*. New York: Vintage Books.

Eysenck, H. J. (1952). The effects of psychotherapy: An evaluation. *Journal of Consulting Psychology, 16*, 319–324.

Garfield, S. L., & Bergin, A. E. (Eds.). (1978, 1986). *Handbook of psychotherapy and behavior change* (2nd & 3rd eds.). New York: Wiley.

Hubble, M. A., Duncan, B. L., & Miller, S. D. (Eds.). (1999). *The heart and soul of change: What works in therapy*. Washington, DC: American Psychological Association.

Lebow, J. (2006). *Research for the psychotherapist: From science to practice*. New York: Routledge.

Luborsky, L. (1969). Critical evaluation of Strupp and Bergin. Research cannot yet influence clinical practice. *International Journal of Psychiatry, 7*, 135–140.

Luborsky, L. (1994). The benefits to the clinician of psychotherapy research: A clinician–researcher's view. In P. F. Talley, H. H. Strupp, & S. F. Butler (Eds.), *Psychotherapy research and practice: Bridging the gap* (pp. 167–180). New York: Basic Books.

Muench, G. A. (1947). An evaluation of nondirective therapy by means of the Rorschach and other tests. *Applied Psychological Monographs, 13*, 1–163.

Norcross, J. C. (Ed.). (2002). *Psychotherapy relationships that work*. New York: Oxford University Press.

Orlinsky, D. E. (1994). Research-based knowledge as the emergent foundation for clinical practice. In P. F. Talley, H. H. Strupp, & S. F. Butler (Eds.), *Psychotherapy research and practice: Bridging the gap* (pp. 99–123). New York: Basic Books.

Orlinsky, D. E. (2006). Comments on the state of psychotherapy research (as I see it). *Psychotherapy Bulletin, 41*, 37–41.

Orlinsky, D. E., & Howard, K. I. (1986). Process and outcome in psychotherapy. In S. L. Garfield & A. E. Bergin (Eds.), *Handbook of psychotherapy and behavior change* (3rd ed., pp. 311–381). New York: Wiley.

Orlinsky, D. E., Rønnestad, M. H., & Willutzki, U. (2004). Fifty years of psychotherapy process-outcome research. In M. J. Lambert (Ed.), *Bergin and Garfield's handbook of psychotherapy and behavior change* (5th ed., pp. 307–389). New York: Wiley.

Raimy, V. C. (1948). Self-reference in counseling interviews. *Journal of Consulting Psychology, 12*, 153–163.

Raskin, N. J. (1949). Analysis of six parallel studies of the therapeutic process. *Journal of Consulting Psychology, 13*, 206–220.

Powdermaker, F. B., & Frank, J. D. (1953). *Group psychotherapy: Strides in methodology of research and therapy*. Cambridge, MA: Harvard University Press.

Rogers, C. R., & Dymond, R. F. (Eds.). (1954). *Psychotherapy and personality change: Co-ordinated research studies in the client-centered approach*. Chicago: University of Chicago Press.

Smith, M. L., Glass, G. V., & Miller, T. I. (1980). *The benefits of psychotherapy*. Baltimore: Johns Hopkins University Press.

Snyder, W. U. (Ed.). (1953). *Group report of a program of research in psychotherapy*. State College: Pennsylvania State University.

Talley, P. F., Strupp, H. H., & Butler, S. F. (Eds.). (1994). *Psychotherapy research and practice: Bridging the gap*. New York: Basic Books.

Wampold, B. E. (2001). *The great psychotherapy debate: Models, methods, and findings*. Mahwah, NJ: Erlbaum.

Wolff, W., & Precker, J. A. (Eds.). (1952). *Success in psychotherapy*. New York: Grune & Stratton.

# PREFACE

It has been 10 years since the first edition of *The Heart and Soul of Change: What Works in Therapy*[1] was published. Many icons of psychotherapy, instrumental to the ideas in this volume, have died: Saul Rosenzweig, Hans Strupp, Klaus Grawe, George Albee, Jerome Frank, Sol Garfield, and Kenneth Howard, to name a few. This book rides on their shoulders, and we hope that it honors these profoundly influential scholars.

Despite the field's love affair with technique, nearly a half century of empirical investigation has revealed that the effectiveness of psychotherapy resides not in the many variables that ostensibly distinguish one approach from another. Instead, the success of treatment is principally found in the factors that all approaches share in common.

The first edition of this volume created a forum for prominent scholars to present the important findings on these common factors to accomplish two purposes: first, to provide an up-to-date account of what is known about what works in therapy; and second, to articulate how a therapy informed by the

---

[1]Hubble, M., Duncan, B., & Miller, S. (Eds.). (1999). *The heart and soul of change: What works in therapy.* Washington DC: American Psychological Association.

common factors might be operationalized in actual practice, beyond the vague generalities about the importance of a good relationship and creating an expectation for change. The response—incredible sales for an edited book and widespread adoption in graduate training programs—was not only gratifying but also a resounding affirmation of the interest in the common factors among clinicians, academics, and researchers alike. We still find it comforting that to many, the research about what works—the common factors—transcends the dogma eat dogma world of competing schools and the siren call for this magic potion or that silver bullet cure.

In the 10 years that have passed, many things have changed and many have remained the same. A new editor, veteran meta-analytic researcher Bruce Wampold, joined our quest to translate what is known for everyday clinical work. We remain committed to following the data wherever they may take us. Just as our thinking evolved from an allegiance to a preferred model to a common factors perspective, we are now thinking about the common factors in a different way. For one thing, this volume brings the psychotherapist back into focus as a key determinant of ultimate treatment outcome—far more important than what the therapist is doing is who the therapist is. For another, gone are the polemic discussions of common versus specific factors. This book seeks a more nuanced perspective on the interdependence among model–technique and the other factors crucial to outcome. Finally, we have embraced the idea that it is the client's response to treatment that counts. Whether a given therapist or approach is effective can only be determined by the specific outcome emerging from each individual client–therapist pairing. The common factors, or any effective psychotherapy, can only be implemented one client at a time on the basis of that unique individual's perceptions of the progress and fit of the therapy and therapist.

The second edition of *The Heart and Soul of Change* describes this turn in our thinking and demonstrates the power of systematic client feedback to address therapist variability, improve effectiveness and efficiency, and legitimize psychotherapy and substance abuse services to third party payers. Hence the new subtitle: *Delivering What Works in Therapy*. Readers familiar with the first edition will encounter the same pragmatic focus but with a larger breadth of coverage: This edition adds chapters on both youth psychotherapy and substance abuse treatment. *Delivering What Works in Therapy* also challenges the reader to maintain a critical edge via scholarly critique of arguably the two most controversial issues of the day—evidence-based practice and pharmacotherapy—not only in separate chapters but also interwoven throughout the other contributions. Readers are encouraged to scratch below the empirical surface of the common beliefs and assumptions that hold sway over professional discourse.

To add a word here about our biases, we have written extensively about the empirical pitfalls of the medical model as it applies to behavioral and emotional problems.[2,3] As this volume attests, we object to the medicalization of psychotherapy because the data do not support it. Consequently, we have eliminated, as much as possible, references to psychotherapy as a medical endeavor viewing clients as patients with illnesses who require treatment from experts administering powerful interventions. Instead, we aspire for an empirically based account of psychotherapeutic services in proportion to the amount of variance attributed to the different factors and for clients to be described in ways other than their diseases, disorders, deficits, disabilities, or dysfunctions; for psychotherapy to be discussed outside of the language of diagnosis, prescriptive treatment, and cure; and for the identity of mental health and substance abuse professionals to reflect the interpersonal nature of the work as well as the consumer's perspective of the outcome of services.

An undertaking of this magnitude requires the efforts of many individuals, always too numerous to mention. In addition to those acknowledged in other publications, we are especially grateful to our contributors, whose scholarship has taken the discussion about the common factors a healthy step forward. And we owe an incalculable debt to you, our readers, whose enthusiastic responses to *The Heart and Soul of Change* continue to inspire us. Finally, we would be remiss if we failed to mention Susan Reynolds, senior acquisitions editor in the Books department at the American Psychological Association, whose belief in and encouragement of this project were instrumental to its fruition.

[2]Duncan, B., & Miller, S., & Sparks, J. (2004). *The heroic client: A revolutionary way to improve effectiveness through client-directed, outcome-informed therapy* (Rev. ed.). San Francisco: Jossey-Bass.
[3]Wampold, B. E. (2001). *The great psychotherapy debate: Models, methods, and findings.* Mahwah, NJ: Erlbaum.

# The HEART & SOUL of CHANGE

## Second Edition

# PROLOGUE: SAUL ROSENZWEIG: THE FOUNDER OF THE COMMON FACTORS

BARRY L. DUNCAN

There is no new thing under the sun
—Ecclesiastes 1:9

On August 9, 2004, Saul Rosenzweig died at the age of 97. Rosenzweig's prolific accomplishments, more than 225 publications, are notable in surprisingly varied contexts: his seminal discussion of experimenter bias (Rosenzweig, 1933), the correspondence with Sigmund Freud (Rosenzweig, 1985), the Picture-Frustration Study (Rosenzweig, 1976), his response to Eysenck's (1952) critique of psychotherapy (Rosenzweig, 1954), and his *New York Times* acclaimed analysis of Freud's visit to the United States (Rosenzweig, 1992). And of course, germane to the current volume, he published the first known proposal for the common factors, "Some Implicit Common Factors in Diverse Methods of Psychotherapy" in 1936 at the ripe old age of 29 (Rosenzweig, 1936).

Following a discussion of the powerful impact of Rosenzweig's seminal contribution on early common factors theorists, Rosenzweig's classic article is reprinted as part of this prologue so the reader may experience firsthand how far four journal pages can reach. The article laid the groundwork for

From "The Founder of Common Factors: A Conversation With Saul Rosenzweig," by B. L. Duncan, 2002, *Journal of Psychotherapy Integration*, 12, 10–31. Copyright 2002 by the American Psychological Association.

common factors and predicted perhaps the most replicated finding in all of psychotherapy—the dodo verdict—a critical issue evaluated throughout this book. Finally, a conversation with Saul Rosenzweig is presented that sheds light on his sources of inspiration for both the common factors and the first invocation of the dodo bird.[1] His first-person account of the historical context (where and how the common factors journey started) enables readers to more fully appreciate what follows in this book: the current empirical case for the common factors as well as their evolution (see chap. 12, this volume).

## THE BIRTH OF THE COMMON FACTORS

In 1936, writing in the *American Journal of Orthopsychiatry*, Rosenzweig observed that no form of psychotherapy or healing is without cures to its credit. Concluding that success is therefore not a reliable guide to the validity of a theory, he suggested that some potent implicit common factors, perhaps more important than the methods purposely used, explained the uniformity of success of seemingly diverse methods. Rosenzweig summarized these common factors in addition to the therapeutic relationship:

> (1) the operation of implicit, unverbalized factors, such as catharsis, and the yet undefined effect of the personality of the good therapist; (2) the formal consistency of the therapeutic ideology as a basis for reintegration; (3) the alternative formulation of psychological events and the interdependence of personality organization as concepts which reduce the effectual importance of mooted differences between one form of psychotherapy and another. (Rosenzweig, 1936, p. 415)

Four years later, an altogether forgotten panel (notable exceptions: Goldfried & Newman, 1992; Sollod, 1981; Weinberger, 1993) assembled several prominent scholars at the 1940 conference of the American Orthopsychiatric Society. This presentation, the "Areas of Agreement in Psychotherapy," was later published in the *American Journal of Orthopsychiatry* (Watson, 1940). The panelists agreed that more similarities existed between approaches than differences and articulated four areas of agreement: objectives are similar, the relationship is central, the responsibility for choice should be with the client, and the focus should be on enlarging the client's understanding of self. Watson concluded the panel with the following:

> If we were to apply to our colleagues the distinction, so important with patients, between what they tell us and what they do, we might find that

---

[1]I had the great fortune to interview Saul Rosenzweig for a commentary I was writing on his classic piece for the *Journal of Psychotherapy Integration* (Duncan, 2002a, 2002b).

agreement is greater in practice than in theory. . . . We have agreed further . . . that our techniques cannot be uniform and rigid, but vary with the age, problems and potentialities of the individual client and with the unique personality of the therapist. . . . A therapist has nothing to offer but himself [sic]. (p. 29)

Although these points alone make the article well worth the read, who participated in the panel is even more compelling. Saul Rosenzweig outlined his implicit common factors, and Carl Rogers presented about areas of agreement in working with children. Rogers highlighted this panel as recommended reading in his first book, *Counseling and Psychotherapy* (1942), and also referenced Rosenzweig's 1936 paper. It is difficult to say how much Rosenzweig's ideas regarding the qualities of a good therapist influenced Rogers, but Rogers often cited Rosenzweig's work and later invited him to present to his colleagues in Chicago (see below).

Not much else was said about common factors until an interesting study by Heine (1953) foreshadowed later comparative investigations. Heine credited the questions raised by Rosenzweig as providing the impetus to conduct a study that compared several of the prevailing methods of the day. Given comparable results, Heine supported Rosenzweig's analysis by concluding that a common factor (or common set of factors) was operating in the different forms of psychotherapy investigated. Heine suggested that theory and technique are less important than the characteristics of the individual applying them, a conclusion that reiterates the 1940 panel's assertions and has since gained much empirical support (see chap. 2 and 10, this volume).

In a similar vein, speaking about the therapist as a common factor, Rosenzweig (1936) noted:

Since no one method of therapy has a monopoly on all the good therapists, another potentially common factor is available to help account for the equal success of avowedly different methods. (p. 413)

Heine (1953) recommended that the field devote itself to developing a single psychotherapy rather than a variety of psychotherapies. Heine's influential study was often referenced by later scholars, as noted below.

Nineteen years after the original article, Paul Hoch echoed Rosenzweig's words, without reference, in a 1955 article:

If we have the opportunity to watch many patients treated by many different therapists using different techniques, we are struck by the divergencies in theory and in practical application and similarity in therapeutic results. . . . There are only two logical conclusions . . . first that the different methods regardless of their theoretical background are equally effective, and that theoretical formulations are not as important as some unclear common factors present in all such therapies. (Hoch, 1955, p. 323)

Rosenzweig said:

> What . . . accounts for the result that apparently diverse forms of
> psychotherapy prove successful in similar cases? Or if they are only appar-
> ently diverse, what do these therapies actually have in common that
> makes them equally successful? . . . [It is justifiable to wonder . . . whether
> the factors that actually are in operation in several different therapies
> may not have much more in common than have the factors alleged to be
> operating. (Rosenzweig, 1936, pp. 412–413)

In 1957, Sol Garfield, champion of a common factors perspective who
also recently passed away, included a 10-page discussion of the common factors in his book, *Introductory Clinical Psychology* (Garfield, 1957). He identified a number of features common to psychotherapy, including a sympathetic
nonmoralizing healer, the emotional and supporting relationship, catharsis,
and the opportunity to gain an understanding of one's problems. Several of
Rosenzweig's articles were referenced in this text, but his common factors
article was not. Garfield (1986) did reference the 1936 article in a discussion
of his evolution to common factors, but he credited Heine (1953) and Rogers
(1942) for the inspiration of his ideas. Heine and Rogers, as noted, were significantly influenced by Rosenzweig.

The same year, Rogers published the profoundly influential paper "The
Necessary and Sufficient Conditions of Therapeutic Personality Change" in
the *Journal of Consulting Psychology* (Rogers, 1957). That article did not reference Rosenzweig. Given the impact of Rogers's 1957 article, his participation
on the 1940 panel and his association with Rosenzweig loom large as unnoticed
but perhaps dramatic events in the development of psychotherapy. Speaking of
the relationship, Rosenzweig made an interesting comment in his 1936 paper
regarding "the indefinable effect of the therapist's personality" (p. 413):

> Observers seem intuitively to sense the characteristics of the good thera-
> pist time and again . . . sometimes being so impressed as almost to believe
> that the personality of the therapist would be *sufficient* [italics added] in
> itself, apart everything else, to account for the cure of many a patient by
> a sort of catalytic effect. (Rosenzweig, 1936, p. 413)

Although the recognition of the importance of the therapeutic relationship was widespread as early as 1940 (see Watson, 1940), this may be the first
report of the "sufficient" nature of the therapist provided variables that were
popularized by Rogers's groundbreaking 1957 article.

If Rosenzweig wrote the first notes of the call to the common factors,
Johns Hopkins University's Jerome Frank composed an entire symphony.
Frank's profound contributions continue to ring true with modern common
factors theorists, as attested in chapters 2 and 5 of this volume. Frank also has
passed away since publication of the first edition, the third common factors

visionary to do so. His 1961 book, *Persuasion and Healing,* was the first entirely devoted to the commonalities cutting across approaches. He incorporated much of Rosenzweig's brief proposal, but articulated a far more expanded theoretical and empirical context, especially regarding the profound effects of expectation and placebo in healing endeavors. In this and later editions (Frank, 1973; Frank & Frank, 1991), Frank placed therapy within the larger family of projects designed to bring about healing. He (joined by his daughter, Julia, in the 1991 edition of this volume) looked for the threads linking such different activities as traditional psychotherapy, group and family therapies, inpatient treatment, drug therapy, medicine, religiomagical healing in nonindustrialized societies, cults, and revivals. It is interesting that Rosenzweig noted (see below) that his historical research of healing in religious and supernatural contexts as a precursor to psychotherapy also fueled his ideas about the common factors.

In his analysis, Frank (1973) concluded that therapy in its various forms should be thought of as "a single entity" (p. 313):

> To put the issue in terms of an analogy, two apparently very different psychotherapies, such as psychoanalysis and systematic desensitization, might be analogous to penicillin and digitalis—totally different pharmacological agents suitable for totally different conditions. On the other hand, the active ingredient of both may be the same, analogous to two compounds marketed under different names, both of which contain aspirin. I believe the second alternative is closer to the mark. (pp. 313–314).

Frank (1973) concluded that psychotherapy can be thought of a single entity that alleviates "demoralization" in much the same way that aspirin relieves pain.

Frank also identified four features shared by all effective therapies: (a) an emotionally charged, confiding relationship with a helping person; (b) a healing setting; (c) a rationale, conceptual scheme, or myth that provides a plausible explanation for the client's symptoms and prescribes a ritual or procedure for resolving them; and (d) a ritual or procedure that requires the active participation of both client and therapist and that is believed by both to be the means of restoring the client's health.

Similarly, Rosenzweig proposed that model particulars or content was unimportant, even suggesting that the truth value of the particulars of an approach was not critical. Rather, it was the formal consistency that mattered:

> Whether the therapist talks in terms of psychoanalysis or Christian Science is from this point of view relatively unimportant as compared with the formal consistency with which the doctrine employed is adhered to, for by virtue of this consistency the patient receives a schema for achieving some sort and degree of personality organization. (Rosenzweig, 1936, p. 414)

Although Frank's common factors bear a resemblance to Rosenzweig's original formulations, especially the notions of a conceptual scheme and alternative explanation as well as the therapeutic relationship, he is not referenced until the 1991 edition. Frank does reference both Rogers (1942) and Heine (1953) in the 1961 edition. Frank's single entity notion seems akin to Heine's idea of developing a psychotherapy. It is curious that both Garfield (1982) and Frank (1982) contributed to Goldfried's (1982) excellent book on common factors, *Converging Themes in Psychotherapy*, which reprinted Rosenzweig's 1936 paper, but neither referenced him.

Picking up on Frank's significant contributions, the 1970s ushered in a more refined definition of the basic ingredients of psychotherapy, an increased empirical argument for the common factors, several notable common factors approaches, and the empirical confirmation of yet another Rosenzweig brainchild: the dodo verdict (Luborsky, Singer, & Luborsky, 1975).

## THE DODO VERDICT

An inspection of Rosenzweig's classic article reveals a quote from *Alice in Wonderland* used as an epigraph (see his explanation for that choice below). Recall that in *Alice in Wonderland* (1865/1962), Lewis Carroll wrote of a race intended to help dry the animals after they were soaked by Alice's tears. The animals ran off helter-skelter in different directions, and the race was soon stopped. The dodo was asked, "Who has won?" And he finally exclaimed the now famous verdict, "Everybody has won, and all must have prizes." The dodo's pronouncement has become not only a metaphor for the state of psychotherapy outcome research but also a symbol of the raging controversy between those who believe in the privileging of specific approaches for specific disorders on the basis of demonstrated efficacy in randomized clinical trials and those who believe that the evidence does not warrant such privileges: the specific ingredients versus common factors debate.

Few discussions of Rosenzweig's article refer to his creative application of Carroll's famous race. The often perfunctory accounts of Rosenzweig's paper have perhaps missed its most profound element: the clever invocation of the dodo's words to describe the equivalence of effectiveness among psychotherapies. Many have credited Luborsky et al. (1975) for its use in their groundbreaking summation of comparative studies of psychotherapy or Frank's invocation of the dodo's judgment in the 1973 edition of *Persuasion and Healing*.

Rosenzweig's article was remarkably clairvoyant: Luborsky et al. (1975) empirically confirmed Rosenzweig's crystal-ball assessment of psychotherapy some 40 years earlier. Rosenzweig not only predicted more than 70 years of data but also, in 1936, presented the classic argument, still used today, for a common factors perspective: Namely, because all approaches appear equal in effectiveness, there must be pantheoretical factors in operation that overshadow any perceived or presumed differences among approaches. In short, he discussed the factors common to therapy as an explanation for the comparable outcomes of varied approaches. His article represents far more than a historical footnote in the evolution of a common factors perspective and deserves far more than an obligatory tip of the cap reference. Luborsky (1995) noted that the 1936 article "deserves a laurel in recognition of its being the first systematic presentation of the idea that common factors across diverse forms of psychotherapy are so omnipresent that comparative treatment studies should show nonsignificant differences in outcomes" (p. 106).

Mark Twain once defined a classic as a book that people praise but do not read. Many have praised Rosenzweig's classic article without experiencing its true profundity. For a whole new generation of mental health and substance abuse professionals with an affinity toward the common factors, here is the article that started it all.

********** 

## SOME IMPLICIT COMMON FACTORS IN DIVERSE FORMS OF PSYCHOTHERAPY[2]

At last the Dodo said, "Everybody has won, and all must have prizes."
—Lewis Carroll, *Alice in Wonderland*

It has often been remarked upon that no form of psychotherapy is without cures to its credit. Proponents of psychoanalysis, treatment by persuasion, Christian Science and any number of other psychotherapeutic ideologies[3] can point to notable successes. The implication of this fact is not, however, univocal. The proud proponent, having achieved success in the cases he mentions, implies, even when he does not say it, that his ideology is thus proved true, all others false. More detached observers, on the other hand, surveying the whole field tend, on logical grounds, to draw a very different conclusion. If such theoretically conflicting procedures, they reason, can lead to success, often even in similar cases, then therapeutic result is not a reliable guide to the validity of theory.

---

[2]From "Some Implicit Common Factors in Diverse Methods of Psychotherapy," by S. Rosenzweig, 1936, *American Journal of Orthopsychiatry*, 6, 412–415. Reprinted with permission of the Foundation for Idiodynamics, Louise Rosenzweig, director.
[3]*Specific* techniques, such as hypnotism, fall outside the intended scope of the present brief discussion. Only such forms of psychotherapy as are based upon a general theory of personality are here being examined.

It takes but little reflection to arrive at the roots of the difficulty from the standpoint of logical deduction. Not only is it sound to believe that the same conclusion cannot follow from opposite premises but when such a contradiction appears, as seems to be true in the present instance, it is justifiable to wonder (1) whether the factors *alleged to be* operating in a given therapy are identical with the factors *that actually are* operating and (2) whether the factors that actually are operating in several different therapies may not have much more in common than have the factors alleged to be operating.

Pursuing this line of inquiry it is soon realized that besides the intentionally utilized methods and their consciously held theoretical foundations, there are inevitably certain *unrecognized factors* in any therapeutic situation—factors that may be even more important than those being purposely employed. It is possible for the procedures consciously utilized by the therapist to have a largely negative value in distracting attention from certain unconscious processes by means of which the therapeutic effect is actually achieved. Thus it might be conceivably argued that psychoanalysis, for example, succeeds, when it does, not so much because of the truth of the psychoanalytic doctrines about genetic development but rather because the analyst, in the practice of his method, quite unwittingly allows the patient to recondition certain inadequate social patterns in terms of the present situation—a phenomenon better explained by Pavlov's than by Freud's theories. Granting for the purpose of argument that this is the case, then the concepts of Freud are far less proved true by the successful analysis of a patient than are those of Pavlov—and therapeutic result achieved cannot uncritically be used as a test of theory advanced!

While this negative conclusion may be satisfying in some measure, it fails to solve the problem inherent in the fact from which it was derived. What, it is still necessary to ask, accounts for the result that apparently diverse forms of psychotherapy prove successful in similar cases? Or if they are only *apparently* diverse, what do these therapies actually have in common that makes them equally successful? In undertaking to answer these questions, it will be assumed for purposes of exposition that all methods of therapy when competently used are equally successful.[4] This assumption is not well-founded, for certain forms of treatment are very likely better suited than others to certain types of cases. For the present, however, this likelihood, as well as the related problem of determining the criteria for applying one method rather than another to a given patient, will be intentionally disregarded.

In seeking the factors common to diverse methods of psychotherapy the foregoing discussion of implicit procedures should be recalled. Such unverbal-

---

[4]It is by no means being overlooked that there is another far more pressing problem that these notes do not consider—how it is that in so many cases all methods of therapy prove equally *unsuccessful*.

ized aspects of the therapeutic relationship as were there illustrated by the concept of social reconditioning may be equally represented in therapies of quite dissimilar guise. The possibility for catharsis constitutes another example of the same sort. With such potent implicit factors in common, externally different methods of therapy may well have approximately equal success.

Very closely related to such implicit factors is the indefinable effect of the therapist's personality. Though long recognized, this effect still presents an unsolved problem. Even the personal qualities of the good therapist elude description for, while the words *stimulating, inspiring,* etc., suggest themselves, they are far from adequate. For all this, observers seem intuitively to sense the characteristics of the good therapist time and again in particular instances, sometimes being so impressed as almost to believe that the personality of the therapist would be sufficient in itself, apart from everything else, to account for the cure of many a patient by a sort of catalytic effect. Since no one method of therapy has a monopoly on all the good therapists, another potentially common factor is available to help account for the equal success of avowedly different methods.

From the standpoint of the *psychological interpretations* given by therapists of different persuasions, another partial solution of the present problem may be offered. If it is true that mental disorder represents a conflict of disintegrated personality constituents, then the unification of these constituents by some systematic ideology, regardless of what that ideology may be, would seem to be a *sine qua non* for a successful therapeutic result. Whether the therapist talks in terms of psychoanalysis or Christian Science is from this point of view relatively unimportant as compared with the formal consistency with which the doctrine employed is adhered to, for by virtue of this consistency the patient receives a schema for achieving some sort and degree of personality organization. The very one-sidedness of an ardently espoused therapeutic doctrine might on these grounds have a favorable effect. Having in common this possibility of providing a systematic basis for reintegration, diverse forms of psychotherapy should tend to be equally successful.

From a somewhat different approach, though still under the general heading of interpretation, another notion contributing to the solution of the problem suggests itself. There are several steps in the argument. In the first place, psychological events are so complex and many-sided in nature that they may be *alternatively formulated* with considerable justification for each alternative. Under these circumstances any interpretation is apt to have a certain amount of truth in it, applying at least from one standpoint or to one aspect of the complex phenomenon being examined. Hence it is often difficult to decide between various interpretations of the same psychological event: they are all relevant, though perhaps to a greater or less degree, and are all therefore worthy of some consideration.

In the second place, personality seems to consist in an *interdependent organization* of various factors, all of them dynamically related.[5] It is impossible to change any significant factor or aspect of this organization without affecting the whole of it for it is all of a piece. If this description is correct, it follows that in attempting to modify the structure of a personality, it would matter relatively little whether the approach was made from the right or the left, at the top or the bottom, so to speak, since a change in the total organization would follow regardless of the particular significant point at which it was attacked.

If, now, a given method of psychotherapy represents but one alternative formulation of the problem presented, it does not need to be completely adequate from every standpoint and may still be *therapeutically* effective. It needs to have merely enough relevance to impress the personality organization at some significant point and so begin the work of rehabilitation. The interdependence of the personality system will communicate this initial effect to the totality. This line of reasoning should, if true, considerably decrease the therapeutic importance of differences in psychological interpretation and so once more contribute to the explanation of how allegedly diverse methods of psychotherapy prove to have about equal success.[6]

In conclusion it may be said that given a therapist who has an effective personality and who consistently adheres in his treatment to a system of concepts which he has mastered and which is in one significant way or another adapted to the problems of the sick personality, then it is of comparatively little consequence what particular method that therapist uses. It is, of course, still necessary to admit the more elementary consideration that in certain types of mental disturbances certain kinds of therapy are indicated as compared with certain others. Were the problem of psychotherapy being considered in detail here, an attempt would be made to show that the therapist should have a repertoire of methods to be drawn upon as needed for the individual case. It would also be important to discuss the intricate psychodynamics of the relationship between the personality of the patient and that of the therapist in order to determine whether a particular sort of patient would not get along best with a therapist having a particular sort of personality. Even with such additions, however, such room would be left for the foregoing general argument based upon the following considerations which apply in common to avowedly diverse methods of psychotherapy: (1) the operation of implicit, universalized factors, such as catharsis, and the as yet undefined

---

[5]The interdependence of the factors is not incompatible with their "disintegration," as may at first glance appear, because factors that are inharmoniously related ("disintegrated") are nevertheless related within the given individual in some measure. The notion of conflict bears out this statement.

[6]The scientific adequacy of the theory of personality upon which a method of therapy is based is another matter. It is, moreover, not at all implied that a more scientifically adequate theory of personality would not give rise to a more effective method of psychotherapy, now or in the future. The point is simply that completer or absolute truth is by no means necessary for therapeutic success.

effect of the personality of the good therapist; (2) the formal consistency of the therapeutic ideology as a basis for reintegration; (3) the alternative formulation of psychological events and the interdependence of personality organization as concepts which reduce the effectual importance of mooted differences between one form of psychotherapy and another.

\*\*\*\*\*\*\*\*\*\*

## A CONVERSATION WITH SAUL ROSENZWEIG

The following conversation occurred at Rosenzweig's office in St. Louis on October 12, 2000.[7]

> *Barry Duncan (BD):* I am very pleased you consented to having me come out here and talk with you. I must have sounded wacky when I called you. Here I am working on this article about your work, and it was just incredible to find out that . . .

> *Saul Rosenzweig (SR):* You thought I might have been in the other world, huh?

> *BD:* Yes, yes.

> *SR:* Then you would have to get a soothsayer or something to communicate with me. [*laughing*] Where do you want to start?

> *BD:* Who or what inspired you to think about or write about implicit common factors? Did you have a professor, or someone that you had discussed the ideas with?

> *SR:* That's a good place to start. Did you notice the wall hanging there? I call it "the panorama of psychotherapy," and I did that as a graduate student at Harvard Psychological Clinic in approximately 1932, when I got my PhD degree, and thereafter when I became a research associate at the clinic with Dr. Henry Murray. You know that name?

> *BD:* Oh, yes.

> *SR:* Well, he was my mentor at that time, my sponsor for my dissertation. So, have you heard of Christiana Morgan?

> *BD:* Yes.

> *SR:* She was the one that really created the TAT [Thematic Apperception Test]. And, of course, it was there that I became interested in the projective techniques, and I studied frustration as part

---

[7]Edited for clarity and space.

of my dissertation. And that interest evolved into the Picture-Frustration Study. . . . Anyway, at the Harvard Psychological Clinic, which started in 1927, I joined the faculty, the staff there, as a research associate. Christiana Morgan was a colleague of mine at the clinic, and she had a hand in this wall hanging. There are some red places in between the pictures, red vermilion. She painted those vermilion red spots. Then I had the border, which is redwood, imported from California. The carvings were put on there by a wood-burning set by an art student that I knew. At the clinic, there was a patient in occupational therapy. His name was John. He was the one who did the framing of those pictures in the glass. It was really a collaborative work.

BD: Yes.

SR: So as they say, the whole story is here. I had an interest in history and psychotherapy from the very beginning of my career, and so that's why I did it. It begins at the left of the top row, starting with the Hindu god of the mind, Indra, resurrecting a young boy. And the next one, which is the Zodiac man, painted by Brown in 1470, taken from Garrison's famous *History of Medicine*. The third one is the confessional, which is a form of therapy, but in the church. Next is the temple of Aesculapius and the scene in Epidaurus. Aesculapius was the god of health and medicine. People used to sleep in this temple in Greece, and they had dreams. And the priests would ask them about their dreams—a predecessor to Freud's interpretation of dreams. Then King Louis X, the fourth picture, of France, applying the royal touch for the cure of diseases. And then there's Jesus, the fifth one, casting out devils. Keep in mind that I am interpreting all these methods of healing as predecessors of psychotherapy. And then the next one is the Egyptian goddess Isis and her son Horus. Isis restored her son to health from a fatal disease. And then the last one at the top is of an American Indian, a medicine man, in action. Then, as you continue, down at the bottom, at the left, that's a picture of Antoine Mesmer, the discoverer of hypnosis, or animal magnetism. And that shows him with a subject at a séance, who had been hypnotized or mesmerized. The people would sit around holding hands, as well as objects that had been soaked in that magnetized water, and were cured of illnesses, including, of course, hysteria. Next comes Pinel, removing the chains from the insane at the Bicetre. And the next one is the revolving chair for treating the insane. Darwin and Cox invented this in the early 19th century. Erasmus Darwin was the grandfather of Charles Darwin and a famous physiologist–poet. And then the next is an amulet, for overcoming the evil eye, and then a reproduction of Rembrandt's painting of David playing before Saul. The biblical story is that Saul was a man of moods and melancholia and David played music, which soothed him. That was the beginning of music therapy. And then the last one is, of course, the etching by Max Pollock of Freud from the *Menorah Journal*. So it's very nice that I can show this "panorama of psychotherapy" to you because it is relevant to our discussion today.

BD: How so?

SR: The common factors came out of my awareness that there was such a variety of methods trying to reach the mind and doing mental tricks of various kinds—like the evil eye, the royal touch, the revolving chair, and so forth. All seemed to have more in common, implicitly, than not. All those precursors to psychotherapy from the panorama bear a resemblance to each other and later forms of healing like psychotherapy.

BD: Through your historical analysis of psychotherapy, you realized the common elements of all forms of influence and healing. That's interesting because Frank used a similar cross-cultural perspective of healing in his discussion of common factors.

SR: Yes, if I wasn't interested in history I wouldn't have arrived at this. That certainly had a lot to do with it. That combined with my own psychotherapy experiences of what seemed to matter.

BD: I am very curious about how you came up with the quote from *Alice in Wonderland*. Everybody thinks that either Frank or Luborsky originally invoked the dodo's judgment, even though Luborsky says in his article in the second line that you did. I hope this interview finally clears this misconception.

SR: Yes, well, Luborsky called it the "dodo verdict." That's what he said, what he did invent. But it was taken from "Some Implicit Common Factors."

BD: How did you come up with that?

SR: Well, I am very interested in literature and creativity. One of the people I studied was Lewis Carroll. Lewis Carroll, of course, wrote the famous *Alice in Wonderland*. He was actually a professor of mathematics at Oxford, and his real name was Charles Dodgson. I have a very special collection of children's literature. So that's how I knew that material inside and out, and the race is one of the famous incidents in that story which seemed to perfectly fit the state of affairs I was discussing in that article.

BD: So the dodo bird came from your avid interest in literature as it applies to your pursuit of understanding creativity.

SR: Yes, oh yes. I studied literature in terms of creativity. In fact, the foundation which I started a few years ago, the Foundation of Idiodynamics, Personality Theory, and Literary Creativity has grown from that interest. I have analyzed, via my idiodynamics, the work of the Henry James Sr. family, Dodgson, and even Freud.

BD: I thought at first that the common factors article just stood by itself. But the more I investigated the more I saw that was a misconception I had formed from only seeing the 1936 article referenced in the common factors literature. That misconception is conveyed in our common factors book, and I will be sure to correct it in the second edition.

SR: Oh sure, that's natural, with a first edition. You always find new things after you have gone to print. I want to emphasize that my thinking evolved from there; That 1936 article was a start of a process that never stopped for me, that took me many different places.

BD: So after the '36 paper, what was the reaction?

SR: Well, I'll tell you a story that characterizes a lot of the reaction: There was a psychiatrist that I worked with at Worcester Hospital, Jacob Kasanin, and he walked in my office holding the issue of the journal in his hand and said only "Fools rush in where angels fear to tread." [*Both laugh.*] I think he meant that it was controversial to challenge the special validity that each psychotherapy believed it held.

BD: It still is, if you can believe that.

SR: Not surprising, really. Psychotherapy models and their followers are more like cults: charismatic leaders with legions of worshippers. [*Both laugh.*]

BD: Next came the 1937 paper "Schools of Psychotherapy: A Complementary Pattern." You seem to take a different angle but in the same direction.

SR: That's right. "Implicit Common Factors" spoke to the commonalities that all approaches shared, and "Schools" spoke to the complementarities that existed among approaches. "Implicit Common Factors" also spoke to complementarities in some ways, especially in the discussion of the many different types of interpretations from differing orientations that can be correct.

BD: In the "Schools" paper, you make a strong case for a relatively simple underlying pattern of complementarity based on each approach's specific representation of a problem, special methodology, and preferential alliance with other sciences. You argue to "unite the warring factions" of psychology through their complementarity and render the disagreements among them as "arbitrary and unnecessary." Not one to avoid controversy, you also said, "Schools have been committing a 'fallacy of arrogation,' i.e., exploiting their concepts by unduly subordinating to them phenomena for which they were not originally intended and for which they are not really adequate." That article has great relevance to today.

SR: Yes, exactly, all of my early articles stressed different types of complementarity. Those early articles led me to idiodynamics, but I didn't use that term until '51. Actually, the first form of complementarity that I discussed was between experimenter and experimentee (Rosenzweig, 1933). The 1936 paper was the second type, and the "Schools" paper was yet another. The "Schools" paper showed that the division of labor among the five then current schools represented a complementary pattern in which a certain type of problem achieved acceptable resolution by methods and concepts appropriate to the problem emphasized. When I wrote that paper, Niels Bohr, the Scandinavian physicist, was an inspiration regarding complementarity. He introduced a similar way to solve seemingly irreconcilable theories in physics. In 1927, the principle of complementarity was formulated as an alternative to Heisenberg's "indeterminacy" and as a new way of reconciling the conflicting conceptions of light as consisting of waves, on one hand, or particles, on the other. To Bohr, both formulations were justified and were equally correct once it was recognized that each was served by a different observational approach. So that notion of complementarity was at the heart of my own thinking.

BD: How did the 1940 panel come together?

SR: Goodwin Watson organized it.

BD: That panel is all but forgotten. You know that two of the three references I found to it, Carl Rogers is not even mentioned, and in one of the references, you are not mentioned.

SR: Yes, yes. Things fall through the cracks often, only to resurface later.

BD: You elaborated on the importance of the faith of the client in the therapist and the method and the notion of fitness. You said that the content of the interpretation or approach was secondary to the common factors and that the correctness actually had more to do with the fitness for a specific client.

SR: Yes, and that actually was one of the conclusions of the panel, about the uniqueness of the individual. So the fit of the interpretation or method is obviously of great importance, more so than its correctness.

BD: Do you recall your interactions with Carl Rogers? Rogers gives a fair amount of emphasis to the impact of that panel on his thinking.

SR: Yes, I remember one time when I visited at his invitation, he was in Chicago at the time and I gave a talk. That must have been like 1945.

BD: Rogers referenced you and the panel in his 1942 book, his first book, and then he referenced you in later works as well, so I think that your view of common factors were an influence on him, and perhaps your interest in the individual reinforced his ideas as well.

SR: Oh yeah, he was interested in those ideas.

BD: So you moved on from there and laid more groundwork for idio-dynamics through your analysis of Murray, Allport, and Lewin and again with an emphasis on complementarity. You were always moving on to new projects, taking your ideas to the next level, and expanding into new areas, but continually weaving in comple-mentarity, history, and literature.

SR: Yes, that's accurate. There actually [were] a couple of other common factors works. A 1938 paper, "A Dynamic Interpretation of Psychotherapy Oriented Towards Research" published in *Psychia-try: Journal of the Biology and Pathology of Interpersonal Relations*.

BD: In that paper you elaborate, like your 1940 panel presentation, more on the faith of the client in the therapist and emphasize the importance of not only recognizing common factors but also researching them. Prophetic words indeed.

SR: The other one is a book I put together in 1951 called *Facets of Psychotherapy*, which brought my collected papers about common factors together as well as other ideas I had about psychotherapy. It went through various revisions and title changes, but it ultimately died in committee so to speak.

BD: Well, you went on to the next thing and didn't want to go back.

SR: That's it, that's exactly it. By the time I got to the next thing, I saw the other as being over with.

BD: That book, *Facets of Psychotherapy*, would have predated all the famous books about common factors, like Jerome Frank's, which came out in '61.

SR: Yes, yes. Well, that is the way it works.

BD: So one thing that I am painting here, and I realize that it's me doing the painting, is that all the common factors roads led back to you in some way or another. I don't know if you are familiar with the trivia game about Kevin Bacon, the actor. The game is called Six Degrees of Kevin Bacon. The theme of the game is to trace any actor to a movie with Kevin Bacon within six connections. So one thing that I am getting from my investigation of the literature and my discussion with you is that many of the people we typically associate with common factors have some connection to you. Like Jerome Frank.

SR: Yes, I went to Harvard with him and had associations with him.

BD: Carl Rogers.

SR: I presented with Carl Rogers in 1940 and spoke to his group in 1945.

BD: Sol Garfield.

SR: He was here at Washington University. He is professor emeritus also.

BD: And you knew Paul Hoch as well.

SR: Yes, well actually those things, I mean people interacted but that doesn't mean that they read everything that I published.

BD: True. So the fact that there is a gap in referencing you is not really a problem for you.

SR: No, because that is the way that it works. I don't think that the citation of my work is that important. A lot of the same influences that influenced me influenced them, except, perhaps, that they didn't have the same interest in history and literature, which brought me to many different places. But I don't like to stress that because I don't know that it's that important, and these people wound up publishing a lot more on the common factors topic than me. And a lot of times, people read things and take things in and forget where ideas come from. That's natural.

BD: Okay, but historically it's important because it seems that after a lull in discussion about common factors, a whole new generation of common factors theorists started writing and saying many things that you said.

SR: That was true even more so about my first paper, the 1933 paper. That paper was published in *The Psychological Review* and delineated the influences between the experimenter and the experimentee. I pointed out the biases of the experimental relationship, which were later explored by Orne and Rosenthal regarding demand characteristics and experimental bias. Those were discovered separately by others, and they didn't cite my paper either.

BD: Okay.

SR: But Rosenthal was very aware of that and called me about 2 years ago. He said that he was just going to give a speech to accept an award from the Society of Experimental Social Psychology. He said that he wanted me to know that at the beginning of the speech he was going to give me credit, that I should really be getting the award.

BD: Well, he could send you the award. [*Both laugh.*]

SR: Well, like I said, it has never really been that important to me, never has been. By the time someone was not referencing me, I was on to the next thing. This isn't about citations to me.

BD: It's fascinating that you wrote two papers in the 30s that were very influential, but initially unrecognized, and others get credit, and then the field finally starts recognizing you.

SR: Well, often people read something that interests them and then they forget the source. That's natural, that's the way things go. And then sometimes people don't cite what came before because they think it lessens their own contribution. . . . Actually, the way the universe evolves, in the end, what will it matter anyway, who said what and when, when I am dead and buried? My passion lies in my current work. The joy is in the moment of discovery. . . . And maybe, somewhere down the line, someone will pick up on it—if they reference me fine, if not, that is the way it goes. I doubt if I'll notice when it is all said and done.

## CONCLUSION

As you experience the evolution of a common factors perspective depicted in this volume, you are invited to reflect on Rosenzweig's seminal article, how it inspired the early theorists most often revered by later common factors visionaries, and how the ideas still strongly resonate among today's researchers and scholars.

To his memory and in his honor, this book is dedicated to the founder of common factors, Saul Rosenzweig: Someone did pick up your ideas, and we are forever grateful.

## REFERENCES

Duncan, B. L. (2002a). The founder of common factors: A conversation with Saul Rosenzweig. *Journal of Psychotherapy Integration, 12,* 10–31.

Duncan, B. L. (2002b). The legacy of Saul Rosenzweig: The profundity of the dodo bird. *Journal of Psychotherapy Integration, 12,* 32–57.

Eysenck, H. (1952). The effects of psychotherapy: An evaluation. *Journal of Consulting Psychology, 16,* 319–324.

Frank, J. D. (1961). *Persuasion and healing*. Baltimore: Johns Hopkins University Press.

Frank, J. D. (1973). *Persuasion and healing* (2nd ed.) Baltimore: Johns Hopkins University Press.

Frank, J. D. (1982). Psychotherapy in America today. In M. R. Goldfried (Ed.), *Converging themes in psychotherapy* (pp. 78–94). New York: Springer Publishing Company.

Frank, J. D., & Frank, J. B. (1991). *Persuasion and healing* (3rd ed.). Baltimore: Johns Hopkins University Press.

Garfield, S. L. (1957). *Introductory clinical psychology*. New York: Macmillan.

Garfield, S. L. (1982). What are the therapeutic variables in psychotherapy? In M. R. Goldfried (Ed.), *Converging themes in psychotherapy* (pp. 135–142). New York: Springer Publishing Company.

Garfield, S. L. (1986). An eclectic psychotherapy. In J.C. Norcross (Ed.), *Handbook of eclectic psychotherapy* (pp. 132–162). New York: Brunner/Mazel.

Goldfried, M. R. (1982). *Converging themes in psychotherapy*. New York: Springer.

Goldfried, M. R., & Newman, C. F. (1992). A history of psychotherapy integration. In J. C. Norcross & M. R. Goldfried (Eds.), *Handbook of psychotherapy integration* (pp. 46–93). New York: Basic.

Heine, R. W. (1953). A comparison of patients' reports on psychotherapeutic experience with psychoanalytic, nondirective and Adlerian therapists. *American Journal of Psychotherapy, 7,* 16–23.

Hoch, P. (1955). Aims and limitations of psychotherapy. *American Journal of Psychiatry, 112,* 321–327.

Luborsky, L. (1995). Are common factors across different psychotherapies the main explanation for the Dodo bird verdict that "everyone has won so all must have prizes"? *Clinical Psychology: Science and Practice, 2,* 106–109.

Luborsky, L., Singer, B., & Luborsky, L. (1975). Comparative studies of psychotherapies: Is it true that "everyone has won and all must have prizes"? *Archives of General Psychiatry, 32,* 995–1008.

Rogers, C. (1942). *Counseling and psychotherapy*. Boston: Houghton Mifflin.

Rogers, C. (1957). The necessary and sufficient conditions of therapeutic personality change. *Journal of Consulting Psychology, 21,* 95–103.

Rosenzweig, S. (1933). The experimental situation as a psychological problem. *Psychological Review, 40,* 337–354.

Rosenzweig, S. (1936). Some implicit common factors in diverse methods of psychotherapy. *American Journal of Orthopsychiatry, 6,* 412–415.

Rosenzweig, S. (1937). Schools of psychology: A complementary pattern. *Philosophy of Science, 4,* 96–106.

Rosenzweig, S. (1938). A dynamic interpretation of psychotherapy oriented towards research. *Psychiatry, 1,* 521–526.

Rosenzweig, S. (1951). *Facets of psychotherapy*. Unpublished manuscript.

Rosenzweig, S. (1954). A transvaluation of psychotherapy: A reply to Hans Eysenck. *Journal of Abnormal and Social Psychology, 49*, 298–304.

Rosenzweig, S. (1976). Aggressive behavior and the Rosenzweig Picture-Frustration (P-F) Study. *Journal of Clinical Psychology, 32*, 885–891.

Rosenzweig, S. (1985). Freud and experimental psychology: The emergence of idiodynamics. In S. Koch & D. Leary (Eds.), *A century of psychology as science* (pp. 135–207). New York: McGraw-Hill.

Rosenzweig, S. (1992). *Freud, Jung, and Hall the king-maker: The expedition to America (1909)*. Seattle: Hogrefe & Huber.

Sollod, B. (1981). Goodwin Watson's 1940 conference. *American Psychologist, 36*, 1546–1547.

Watson, G. (1940). Areas of agreement in psychotherapy. *American Journal of Orthopsychiatry, 10*, 698–709.

Weinberger, J. (1993). Common factors in psychotherapy. In J. R. Gold & G. Stricker (Eds.), *Comprehensive handbook of psychotherapy integration* (pp. 43–56). New York: Plenum Press.

# 1

# INTRODUCTION

MARK A. HUBBLE, BARRY L. DUNCAN,
SCOTT D. MILLER, AND BRUCE E. WAMPOLD

It was the best of times, it was the worst of times, it was the age of wisdom, it was the age of foolishness, it was the epoch of belief, it was the epoch of incredulity.

—Charles Dickens, *A Tale of Two Cities*

Dickens, starting his celebrated novel, used the rhetorical device called *anaphora:* the repetition of a word or words at the beginning of two or more successive clauses or sentences. In so doing, he created a cadence that not only makes the passage more memorable—some might say immortal—in the annals of literature but also intensifies the emotions he intends to evoke in his readers. *A Tale of Two Cities*, as the opening foreshadows is in part a story of dualities, set in a revolution at a defining moment in history. For many, this moment meant opportunity, hope, a promise of change and modernization, and a long-awaited shift in authority and control from the privileged to those disenfranchised. For others, it was nothing more than turmoil, uncertainty, loss of power, folly, the fall of the old order, and financial ruin.

At first blush, citing Dickens's reasoned use of language and the French Revolution might be seen as far removed from contemporary psychotherapy and a singular approach to introducing the second edition of *The Heart and Soul of Change*. Of course, students of the work of the late psychiatrist and prominent exponent of common factors, Jerome Frank (1961, 1973), and that of Frank and his daughter Julia (Frank & Frank, 1991), would not find any reference to rhetoric out of place in the present context. Frank maintained that psychotherapists and rhetoricians both rely on the stimulation of emotions and additional, shared methods to persuade and influence others to achieve improvements in personal well-being (Frank & Frank, 1991, p. 68). As in the first edition, how therapists, in partnership with their clients, achieve what they do is at the very center of this volume.

The struggles experienced and endured in the profession of psychotherapy hardly compare with the great adventure called the French Revolution. Yet, it is true that in this period of our history, it is the "best of times" and the "worst of times." This is neither a cliché nor a literary technique. Over the past decade, advances in knowledge and social changes congenial to the practice of psychotherapy are contrasted to instability, monetary anxieties, and a crisis of confidence. To date, the solutions proposed to address this dilemma are falling far from the mark. How this state of affairs has come about and what it bodes for our future is a matter of considerable debate. We are at the point that knowing what works in therapy is not enough. Delivering what works, the subtitle of this edition, is the next revolutionary step. In stark terms, taking this step is critical both for the continued success of psychotherapy as a profession and for the clients we serve.

This introductory chapter begins with a summary of the current status of the field of psychotherapy: the encouraging developments (the best of times) and the areas of concern (the worst of times). We then present briefly an integrated model of the common factors. The ensuing chapters elucidate its structure. In so doing, we avoid the dichotomy of common versus specific factors, to the extent possible, to emphasize aspects of psychotherapy that are responsible for the benefits clients experience. Our principal intent in this volume is to focus on what is therapeutic and how to deliver what works for each and every client. It is proposed that practice-based evidence brings accountability to the practice of psychotherapy and improves the quality of services.


THE BEST OF TIMES

A discussion of the circumstances—fortunate or favorable for the field—comes first. It is by no means exhaustive or intended as comprehensive, and the order of the review is not determinative of importance. Rather, it summarizes the major positive changes seen since the publication of the first edition of *The Heart and Soul of Change* (Hubble, Duncan, & Miller, 1999b).

**The Decline of "Model Mania"**

If anything can be said of psychotherapy, it is maturing. The days when models and theories arrived and were pursued with all the alacrity that only the latest designer drugs could excite on the streets are over. New therapeutic approaches are still emerging, but the fire for the novel, different, and exotic therapies has for the most part been extinguished.

The University of Chicago's David Orlinsky has provided insight into the reasons for a downturn in model development. Citing Thomas Kuhn, author of *The Structure of Scientific Revolutions* (1970), Orlinsky (2006) suggested that psychotherapy has moved from the earliest stage of science, termed *preparadigmatic*, to the next, termed *normal science*. Thirty years ago, Orlinsky and Howard (1978) tendered that "the difficulties encountered in [the] earliest stage of science arise not from the absence of a model for research, but from the multiplicity of basic models dividing the allegiances of researchers" (p. 283). When the foregoing observation was made, *schoolism*—that is, immersion in and loyalty to a therapeutic orientation (be it psychoanalytic, behavioral, cognitive, etc.)—was the rule of the day. Those entering the field at that time tended to "work within one or another of these competing orientations, according to personal preference and the historical accidents of their training and work environs" (Orlinsky & Howard, 1978, p. 283). It is not surprising that debates were rampant and discourse was of the puerile "mine's better" sort. In this period, Strupp (1978) suggested that a newcomer's first impression of modern psychotherapy was bound to be bewilderment. One would observe "a welter of theories and practices that seemingly have little in common . . . ; a mélange of practitioners whose philosophical leanings, training, and activities are grossly divergent . . . ." (p. 3). So much disagreement provided fertile ground for the sincere, the ambitious, or the merely narcissistic to advance new therapies and inflate assertions of their effectiveness.

Gradually, the field of psychotherapy has "settled down," for lack of any better way to characterize this change. In particular, with the great "battle of the brands" (Hubble, Duncan, & Miller, 1999c, p. 5) waning, Orlinsky (2006) posited that the profession has entered a stage of "normal science":

> Research by and large has become devoted to incrementally and systematically working out the details of a general "paradigm" that is widely accepted and largely unquestioned. The research paradigm or standard model involves the study of (a) manualized therapeutic procedures (b) for specific types of disorder (c) in particular treatment settings and conditions. This is very different from the field that I described three decades ago (Orlinsky & Howard, 1978) as "pre-paradigmatic."(p. 2).

His assessment of this evolution, however, does not imply endorsement. Orlinksy (2006) made abundantly clear in his essay that despite an "implicit paradigmatic consensus," as the turnaround in the science might imply, the field is at risk of trapping itself in a "constricted and unrealistic model" (p. 2). For the purposes of the present discussion, it is sufficient to say that this phase or current instantiation of normal science has helped quash model propagation. (Further elaboration and critiques of this "unrealistic model"—as embodied in much of the empirically supported treatment movement—are found throughout this volume, with a pointed and detailed evaluation provided by Wampold in chap. 2.) Even so, the attenuation of proliferation does not reduce the threat that one existing model, say cognitive–behavioral treatments, might be privileged over other, well-established treatments, such as humanistic and psychodynamic approaches (Wampold & Bhati, 2004).

## No More Stigma

Concomitant with the profession standing down from its faddist pursuit of new treatments, another welcome change has come about. Specifically, the stigma associated with psychotherapy and psychological complaints has significantly decreased (Slife, Williams, & Barlow, 2001). A recent survey by the American Psychological Association (APA) attests to this fact (Penn, Schoen, & Berland Associates, 2004). When queried in the APA's 2004 poll, more than 9 in 10 Americans (91%) said they were likely to consult a mental health professional or recommend that a family member do so if they or a family member were experiencing a problem. The same percentage stated they would opt for a mental health professional who would emphasize talk therapy as a first course of action rather than medication. Of the respondents, 30% said they would be concerned about others finding out if they had consulted with a mental health professional, and only 20% identified stigma as a very important reason for not choosing to seek assistance. Of 12 possible reasons for not seeing a mental health professional, stigma and concerns about others' opinions ranked, in order, 11th and 12th. Lack of insurance coverage and cost of treatment were at the top of the list.

The "Therapy in America 2004" Harris Poll, acclaimed as the first of its kind to examine consumer trends and attitudes toward mental health treatment in this country, yielded similar findings (Harris Poll, 2004). On the basis of these results, the sponsors (*Psychology Today* and PacifiCare Behavioral Health) concluded that psychologically informed treatment had become an important part of American life. In effect, psychotherapy had gone mainstream, as evidenced by the following results. First, more than 1 in 4 American adults (27% of adults, or an estimated 59 million people) had received treatment for a mental health problem in the 2 years preceding the poll, through talk therapy, medication, or a combination of the two. Almost half of those surveyed (49%) knew someone who has been in treatment, and approximately two thirds (61%) said they did not view the choice to receive therapy as a mark of character weakness. Close to 4 out of 5 (79%) respondents believed that if a coworker were in therapy it would make no difference in his or her ability to do the job, and 7% of respondents said it would actually make the coworker better able to do the job. Forty percent of adults thought that their parents would have benefited from therapy. As to stigma, just 22% expressed the fear that therapy would go on their "record," and 19% were concerned that family or friends could find out if they attended therapy.

## The Profession Grows and Diversifies

Hand in hand with psychotherapy's greater acceptance in society, more and more people are entering the mental health professions. Since the publication of the first edition of this volume, the number of mental health practitioners has nearly doubled. The latest estimate pins the total at more than 800,000 (see chap. 9, this volume), with an additional 200,000 in the substance abuse field (Mulvey, Hubbard, & Hayashi, 2003). With this increase, the demographics are changing. In psychology, for example, women are becoming the majority, a development seen in other mental health professions and not only in the United States but also in Europe and Latin America. The entry of minorities into psychology and the other professions has grown as well, which reflects a change to be more representative of the culture at large. For example, the 2008 report from the APA Commission on Ethnic Minority Recruitment, Retention, and Training in Psychology indicated that between 1998 and 2003, minority student affiliate membership increased by 28.7% (APA, Office of Ethnic Minority Affairs, 2008). Additionally, between 1996 and 2004, ethnic minority recipients of master's degrees in psychology increased by 90.8%, and ethnic minority doctoral recipients in psychology increased by 16.6%. Whether these changes in the overall numbers of clinicians, including the composition of the workforce, speak to an affirmation of psychotherapy or to perceived opportunities for a career, we see here further evidence of therapy viewed as a viable and vital profession.

## It Works

More good news: Psychotherapy continues to prove its effectiveness. The weight of quantitative studies consistently produces an effect size of about 0.8 standard deviations, which means the average treated person is better off than 80% of those who do not have the benefit of treatment (see chap.2, this volume; Lambert & Ogles, 2004; Wampold, 2007). These substantial benefits extend from the laboratory to everyday practice. For example, Minami et al. (2008) found clinicians in a managed care context attained effects that were comparable with those reported in randomized clinical trials for the treatment of depression. Furthermore, a real world study in the United Kingdom (Stiles, Barkham, Mellor-Clark, & Connell, 2008) comparing cognitive–behavioral therapy (CBT), psychodynamic therapy, and person-centered therapy as routinely practiced reported large effects comparable to those attained in clinical trials.

When such findings are contrasted with results widely heralded as advances in the medical arena, psychotherapy yields significant benefits hand over fist. Rosenthal (1990) pointed out, for instance, that the large-scale clinical trial of aspirin as a prophylaxis for heart attacks produced an effect size of .03 (compared with .80 for psychotherapy as a treatment for mental health problems). It is interesting that the magnitude of the effect was thought to be so astonishing that the trial was stopped prematurely because it was decided that delivering the placebo was unethical. Such findings are not the result of cherry-picking studies from the literature. In medicine, comparatively meager outcomes are the rule rather than the exception (e.g., statins for reducing heart attacks; Carey, 2008; Lambert et al., 2003; see also Wampold, 2007, and chap. 2 of this volume).

## Common Factors Come of Age

From the very beginning of psychotherapy, speculation has abounded on what causes change. With some notable exceptions (e.g., Allen Bergin, Jerome Frank, Sol Garfield, Michael J. Lambert, Saul Rosenzweig), most of the discourse has championed methods derived from theoretical approaches. The abiding faith that specific treatments that target particular psychological disorders—a kind of psychological formulary—have been or will be developed is remarkably strong. And why not? The prospect of having on hand a special psychological intervention for a given problem is very appealing (Hubble & Miller, 2004). Also, that therapists might possess the equivalent of a pill for emotional distress is one that resonates with the public and policymakers, both in government and in the insurance industry. Notwithstanding, after more than 40 years of research, evidence that specific ingredients are needed for resolving particular disorders remains conspicuously missing. The conclusion is inescapable: "Psychotherapy does not work in the same way as medicine" (Miller, Duncan, & Hubble, 2005, p. 22; see also Wampold, 2001, 2007; and chap. 2, this volume). Bluntly put, the existence of specific psychological treatments for specific disorders is a myth.

By contrast, the empirical case for the common factors is compelling. In professional parlance, *common factors* refer to ingredients or elements that exist in all forms of psychotherapy. These shared, curative factors drive the engine of therapy. The body of research amassed on the subject since the publication of the first edition of *The Heart and Soul of Change* affirms that a core group of factors shared by all treatment approaches is responsible for change. It also calls for a major reconceptualization of psychotherapy, with particular emphasis on what constitutes the pantheoretical ingredients, how they are structured, and the way in which they interact to foster positive outcomes. Owing to the importance of these developments, an entire section (What Works in Therapy Redux) is devoted to their discussion later in this chapter.

## Evidence-Based Practice Defined

Amid the evidence-based practice movement in medicine and other health professions, APA President Ronald Levant appointed the Presidential Task Force on Evidence-Based Practice (hereafter Task Force) in 2005. The Task Force (2006) defined *evidenced based practice* in psychology as "the integration of the best available research with clinical expertise in the context of patient characteristics, culture, and preferences" (p. 273). The APA policy reflected the "best of times" because it recognized the importance of clinical expertise, defined *evidence* broadly, and considered the client's contribution.

The first part of the definition regarding best research evidence was constructed to include "scientific results related to intervention strategies, assessment, clinical problems, and patient populations in laboratory and field settings as well as to clinically relevant results of basic research in psychology and related fields" (Task Force, 2006, p. 274). Of importance, primacy was not given to randomized clinical trials aimed at establishing the superiority of a particular treatment, as has been the standard in establishing empirically supported treatments, and the types of research that are used to investigate the importance of the common factors were honored.

Evidence-based practice recognizes the therapist as a critical element in the therapeutic equation through the importance of clinical expertise. That is, interpersonal skill—combined with the competence attained through education, training, and experience—forms an essential part of psychotherapy. Clinical expertise also includes using the best research evidence in practice. One purpose of this volume is to show how research evidence can lead to better outcomes in psychotherapy.

The third component of the definition recognizes the importance of the client's characteristics, culture, and preferences. This entails what the client brings to the therapeutic stage, as well as the fit of any intervention with the client's expectations. As indicated in the APA policy, "Services are most effective when responsive to the [client's] specific problems, strengths, personality, sociocultural context, and preferences" (Task Force, 2006, p. 278). As in the prior edition, this volume emphasizes the client as a critical part of the equation. The Task Force added that "the application of research evidence to a given patient always involves probabilistic inferences. Therefore, ongoing monitoring of patient progress and adjustment of treatment as needed are essential" (Task Force, 2006, p. 280).

Proponents representing both sides of the common versus specific factors debate recognized that outcome is not guaranteed, regardless of evidentiary support of a given technique or the expertise of the therapist. Monitoring outcome and adjusting accordingly on the basis of client feedback—practice-based evidence—must become routine. Monitoring and feedback are primary emphases of this volume.


## THE WORST OF TIMES

The suggestion that something could be amiss for professional psychotherapy must strike the reasonable person as preposterous. The field's compulsive fascination for the new and different has ended, and for many, the stigma associated with using mental health services is a relic—gone and mostly forgotten. The ranks of the profession are growing. Therapy works as well, if not better, than any other intervention aimed at promoting health and well-being. All who do therapy, or consider themselves friends of the profession, should feel buoyant, flushed with optimism, and proud of the many accomplishments of psychotherapy as a profession.

Owing to these encouraging developments, is it right to conclude psychotherapy has entered a golden age? Surely, with the discipline's greater maturity and certainty about the results of therapy and, for that matter, what works, clinicians are enjoying respect and prosperity. For the most part, it seems, therapists have the freedom to practice how they want and when and where they choose. This is an illusion, however; the mood among many therapists, far from upbeat, is best captured in one word: despair.

### Psychotherapy as a Viable Profession

In the 1990s, reports emerged about the declining incomes of psychologists. A survey conducted under the auspices of *The National Psychologist* (Saeman, 1998), for instance, determined that the average income in this group had plunged notably in the preceding 30-month period. In that polling, the majority of respondents also viewed their future job prospects as negative and would not recommend that their son or daughter try psychology as a career. Leon Vandecreek (2005), then president of Division 29 of the APA (Psychotherapy), later wrote that during the past 15 years, practitioners had seen their income levels turn down and the opportunities for employment in traditional practice shrink. In the same year, Norcross (2005) documented decreased incomes for private practitioners. For those acknowledging a decline, "the mean and median reduction in net income was 15%" (Norcross, 2005, p. 665). National surveys yielded similar results (Minami & Wampold, 2008).

Managed care and the tight-fisted financial policies of third-party payers are often cited as the usual suspects behind psychotherapists' financial woes. Doubtless, their impact is a reality, keenly felt throughout the health care industry. Nonetheless, as much as those nefarious "bean counters" might provide an easy enemy to rally against, the answer does not conveniently end there. Changes in demographics and the sheer size of the therapist workforce are contributory. Regarding the latter, as much as the profession has grown, the profession may have grown too much (see chap. 10, this volume). In short, there are more clinicians than are needed. Combined with flat utilization rates, the supply of therapists far exceeds demand, creating unrelenting downward pressures on reimbursement. The Therapy in America Survey (Harris Poll, 2004) also revealed that among those who needed treatment but chose not to pursue it, doubt about its efficacy was cited as the deciding factor after cost. If that were not enough, the APA's 2004 Survey (Penn, Schoen, & Berland Associates, 2004; a comprehensive, nationally representative telephone study) found that 78% polled identified lack of confidence in the outcome as the major reason for not seeking treatment—nearly 8 out of 10—and this figure was up 1% from the 2000 APA Survey. In comparison, only 20% identified stigma.

These data may explain why Americans are choosing to spend billions on alternative health care remedies rather than psychotherapy (Duncan, Miller, & Sparks, 2004). The data may also account for why nearly half of those who begin psychotherapy quit (Wierzbicki & Pekarik, 1993). Like it or not, this is the perception of a large segment of consumers: Psychotherapy is unable to fulfill the need for change.

These adverse findings are coinciding with other events in the mental health marketplace, which are all potentially unfriendly to the practice of psychotherapy. For one, here and abroad, and more than at any previous time in the history of the field, policymakers and payers are insisting that to be paid, therapists and the systems of care in which they operate must "deliver the goods." As Hubble, Duncan, and Miller (1999b) predicted more than a decade ago, accountability is the watchword of the day, and real returns on investment are the guiding metric. The chickens have since come home to roost. This goes beyond the mere cost-cutting and containment methods of managed care. Those who underwrite mental health services want proof. They are not willing to listen to the expert claims of the mental health guilds and their officers, especially whiny complaints that practitioners are being treated unfairly or insufficiently reimbursed for their fine work. The assertion that overall psychotherapy has proven its effectiveness year after year, study after study, is also not enough. In all, it is as though the Missouri state motto has become the mantra of the industry: "Show me."

## Underutilization

Clearly, psychotherapy is an effective treatment for psychological distress. But are clients receiving the mental health services they need? Nationally, about 20% of the population obtains some service for emotional or substance abuse problems (Minami & Wampold, 2008). However, many presenting with what would be classified as a mental disorder (e.g., a *Diagnostic and Statistical Manual of Mental Disorders* diagnosis) do not receive any mental health treatment, and those who do are often treated in the medical system (i.e., with psychotropic medication, chiefly by primary care physicians). It is estimated that of those with psychological or behavioral problems, less than 16% are seen by clinicians who would offer psychotherapy (Minami & Wampold, 2008).

On the basis of national survey, Wang et al. (2005) noted that "most people with mental disorders in the United States remain either untreated or poorly treated" (p. 629). Wang et al. also reported that the problem is worse for clients most in need: "Unmet need for treatment is greatest in traditionally underserved groups, including elderly persons, racial–ethnic minorities, those with low incomes, those without insurance, and residents of rural areas" (p. 629). These findings give little cause to be sanguine.

## Therapist Competency

As will be discussed later in this chapter and in several subsequent chapters, much of the variability in outcomes in therapy is due to the therapist (Kim, Wampold, & Bolt, 2006; Okiishi, Lambert, Nielsen, & Ogles, 2003; Wampold & Brown, 2005). This is a result found in day-to-day practice and in clinical trials in which therapists are first selected for their skill and then later receive training with ongoing supervision. Although it is not surprising that therapists should vary considerably in their abilities, the disturbing news is that the poorest performing therapists consistently deliver a quality of service that would be classified as second rate. Indeed, Okiishi et al. (2003) noted that "therapists whose clients showed the slowest rate of improvement actually showed an average increase in symptoms among their clients" (p. 361). Wampold and Brown (2005) found that approximately one fifth of clients receiving care from the lowest quartile of therapists achieve a reliable change in their level of functioning. This may also explain why many clients who begin therapy drop out before experiencing significant benefit. In this volume, much attention is given to the proposition that to improve outcomes, effort should be directed to the person of the therapist.

In conclusion, it is safe to say that the tide is slowly beginning to turn but the ship remains at risk of going under. Will the profession reach safe harbor before sinking? Fortunately, science and a little common sense are showing the way. The profession has the means to (a) instill trust in the public that therapy works, (b) improve results, and (c) be accountable. To these issues we now turn.

## WHAT WORKS IN THERAPY REDUX

Proving that psychotherapy is deserving of the public's confidence will not come from more attempts to design the "right" treatment. No "right" treatment exists anyway. The data are unequivocal: All treatment approaches have won, and all deserve prizes. It is time to bury once and for all the doctrine of specificity—the idea that specific treatments have differential effects for specific disorders. As Wampold (2001) reported, "Research designs that are able to isolate and establish the relationship between specific ingredients and outcomes . . . have failed to find a scintilla of evidence that any specific ingredient is necessary for therapeutic change" (p. 204; see also Ahn & Wampold, 2001; Wampold & Bhati, 2004; Wampold, 2007). For this reason, the public must learn how psychotherapy really works. Here again, the evidence is indisputable: Change as a result of psychotherapy derives from key ingredients or elements that transcend all approaches. Sharing such findings will foster the public's trust. Even more, such sharing is a professional duty owed to the consumers of psychological services.

Lambert (1986, 1992), following an extensive review of outcome research spanning decades, identified four therapeutic factors. He ranked their importance on the basis of their estimated percentage-wise contribution to outcome. The four factors were extratherapeutic variables (40%); common factors (30%); hope, expectancy, and placebo (15%); and model or technique (15%). Conceding that the percentages were not derived from a strict statistical analysis, he suggested that they embody what studies indicated at the time about treatment outcome. The first edition of this volume used Lambert's proposal as a framework for the common factors but with modification. His *common factors* were amended to *relationship factors*, a change that reflected how he actually described these variables in his works (i.e., "empathy, warmth, acceptance, encouragement of risk taking, etc." [1992, p. 97]).

As previewed earlier in this chapter (in the section Common Factors Come of Age), research findings published since the first edition of *The Heart and Soul of Change* necessitate major revisions in the conceptualization of the factors responsible for change. Specifically, data accrued from meta-analytic studies call for another look at how these elements interact and contribute to success. A reassessment of what factors to include is also required. Of singular import, Wampold's (2001) investigation of psychotherapy outcome, which serves as the foundation for the current volume, extended the understanding of the common factors—broadening an appreciation of the potency of client, therapist, and alliance factors—while elucidating the limited impact of model differences. His analysis revealed that the differences among models accounted for only 1% of the variance of outcome, dramatically reducing Lambert's (1986, 1992) estimate of the contribution of specific effects.

There is more. The simple pie chart used to depict the relationship among the factors (Asay & Lambert, 1999; Hubble et al., 1999c) allocated to each an invariant or fixed percentage, implying that the factors were independent and the percentages additive. This apportionment of percentages also suggested that the factors were, or could be, rendered as discrete elements and thus individually operationalized. It is not surprising that over time the empirically unsubstantiated logic of specificity came to be applied to the common factors. It was as though they could be distilled into a treatment model, used to create techniques, and then administered to the client. From this point of view, if one wants a good outcome add a little more therapist–client alliance (a potent therapeutic factor), and this is how to do it: Be a good listener, reflect, nod, smile, and maintain eye contact; offer a tissue; validate; and serve coffee, tea, or bottled water. Similarly, as an antidote to despair, add client and extratherapeutic factors. Mix in two parts client strengths and a pinch of social support, all the while being sensitive to the client's stage of change.

In reality, the common factors are not invariant, proportionally fixed, or neatly additive. Far from it, they are interdependent, fluid, and dynamic. Unlike a manufacturing operation, with linear inputs and predictable outputs, therapy is a reciprocal process, in which the inputs are changed in and by the participants' interaction. In short, the role and degree of the influence of any one factor are dependent on the context: who is involved; what takes place between therapist and client; when and where the therapeutic interaction occurs; and ultimately, from whose point of view these matters are considered. Much like raw materials in nature, the common factors exist in an unprocessed or minimally processed state and must be used or acted on to create a product or structure. The eventual form a treatment assumes is thus entirely dependent on the materials available; the skills of the artisan; and most important, the desires and preferences of the end user.

To illustrate, any treatment involves specific components (e.g., reality testing in CBT), but the manner in which they unfold or are manifested depends on the interaction between therapist and client. In this respect, the therapist and client produce the treatment collaboratively. A CBT provided by an empathic and skilled therapist to a motivated client, with sufficient social support and cultural sensitivity, is considerably different from a CBT provided in a context in which those factors do not exist.

The first edition of *The Heart and Soul of Change* anticipated the transition from discrete common factors to interdependent factors that are mobilized by the delivery of a treatment. Hubble et al. (1999a) asserted that in contrast with the tradition of separating models and techniques from the common factors . . . theoretical models and their related techniques are included here as part of the family of common factors . . . models and techniques help provide therapists with replicable and structured ways for developing and practicing the values, attitudes, and behaviors consistent with the core ingredients of effective therapy. This nontraditional role for models and techniques suggests that their principal contribution to therapy comes about by enhancing the potency of the other common factors. . . . A way to view techniques is to see them as something akin to a magnifying glass. *They bring together, focus, and concentrate the forces of change, narrow them to a point in place and time, and cause them to ignite into action* [italics added]. (pp. 421–422)

## The Common Factors in Context

What the latest science has to say about the common factors comes next. In particular, we briefly discuss four elements: client and extratherapeutic factors, models and techniques, therapists, and therapeutic relationship or alliance. Although presented sequentially, bear in mind that they cause and are caused by each other, exerting their benefits through their joint and inseparable emergence over the course of therapy. It may well be that the specific ingredients of particular therapies are related to outcomes and yet, that contribution is negligible (i.e., less than 1% of the variability; Wampold et al., 1997) compared with the potency of the common factors working together.

### Client and Extratherapeutic Factors

These factors encompass all that affects improvement independent of treatment. As any therapist knows, clients come to therapy with varying degrees of motivation and with varying degrees of internal and external resources. Once clients are in therapy, events beyond the control of the therapist and the client occur, and these events influence the outcome of therapy. Research has demonstrated the importance of clients' readiness for change, strengths, resources, level of functioning before treatment, existing social support network, socioeconomic status, personal motivations, and life events.

As discussed in chapter 3 of this volume, in many ways clients are the most neglected therapeutic factor in studies of psychotherapy. Descriptions of consumers are frequently circumscribed, limited to portrayals as the poster children of dysfunction. It is more realistic to describe clients as people who are having trouble in life, have made valiant attempts to change, and use therapy constructively (Bohart & Tallman, 1999; Duncan et al., 2004; Hubble & Miller, 2004; Linley & Joseph, 2004; Seligman, 2002). The latest data challenge the field to leave behind the belief that therapy is reducible to a set of diagnostic or classification schemes and formulaic practices. To quote Lambert, Garfield, and Bergin (2004), "Clients are not inert objects or diagnostic categories on whom techniques are administered. They are not dependent variables on which independent variables operate . . . people are agentive beings who are effective forces in the complex of causal events" (p. 814).

As basic as it is to adjust therapy to the client—a complete commitment to "starting where the client is at"—it is critically important. In practical terms, without preconceptions, this means organizing clinical services to clients: who they are, what they want, and what constitutes and influences the circumstances of their lives. It also means that assessments of the quality and the outcome must come from the client, the ultimate beneficiary of the service. The field can no longer assume that therapists know what is best independent of consumers. As later chapters show, regardless of the theoretical orientation, therapies that include the client's ongoing evaluation of progress, as well as feedback to the participants with that information, achieve significantly superior results.

*Models and Techniques*

Over the past decade, while the profession as a whole has confined its search for what works to a handful of specific treatments for a circumscribed set of disorders, the editors' understanding of the role of models and techniques has evolved in a major way. Since the first formulation of the common factors, any discussion of models was considered separately from the contribution of placebo, hope, and expectancy (see Asay & Lambert, 1999; Hubble et al., 1999b; Lambert, 1986; Miller, Duncan, & Hubble, 1997). The latest evidence indicates that this division is no longer warranted. Models achieve their effects in large part, if not completely, through the activation and operation of placebo, hope, and expectancy. In fact, when a placebo or technically inert condition is offered in a manner that fosters positive expectations for improvement, it reliably produces effects almost as large as a bona fide treatment (Wampold, 2007). Studies further show that when researchers and practitioner's allegiance to a method is added, the variability attributable to differences in models is almost, if not entirely, explained (see, e.g., Miller, Wampold, & Varhely, 2008).

At the core, model or technique factors induce positive expectations and assist the client's participation in healthy and helpful actions. Common to all treatments, they offer the client an appropriate explanation for his or her difficulties and set forth strategies for problem resolution (Frank & Frank, 1991; Wampold, 2007). Because comparisons of therapy techniques have found little differential efficacy, they may all be understood as healing rituals— technically inert, but nonetheless powerful, organized methods for enhancing expectations of change—the so-called and perhaps poorly named *placebo factors*. That they are not specifically curative should not be construed to imply anything goes in a therapy. Packaging is important. In fact, studies conducted have indicated that a good predictor of a negative outcome is a lack of structure and focus in treatment (e.g., Lambert & Bergin, 1994; Mohl, 1995; Sachs, 1983).

Owing to these findings, we conclude that what happens (whether a clinician is confronting negative cognitive schema, addressing family boundaries, or interpreting transference) is less important than the degree to which any particular activity is consistent with the therapist's beliefs and values (allegiances) while concurrently fostering the client's hope (expectations). Allegiance and expectancy are two sides of the same coin: the faith of both the therapist and the client in the restorative power and credibility of the therapy's rationale and related rituals. Though rarely viewed in this way, models and techniques work best when they engage and inspire the participants.

## The Therapeutic Relationship/Alliance

Of those factors directly related to treatment outcome, one of the largest contributors to outcome is the therapeutic relationship, which encompasses a wide range of variables found among therapies, no matter the therapist's theoretical persuasion. Therapist-provided variables, especially the core conditions popularized by Rogers (1957), have not only been empirically supported but are also remarkably consistent in client reports of successful therapy (Norcross & Lambert, 2005).

Evidence regarding the power of the alliance is reflected in more than 1,000 findings (Orlinsky, Rønnestad, & Willutzki, 2004). Researchers repeatedly have found that a *positive alliance*—that is, a partnership between the client and therapist to achieve the client's goals (Bordin, 1979)—is one of the best predictors of outcome (see chap. 4, this volume; Horvath & Symonds, 1991; Martin, Garske, & Davis, 2000). Depending on which study is cited, the amount of change attributable to the alliance is five to seven times greater than that of specific models or techniques (Horvath & Symonds, 1991; Martin et al., 2000; Wampold, 2001).

Consider several other interrelated findings. First, studies indicate that clients' evaluations of the alliance are better predictors of outcome than therapists' (Bachelor & Horvath, 1999). Second, little or no correlation exists between the length of treatment and the strength of the alliance. Third, the alliance is predictive of outcome across different types of therapy and is even predictive of outcome in psychopharmacotherapy. And finally, alliance formation at the initiation of therapy is predictive of outcome and not merely an artifact of improvement (Baldwin, Wampold, & Imel, 2007; Horvath & Symonds, 1991).

The alliance, however, is not independent of other factors. Clients come to therapy with an attachment history and varying capacities to form a relationship with the therapist. However, it is the therapist's ability to forge a collaborative relationship with the client that is predictive of outcome (Baldwin et al., 2007). Because the alliance involves agreement about the tasks and goals of therapy, it is not really possible to form an adequate alliance without a treatment; that is, the alliance comes about within the context of the treatment. The therapist needs to present a cogent rationale to the client, offer an adequate explanation for the presenting problems, and implement a set of procedures consistent with the rationale and explanation to develop properly a working alliance.

Taken together, these data, yet again, point to the importance of starting where the client is. Therapists cannot presume that given enough time a good alliance will develop. Instead, they must ensure that from the first moments of the therapeutic encounter, the client is experiencing the relationship as meaningful and positive. The simplest course of action is to solicit the client's perspective regarding the relationship (see chaps. 4 and 8).

*Therapist Factors*

In this volume, a new addition to the list of curative factors is the person of the therapist. That the therapist was previously overlooked turns out to be a particularly egregious omission. Available evidence documents that the therapist is the most robust predictor of outcome of any factor ever studied. As Wampold (2005) summarized, "The variance of outcomes due to therapists (8%–9%) is larger than the variability among treatments (0%–1%), the alliance (5%), and the superiority of an empirically supported treatment to a placebo treatment (0%–4%)" (p. 204).

Research confirms what everybody knows but at the same time is unwilling to acknowledge or explore: Some therapists are more effective than others. Clients of the most effective therapists, for instance, experience 50% less dropout and 50% more improvement than those seen by average clinicians. Many variables widely and enthusiastically believed to be determinative (e.g., age, gender, years of experience, professional discipline, degree, training, licensure, theoretical orientation, amount of supervision, personal therapy, specific or general competence, use of evidence-based methods) do not account for the variability among practitioners (Beutler et al., 2004; Miller, Hubble, & Duncan, 2007). Unfortunately, the characteristics or actions of the most effective therapists are not really known (Beutler et al., 2004), but the evidence suggests that better therapists use the common factors to achieve better outcomes. Take, for example, the alliance. Baldwin et al. (2007) found that variability among therapists in terms of outcome was explained by the therapists' contributions to the alliance; that is, better therapists formed better alliances with a range of clients. This finding suggests that helping therapists in building relationships may represent an arena for influencing outcome due to the therapist. Several chapters in this volume (8, 9, 10, 11, 12, and 14) address how systematic client feedback can improve individual therapist performance.

## MOVING FROM WHAT WORKS TO DELIVERING WHAT WORKS

Understanding and disseminating the science of the common, therapeutic factors—how therapy really works—can go a long way toward restoring public confidence. It does not, however, address the issue of accountability. Meeting that challenge requires a major shift in the traditional way psychotherapy has been conducted and researched. It is no longer a matter of which therapeutic approach is best. Rather, it is about showing that a treatment, conducted by a given therapist with particular client at specific time and place, yielded positive results. A little reflection reveals that what payers and consumers want is the "right" outcome. They could not care less how it comes about, they simply want it. In this case, "right" means that a treatment worked and that the money paid was well spent.

Building a practice around the right outcome is not difficult. It is part of the culture; people are accustomed to it and expect it. It is the way businesses are successful. They begin with the customers and concentrate on their needs. Then, they concern themselves with the delivery of what the customer wants (Levitt, 1975; Miller, Duncan, & Hubble, 2004). Those who succeed in a competitive market stay results driven and people focused; work with their customers to create enduring partnerships; and, when required, are ready to act as champions for their customers.

Within the profession, researchers are already making the shift. They are setting aside evidence-based practice, in which the emphasis is placed on the treatment itself, in favor of *practice-based evidence* (Anker, Duncan, & Sparks, 2009; Barkham et al., 2001; Duncan et al., 2004; Miller et al., 2005). In practical terms, this means not only gathering data on how treatment is working for a particular client and therapist pairing but also then providing feedback to the therapist about the client's improvement (Howard, Moras, Brill, Matinovich, & Lutz, 1996). The results are impressive (Anker et al., 2009; Lambert, 2005; Miller, Duncan, Brown, Sorrell, & Chalk, 2006). The combination of measuring progress (i.e., *monitoring*) and providing feedback consistently yields clinically significant change, with treatment effects outstripping whatever has been seen in the so-called empirically supported psychotherapy literature. Rates of deterioration are cut in half, as is dropout. Include feedback about the client's formal assessment of the relationship, and the client is less likely to deteriorate, more likely to stay longer, and twice as likely to achieve a clinically significant change (see chaps. 8, 10, 11, 12, and 13, this volume).

Feedback also allows psychotherapy to be individualized taking into account treatment response and client preference. Client-based feedback, therefore, remedies any rigid interpretation of the common factors, enabling a reliable and valid method of tailoring services to the individual. It allows the therapeutic factors to be delivered to one client at a time.

Monitoring combined with feedback is a simple method, divorced of theoretical baggage, for providing accountability. The results are apparent to all who have an interest in the outcome: therapists, consumers, administrators, and payers. Accepting the premise that therapeutic factors constitute the engine of change, then monitoring and feedback offers the means to deliver them. Many are anxious about the future and deservedly so. At the same time, the profession has the opportunity to establish itself in its own right. Psychotherapy works. It works. Therapists now have the ability to show it and the means to banish the despair in the workforce. The challenge is to put it into practice.

In the end, monitoring outcomes may provide a common ground for those who advocate empirically supported treatments and those who espouse the importance of the common factors. Improvement in the results attained by clients in actual practice is and should be the shared goal. Leaving behind the polemic of what is specific or common, this edition of *The Heart and Soul of Change* focuses on methods for promoting excellent outcomes across all systems of care. In short, we want the best for those who seek help from psychotherapists.


ORGANIZATION

*The Heart and Soul of Change, Second Edition: Delivering What Works in Therapy* is intended, as was the first edition, as a crossover work for researchers, teachers, students, and practitioners. Each chapter provides thorough coverage of the research on the topic under review. Plus, the chapters specify the day-to-day implications of the latest research findings. As before, all chapters end with questions from the editors and the contributors' responses. These questions, requesting further reflection, provide the authors an opportunity to candidly discuss the implications raised in their work. The organization of the book follows, with synopses of each chapter.

The book is divided into four parts. Part I, What Works and What Does Not, consists of six chapters. In chapter 2, Wampold reviews the evidence regarding the efficacy of psychotherapy, contrasting the medical model with a common factors paradigm and setting the stage for the rest of the book. In chapter 3, Bohart and Tallman argue that despite their powerful contribution to treatment outcome, clients are without doubt the most neglected therapeutic factor in studies of psychotherapy. Norcross follows in chapter 4 with a discussion of the importance of the therapeutic relationship and the research that supports this factor. Rounding out the common factors covered in this section, Anderson, Lunnen, and Ogles, in chapter 5, thoughtfully address the role of models and techniques, arguing convincingly that the power of treatments resides largely in the provision of a credible myth and a healing ritual.

The next two chapters in Part I challenge popular claims about psychotherapy and psychopharmacology. In chapter 6, Littell provides a practical template and examples for scrutinizing the claims regarding the superior efficacy of empirically supported treatments. Sparks, Duncan, Cohen, and Antonuccio, in chapter 7, demonstrate that drug effectiveness is overstated and variables other than the psychoactive properties of medications account for a significant portion of the outcomes. Like Littell, the authors provide a method for evaluating the claims of psychopharmacotherapy.

Part II, Delivering What Works, covers the newest common factor: the therapist. It also describes how the field can shift toward practice-based evidence. In the first of three chapters in this section, Lambert (chap. 8) answers the question he and his colleagues posed in an influential previous article (Lambert et al., 2003): Is it time for psychotherapists to routinely track outcome? He reviews the evidence about client feedback, making a strong case for an affirmative reply. Lambert also surveys available systems of outcome management. Building on a review of therapist variability and current trends in managed care, Brown and Minami (chap. 9) assert that achieved outcome is emerging as the ultimate arbiter of reimbursement. They make the provocative argument that therapist variability points to a need to validate psychotherapists, not psychotherapies. Bohanske and Franczak (chap. 10) uniquely combine the consumer and recovery movements to present an innovative application of the common factors in public behavioral health. They demonstrate through the experiences of two large community behavioral health organizations that transformation of public behavioral health can occur when a consumer-directed, outcome-informed infrastructure is in place.

Part III, Special Populations, reviews the common factors and their application with diverse groups and differing modalities of service. Kelley, Bickman, and Norwood (chap. 11) cover child and adolescent therapies; Sparks and Duncan (chap. 12) address marriage and family therapies; and Mee-Lee, McLellan, and Miller (chap. 13) discuss addiction services.

Finally, Part IV, Conclusions, contains the last chapter: In it we distill the implications from all the contributors. The final chapter also comments on the exciting findings emerging from practice-based evidence and explores the new frontier of therapist variability. Identifying the best from the rest and studying how they do therapy provides insight into what makes for excellence as a therapist. Finally, we speculate on what the future might hold, and although caution is warranted, hope is in the forecast.

## REFERENCES

Ahn, H., & Wampold, B. E. (2001). A meta-analysis of component studies: Where is the evidence for the specificity of psychotherapy? *Journal of Counseling Psychology, 48,* 251–257.

Anker, M. G., Duncan, B. L., Sparks, J. A. (2009). Using client feedback to improve couple outcomes. A randomized clinical trial in a naturalistic setting. *Journal of Consulting and Clinical Psychology, 77,* 693–704.

American Psychological Association, Office of Ethnic Minority Affairs. (2008). *A portrait of success and challenge—Progress report: 1997-2005.* Washington, DC: Author. Retrieved March 22, 2007, from http://www.apa.org/pi/oema/CEMRRAT_progress_report_success_challenges.pdf

American Psychological Association Presidential Task Force on Evidence-Based Practice. (2006). Evidence-based practice in psychology. *American Psychologist, 61,* 271–285.

Asay, T. P., and Lambert, M. J. (1999). The empirical case for the common factors in therapy: Quantitative findings. In M. A. Hubble, B. L. Duncan, & S. D. Miller (Eds.), *The heart and soul of change: What works in therapy* (pp. 33–56). Washington, DC: American Psychological Association.

Bachelor, A., & Horvath, A. (1999). The therapeutic relationship. In M. A. Hubble, B. L. Duncan, & S. D. Miller (Eds.), *The heart and soul of change: What works in therapy* (pp. 133-178). Washington, DC: American Psychological Association.

Baldwin, S. A., Wampold, B. E., & Imel, Z. E. (2007). Untangling the alliance–outcome correlation: Exploring the relative importance of therapist and patient variability in the alliance. *Journal of Consulting and Clinical Psychology, 75,* 842–852.

Barkham, M., Margison, F., Leach, C., Lucock, M., Mellor-Clark, J., Evans, C., et al. (2001). Service profiling and outcome benchmarking using the CORE-OM: Toward practice based evidence in the psychological therapies. *Journal of Consulting and Clinical Psychology, 69,* 184–196.

Beutler, L.E., Malik, M., Alimohamed, S., Harwood, T. M., Talebi, H., Noble, S., et al. (2004). Therapist variables. In M. J. Lambert (Ed.), *Bergin and Garfield's handbook of psychotherapy and behavior change* (5th ed., pp. 227–306). New York: Wiley.

Bohart, A. C., & Tallman, K. (1999). *How clients make therapy work: The process of active self-healing.* Washington, DC: American Psychological Association.

Bordin, E. S. (1979). The generalizability of the psychoanalytic concept of the working alliance. *Psychotherapy, 16,* 252–260.

Carey, J. (2008, January 28). Do cholesterol drugs do any good? *Business Week*. Retrieved April 3, 2009, from http://www.businessweek.com/magazine/content/08_04/b4068052092994htm?chan=magazine+channel_top+stories

Duncan, B. L., Miller. S. D., & Sparks, J. (2004). *The heroic client: A revolutionary way to improve effectiveness through client directed outcome informed therapy* (Rev. ed.). San Francisco: Jossey-Bass.

Frank, J. D. (1961). *Persuasion and healing: A comparative study of psychotherapy*. Baltimore, MD: Johns Hopkins University Press.

Frank, J. D. (1973). *Persuasion and healing: A comparative study of psychotherapy* (2nd ed.) Baltimore, MD: Johns Hopkins University Press.

Frank, J. D., & Frank, J. B. (1991). *Persuasion and healing* (3rd ed.). Baltimore: Johns Hopkins University Press.

Harris Poll. (2004). *Therapy in America: A poll sponsored by Psychology Today and PacifiCare*. Retrieved May 11, 2007, from http://www.harrisinteractive.com/services/pubs/pacificare_behavioral_health_psychology_today.pdf

Horvath, A. O., & Symonds, B. D. (1991). Relation between working alliance and outcome in psychotherapy: A meta-analysis. *Journal of Counseling Psychology, 38*, 139–149.

Howard, K. I, Moras, K., Brill, P. L., Martinovich, Z., & Lutz, W. (1996). Evaluation of psychotherapy: Efficacy, effectiveness, and patient progress. *American Psychologist, 51*, 1059–1064.

Hubble, M. A., Duncan, B. L., & Miller, S. D. (1999a). Directing attention to what works. In M. A. Hubble, B. L. Duncan, & S. D. Miller (Eds.), *The heart and soul of change: What works in therapy* (pp. 407–448). Washington, DC: American Psychological Association.

Hubble, M. A., Duncan, B. L., & Miller, S. D. (1999b). *The heart and soul of change: what works in therapy*. Washington, DC: American Psychological Association.

Hubble, M. A., Duncan, B. L., & Miller, S. D. (1999c). Introduction. In M. A. Hubble, B. L. Duncan, & S. D. Miller (Eds.), *The heart and soul of change: What works in therapy* (pp. 1–19). Washington, DC: American Psychological Association.

Hubble, M. A., & Miller, S. D. (2004). The client: Psychotherapy's missing link for promoting a positive psychology. In P. A. Linley & S. Joseph (Eds.), *Positive psychology in practice* (pp. 335–353). Hoboken, NJ: Wiley.

Kim, D. M., Wampold, B. E., & Bolt, D. M. (2006). Therapist effects in psychotherapy: A random effects modeling of the NIMH TDCRP data. *Psychotherapy Research, 16*, 161–172.

Kuhn, T. S. (1970). *The structure of scientific revolutions* (2nd ed.). Chicago: University of Chicago Press.

Lambert, M. J. (1986). Implications of psychotherapy outcome research for eclectic psychotherapy. In J. C. Norcross (Ed.), *Handbook of eclectic psychotherapy* (pp. 436–462). New York: Brunner/Mazel.

Lambert, M. J. (1992). Implications of psychotherapy outcome research for psychotherapy integration. In J. C. Norcross & M. R. Goldfried (Eds.), *Handbook of psychotherapy integration* (pp. 94–129). New York: Basic Books.

Lambert, M. J. (2005). Enhancing psychotherapy outcome through feedback. *Journal of Clinical Psychology: In Session, 61*, 141–217.

Lambert, M. J., & Bergin, A. E. (1994). The effectiveness of psychotherapy. In A. E. Bergin & S. L. Garfield (Eds.), *Handbook of psychotherapy and behavior change* (4th ed., pp. 143–189). New York: Wiley.

Lambert, M. J., Garfield, S. L., & Bergin, A. E. (2004). Overview, trends, and future issues. In M. J. Lambert (Ed.), *Bergin and Garfield's handbook of psychotherapy and behavior change* (5th ed., pp. 805–819). New York: Wiley.

Lambert, M. J., & Ogles, B. (2004). The efficacy and effectiveness of psychotherapy. In M. J. Lambert (Ed.), *Bergin and Garfield's handbook of psychotherapy and behavior change* (5th ed., pp. 139–193). New York: Wiley.

Lambert, M. J., Whipple, J. L., Hawkins, E. J., Vermeersch, D. A., Nielsen, S. L., & Smart, D.W. (2003). Is it time for clinicians routinely to track patient outcome? A meta-analysis. *Clinical Psychology, 10*, 288–301.

Levitt, T. (1975, September–October). Marketing myopia. *Harvard Business Review*, pp. 19–31.

Linley, P.A., & Joseph, S. (2004). *Positive psychology in practice*. Hoboken, NJ: Wiley.

Martin, D. J., Garske, J. P., & Davis, M. K. (2000). Relation of the therapeutic alliance with outcome and other variables: A meta-analytic review. *Journal of Consulting and Clinical Psychology, 68*, 438–450.

Miller, S. D., Duncan, B. L., Brown, J., Sorrell, R., & Chalk, B. (2006). Using outcome to inform and improve treatment outcomes. *Journal of Brief Therapy, 5*, 5–22.

Miller, S. D., Duncan, B. L., & Hubble, M. A. (1997). *Escape from Babel: Toward a unifying language for psychotherapy practice*. New York: Norton.

Miller, S. D., Duncan, B. L., & Hubble, M. A. (2004). Beyond integration: The triumph of outcome over process in clinical practice. *Psychotherapy in Australia, 10*(2), 20–37.

Miller, S. D., Duncan, B. L., & Hubble, M. A. (2005). Outcome informed clinical work. In J. Norcross & M. Goldfried (Eds.), *Handbook of psychotherapy integration* (2nd ed., pp. 84–102). New York: Oxford University Press.

Miller, S. D., Hubble, M. A., & Duncan, B. L. (2007). Supershrinks. *Psychotherapy Networker, 31*(6), 26–35, 56.

Miller, S. D., Wampold, B. & Varhely, K. (2008). Direct comparisons of treatment modalities for youth disorders: A meta-analysis. *Psychotherapy Research, 18*(1), 5–14.

Minami, T., & Wampold, B. E. (2008). Adult psychotherapy in the real world. In W. B. Walsh (Ed.), *Biennial review of counseling psychology* (Vol. 1, pp. 27–45). New York: Taylor & Francis.

Minami, T., Wampold, B. E., Serlin, R. C., Hamilton, E. G., Brown, G. S., & Kircher, J. C. (2008). Benchmarking the effectiveness of psychotherapy treatment for adult depression in a managed care environment: A preliminary study. *Journal of Consulting and Clinical Psychology, 76*, 116–24.

Mohl, D.C. (1995). Negative outcome in psychotherapy: A critical review. *Clinical Psychology, 2*, 1–27.

Mulvey, K. Hubbard S., & Hayashi, S. (2003). A national study of the substance abuse treatment workforce. *Journal of Substance Abuse Treatment. 24*, 51–57.

Norcross, J. C. (2005). Psychologists' fees and incomes. In G. P. Koocher, J. C. Norcross, & S. S. Hill III (Eds.), *Psychologists' desk reference* (2nd ed., pp. 662–665). New York: Oxford University Press.

Norcross, J. C., & Lambert, M. J. (2005). The therapy relationship. In J. C. Norcross, L. E. Beutler, & R. F. Levant (Eds.), *Evidence-based practices in mental health: Debate and dialogue on the fundamental questions* (pp. 208–217). Washington, DC: American Psychological Association.

Okiishi, J., Lambert, M. J., Nielsen, S. L., & Ogles, B. M. (2003). Waiting for supershrink: An empirical analysis of therapist effects. *Clinical Psychology & Psychotherapy, 10*, 361–373.

Orlinsky, D. E. (2006). Comments on the state of psychotherapy research (as I see it). *Psychotherapy Bulletin, 41*, 37–41.

Orlinsky, D. E., & Howard, K. (1978). The relation of process to outcome in psychotherapy. In S. L. Garfield & A. E. Bergin (Eds.), *Handbook of psychotherapy and behavior change* (2nd ed., pp. 282–330). New York: Wiley.

Orlinsky, D. E., Rønnestad, M. H., & Willutzki, U. (2004). Fifty years of process–outcome research: Continuity and change. In M. J. Lambert (Ed.), *Bergin and Garfield's handbook of psychotherapy and behavior change* (5th ed., pp. 307–390). New York: Wiley.

Penn, Schoen, & Berland Associates. (2004, February 11). *Survey for the American Psychological Association*. Unpublished data.

Rogers, C. (1957). The necessary and sufficient conditions of therapeutic personality change. *Journal of Consulting Psychology, 21*, 95–103.

Rosenthal, R. (1990). How are we doing in soft psychology? *American Psychologist, 45*, 775–777.

Sachs, J. S. (1983). Negative factors in brief psychotherapy: An empirical assessment. *Journal of Consulting and Clinical Psychology, 51*, 557–564.

Saeman, H. (1998). Average income of psychologists has dropped notably, survey shows. *The National Psychologist, 1*(4). Retrieved September 29, 2007, from http://nationalpsychologist.com/articles/art7981.htm

Seligman, M. E. P. (2002). *Authentic happiness*. New York: Free Press.

Slife, B. D., Williams, R. N., & Barlow, S. H. (2001). *Critical issues in psychotherapy: Translating new ideas into practice*. Thousand Oaks, CA: Sage.

Stiles, W. B., Barkham, M., Mellor-Clark, J., & Connell, J. (2008). Effectiveness of cognitive–behavioural, person-centred, and psychodynamic therapies in UK primary-care routine practice: Replication in a larger sample. *Psychological Medicine, 38,* 677–688.

Strupp, H. H. (1978). The therapist's theoretical orientation: An overrated variable. *Psychotherapy: Theory, Research and Practice, 15,* 314–317.

Vandecreek, L. (2005). President's column. *Psychotherapy Bulletin, 40,* 2–3.

Wampold, B. E. (2001). *The great psychotherapy debate: Models, methods, and findings.* Mahwah, NJ: Erlbaum.

Wampold, B. E. (2005). The psychotherapist. In J. C. Norcross, L. E. Beutler, & R. F. Levant (Eds.), *Evidence-based practices in mental health: Debate and dialogue on the fundamental questions* (pp. 200–207). Washington, DC: American Psychological Association.

Wampold, B. E. (2007). Psychotherapy: The humanistic (and effective) treatment. *American Psychologist, 62,* 857–873.

Wampold, B. E. & Bhati, K. S. (2004). Attending to the omissions: A historical examination of the evidenced-based practice movement. *Professional Psychology: Research and Practice, 35,* 563–570.

Wampold, B. E., & Brown, G. (2005). Estimating therapist variability in outcomes attributable to therapists: A naturalistic study of outcomes in managed care. *Journal of Consulting and Clinical Psychology, 73,* 914–923.

Wampold, B. E., Mondin, G. W., Moody, M., Stich, F., Benson, K., & Ahn, H. (1997). A meta-analysis of outcome studies comparing bona fide psychotherapies: Empirically, "all must have prizes." *Psychological Bulletin, 122,* 203–215.

Wang, P. S., Lane, M., Olfson, M., Pincus, H. A., Wells, K. B., & Kessler, R. C. (2005). Twelve-month use of mental health services in the United States: Results from the National Comorbidity Survey Replication. *Archives of General Psychiatry, 62,* 629–640.

Wierzbicki, M., & Pekarik, G. (1993). A meta-analysis of psychotherapy dropout. *Professional Psychology: Research and Practice, 24,* 190–195.

# I

# WHAT WORKS AND WHAT DOES NOT: THE EMPIRICAL FOUNDATIONS FOR THE COMMON FACTORS

# 2

# THE RESEARCH EVIDENCE FOR THE COMMON FACTORS MODELS: A HISTORICALLY SITUATED PERSPECTIVE

BRUCE E. WAMPOLD

Daring as it is to investigate the unknown, even more so it is to question the known.

—Kaspar

The development of psychotherapy as a modern treatment is complex. One strand of this development has been closely intertwined with the development of modern medicine since the late 19th century; this strand appears to be the most apparent in scientific discussions of psychotherapy. However, another strand—embedded more in culture, humanism, and traditional healing practices—has been present since the origins of psychotherapy, and although it is tenaciously holding fast, it is often not apparent. Indeed, this later strand may form the core of the psychotherapy rope and be the hidden source of strength.

In this chapter, a brief history of psychotherapy is presented to show the influence of modern medicine on the development of psychotherapy (the first strand) and to demonstrate that other influences (the second strand) have been ever present, although frequently ignored. The research evidence is presented to demonstrate that the medical model that is the fabric of the medical strand of psychotherapy is not generally supported, whereas the contextual model, which emanates from the second strand, is supported by this evidence. Finally, there is a brief synopsis of the factors involved in the second strand. This common factor strand forms the basis of this book.

49

# BRIEF HISTORY OF PSYCHOTHERAPY

This brief history reviews the origins of a medical model of psychotherapy and the origins of a contextual model, with as much emphasis on what was omitted as what transpired. As will be clear, what is omitted is often more important than what is apparent in the development of psychotherapy as a profession.

## First Strand: Medical Model

From the middle to the end of the 19th century, medicine, attempting to cast aside the shackles of practices predominated by myth (Harrington, 2008; A. K. Shapiro & Shapiro, 1997), increasingly concentrated on the physio-chemical causes of illness. Because medicine was not yet dominant, an increasing number of Americans during this period turned toward practices that healed through the mind and contained aspects of spirituality and religion, the most popular of which were Christian Science and the New Thought movement (Caplan, 1998; Taylor, 1999). At first, medicine deliberately dismissed these movements, for the most part, as unscientific attempts to cure illnesses, whether physical or mental. Legitimacy lagged behind popularity, but gradually the involvement of American psychologists lent credibility to the idea of talk therapy as distinct from the religious movements. The Boston School of Psychopathology, which was initiated in 1859 and included the psychologists William James and G. Stanley Hall as well as neurologists and psychiatrists, was followed by the Emmanuel Movement, which was initiated in 1906 as a collaboration between physicians who recognized the importance of the psyche and Christian ministers who recognized the moral aspect to behavior (Caplan, 1998; Taylor, 1999).

Medicine was particularly threatened by treatments provided by non-physicians for physical as well as mental distress and exerted its professional privilege to conduct psychotherapy (Caplan, 1998; Wampold, 2001a). The sentiment was expressed by prominent physician John K. Mitchell, "Most earnestly should we insist that the *treatment* of a patient, whether it be surgical, medical, or psychic, should for the safety of the public, be in the hands of a doctor" (Caplan, 1998, p. 143). Conspicuously missing at the origins of psychotherapy as a medical practice was a scientific explanation—that was provided by Sigmund Freud in his lectures at Clark University in 1909. Within 6 years of these lectures, psychoanalysis had become the predominant form of psychotherapy in the United States: "Psychoanalysis appeared to be more proper and civilized than mind cure, more scientific than Christian Science and positive thinking, and more medical than advertising" (Cushman, 1992). Moreover, the practice of psychotherapy in the United

States was restricted in those years to physicians for the most part (Frank, 1992; VandenBos, Cummings, & DeLeon, 1992), which shows that at the origins of psychotherapy there existed a cozy relationship with medicine. The cozy relationship between psychotherapy and medicine has varied by country and over time. To be certain, however, the manner in which psychotherapy is understood and delivered reflects a history closely entwined with medicine.

Although psychoanalytic theory provided medicine with what was at the time a scientific explanation for mental disorders,[1] the validity of the theory quickly was challenged by emergent behaviorists. On the basis of the experimental work of Thorndike, Pavlov, and Skinner, various behavioral treatments were developed, notably systematic desensitization (Wolpe, 1958). This and subsequent behavioral treatments were categorized as scientific because they were based purportedly on learning theory, which emanated from scientific and empirical psychology (Eysenck, 1961, 1966; Fishman & Franks, 1992) rather than from the mentalistic and decidedly theoretical concepts posited by Freud and other psychoanalysts.

It is interesting that behaviorists presented their techniques as distinct from a medical model, in the sense that they claimed that mental disorders were the result of learning (i.e., an interaction with the environment) rather than the result of biology. Nevertheless, at a higher level of abstraction, behavioral treatments conform to the medical model (Wampold, 2001b), as they are composed of five crucial components. First, there is a disorder, problem, or complaint (e.g., the client is suffering from intrusive thoughts, distractibility, and depression). Second, there is an explanation for the problems; in medicine the explanation would be biological (e.g., the patient's stomach pain was an ulcer caused by bacteria), whereas in psychotherapy the explanation would be psychological (e.g., the patient's insomnia is the result of traumatic experiences). Third, there exist mechanisms of change that are consistent with the theoretical explanation for the disorder (e.g., extinction). Fourth, the mechanisms of change suggest that particular therapeutic actions should be used (e.g., prolonged exposure). Fifth, and most important, the therapeutic action is responsible for the benefits of the psychotherapy and not other factors, such as the alliance with the therapist (i.e., the decrease in symptoms was caused by prolonged exposure and not other therapeutic actions or conditions). The last component, which is referred to as *specificity*, is in many ways the hallmark of medicine (Wampold, 2001b). After all, Franz Anton Mesmer was not exposed as a charlatan because his treatments were not effective but because the purportedly causal mechanism (viz., animal magnetism) was not responsible for the

---

[1]In this chapter, the term *disorder* is used because research on mental health services is organized around that concept. However, the term is affiliated with a medical model and is not descriptive of many models of psychotherapy. Indeed, the diagnostic systems used to identify disorders are flawed, as discussed briefly later in this chapter.

improvement experienced by Mesmer's patients (Wampold & Bhati, 2004). The five-component model (complaint, explanation, mechanism of change, therapeutic ingredients, and specificity), which forms the medical model in medicine as well as psychotherapy, is emblematic not only of behavioral treatments; the advocates of particular treatments for particular disorders typically offer such models in treatments manuals and descriptions of their treatments.

The adoption of a medical model of psychotherapy also necessitates certain methods. The gold standard to establish specificity in medicine is the randomized double-blind placebo control group design, often referred to simply as a randomized clinical trial (RCT). Such designs are required by the Food and Drug Administration (FDA) to demonstrate that the effects of drugs are due to their specific ingredients, rather than to patient expectations, hope, remoralization, or other psychological factors that are independent of the specific ingredients of the drug. In the past few decades, RCTs have similarly become the gold standard in psychotherapy research, at least among those who wish to establish that a particular treatment is efficacious for a particular disorder (Goldfried & Wolfe, 1998).

The notion that therapies need to be validated by the use of RCTs was institutionalized by the Society of Clinical Psychology (Division 12 of the American Psychological Association) in the mid-1990s when the Task Force on Promotion and Dissemination of Psychological Procedures was charged with developing criteria for establishing treatments as empirically validated treatments (which are now called *empirically supported treatments* [ESTs]) and compiling a list of treatments that satisfied the criteria (Task Force on Promotion and Dissemination of Psychological Procedures, 1995). The EST movement clearly aligned psychotherapy and psychotherapy research with the medical establishment. The criteria, which are in most respects indistinguishable from the criteria used by the FDA to approve drugs, clearly oriented psychotherapy to a mental illness: "We do not ask whether a treatment is efficacious; rather, we ask whether it is efficacious for a specific problem" (Chambless & Hollon, 1998). Although use of the *Diagnostic and Statistical Manual of Mental Disorders* (DSM) as the nosology for assigning disorders was not required, Chambless and Hollon (1998) indicated the DSM has "a number of benefits" for determining ESTs (p. 9). Moreover, the notion of specificity is inherent in the criteria for ESTs, as it was important to show that psychotherapeutic treatments were not simply efficacious but added something above and beyond the effects produced by placebo (i.e., what could be achieved by hope, expectation, alliance, or relationship):

> We [The Task Force] believe establishing efficacy in contrast to a waiting list control group is not sufficient. Relying on such evidence would leave psychologists at a serious disadvantage vis-à-vis psychiatrists who can point to numerous double-blind placebo trials to support the valid-

ity of their interventions. (Task Force on Promotion and Dissemination of Psychological Procedures, 1995, p. 5)

It is clear that the development of psychotherapy in the United States has been closely associated with medicine. Indeed, some have argued that psychological treatments (in the main, ESTs), although built on characteristics found in a variety of treatments including "the therapeutic alliance, the induction of positive expectancy of change, and remoralization," contain "specific psychological procedures targeted at the psychopathology at hand" (Barlow, 2004, p. 873). Treatments lacking the specific psychological procedures to which Barlow refers would be designated as *generic psychotherapy*, whereas those containing the ingredients would be referred to as *psychological treatments*. In this conceptualization, the focus is on the particular therapeutic ingredient that is purportedly critical to client change and relegates to an inferior status therapist qualities and actions, the working alliance of the therapist and the client, the client's active participation, and other factors that often are assigned to the common factors. As presented here, however, the status of superiority of treatment method, above all else, may well indeed be a consequence of history rather than of science. Indeed, as the next section discusses, the research evidence has shown convincingly that the particular treatment is relatively unimportant and the combination of therapist, the client, and their work together is critical to the success of psychotherapy.

## Second Strand: Common Factors Models

The strand that is obscured by the medical model of psychotherapy is the one that emphasizes the humanistic interaction of therapist and client. In 1936, Saul Rosenzweig, having observed that advocates of the various psychotherapies all claimed great success, suggested that there were commonalities among various treatments and that these commonalities were responsible for the benefits of psychotherapy. Over the years, a number of luminaries have offered various common factors models, including notably Jerome Frank (Frank & Frank, 1991), Judd Marmor (1962), and Sol Garfield (1995). Although there are differences among the various models presented, they share the principle that the specific ingredients stipulated in various treatments are relatively unimportant and instead give primacy to the engagement of a therapist and client in a healing process. The common factors models emphasize the collaborative work of therapist and client, and thus there is a focus on the therapist, the client, the transaction between them, and the structure of the treatment that is offered.

Despite the pioneering work of Rosenzweig, Frank, Marmor, Garfield, and others, scientific discussions of psychotherapy have been focused most prominently on treatments. As in medicine, the question is, "What treatment is indicated for a given disorder?" This emphasis places the common factors in the background, relegated to a status sometimes expressed as "necessary to deliver the treatment but not sufficient to remediate psychological distress." The thesis of this book is that these common factors are indeed the "heart and soul" of therapy, a conjecture that is fully supported by the research evidence, as demonstrated in this chapter.

## PSYCHOTHERAPY EVIDENCE FOR SPECIFIC INGREDIENTS

The research evidence fails to support the conjecture that the focus on treatment is related to outcome and instead suggests that the common factors, as Rosenzweig (1936) presciently predicted, are critical to successful psychotherapy. Briefly, the research evidence related to several critical questions is reviewed in this section.

### Does Psychotherapy Work?

Healing practices, which have existed since the origins of the human species and which are indigenous to every culture, past and present, have only recently been subjected to scientific scrutiny to determine whether or not they are effective. Of course, the history of modern medicine is closely tied to the empirical documentation that the various medical treatments are effective. Indeed, in a perspicuous way, it has been the documentation of effectiveness that distinguishes modern from premodern medicine; the development of the double-blind randomized placebo control research design in the 1950s allowed researchers to document that various drugs are superior to a placebo that is indistinguishable from the active medication (A. K. Shapiro & Shapiro, 1997; Wampold, 2001b; Wampold & Bhati, 2004). The result has been to establish the effectiveness of many medical drugs and procedures.

The only other healing practice that has been subject to scientific scrutiny that approaches the rigor of modern medicine is psychotherapy, although the journey to scientific establishment has not been without some tortured turns. In the 1950s and 1960s, Hans Eysenck (1952, 1961, 1966) claimed that research demonstrated that psychotherapy—which included for his purposes predominantly psychodynamic and eclectic treatments but not treatments based on learning theory (i.e., behavior therapies)—was not only ineffective but possibly harmful.

It was about 2 decades after Eysenck's original claims about the ineffectiveness of psychotherapy that Mary Lee Smith and Gene Glass (Smith & Glass, 1977; Smith, Glass, & Miller, 1980) used meta-analyses, an emerging statistical technology, to test Eysenck's claim. They examined the extant research that compared psychotherapy with no treatment control groups; the results demonstrated that psychotherapy was, in fact, remarkably effective, yielding an effect size estimate of .80, which has proven to be remarkably robust (Wampold, 2001b).

As with any quantitative index, it is important to understand the practical implications of an effect of this size. Literally, an effect size of .80 means that the average score on whatever outcomes measure (or measures) used to assess functioning (e.g., symptoms, well-being, functioning) of those who receive treatment is 0.8 standard deviation better than the score of those who do not received any treatment. Of course, the practical application of such an interpretation is limited, but there are several ways to convert this index into something more useful (see Wampold, 2001b). An effect size of .80 indicates that the average client receiving a treatment would be better off than about 79% of untreated clients, which should be quite impressive to researchers, clinicians, and clients alike. Another means to understanding an effect is to convert it to an index called the *number needed to treat* (NNT), which is the number of clients who need to receive the treatment to achieve one better outcome than would have been accomplished in the absence of treatment. NNT is becoming the common metric of evidence-based medicine. An effect size of .80 corresponds to an NNT of approximately 3 (Kraemer & Kupfer, 2006), which indicates that three clients need to receive psychotherapy to achieve a better outcome than would have been attained without treatment. Although psychotherapy clearly does not lead to success with every client, psychotherapy compares well with established medical practices. Indeed, psychotherapy is as or more effective than many medical treatments highlighted in reviews of evidence-based practices in medicine, including many interventions in cardiology, geriatric medicine, and asthma as well as aspirin as a prophylaxis for heart attacks, the influenza vaccine, and cataract surgery (Wampold, 2007). Moreover, psychotherapy typically is as effective as drug treatments for emotional problems and is more enduring and creates less resistance to multiple administrations than drugs (Barlow, Gorman, Shear, & Woods, 2000; Hollon, Stewart, & Strunk, 2006; Imel, Malterer, McKay, & Wampold, 2008; Leykin et al., 2007). Finally, clinicians treating depression in a managed care environment achieve outcomes comparable with the outcomes attained in clinical trials of established and evidence-based treatments for depression (Minami et al., 2008).

The answer to the question "Does psychotherapy work?" is a resounding "Yes." Psychotherapeutic treatments have been subjected to rigorous clinical trials, and the benefits are demonstrably large. The effectiveness of psychotherapy exceeds that of many accepted medical practices. Moreover, and important for clients, it appears that psychotherapy delivered in naturalistic settings produces outcomes comparable with the outcomes attained in clinical trials.

Psychotherapy is truly a remarkably effective healing practice. But the next logical question is, "Are some psychotherapies more effective than others, and if so, which ones?"

## Are Some Psychotherapies More Effective Than Others?

In medicine, it is clear that some treatments are more effective than others, and indeed some have been found to be harmful. The notion in medicine, as discussed earlier, is that the critical aspect of a treatment is the specific ingredient; if some of those ingredients are more potent than others, then treatments that rely on the more potent ingredients produce better outcomes than other treatments. As medicine progresses, more effective treatments are developed, and the less effective treatments are discarded; gastric ulcers are now treated with antibiotics rather than acid-neutralizing antacids because it was discovered that ulcers are caused by bacteria living in the gut.

A medical model of psychotherapy predicts that some types of psychotherapies will be more effective than others because superior specific ingredients will result in better outcomes. This actually was the point of Eysenck's (1952, 1961, 1966) denunciation of psychotherapy: He was claiming that psychotherapy (meaning psychodynamic, humanistic, and eclectic, primarily) were ineffective or harmful, whereas scientifically designed treatments (which to his reckoning were behavioral treatments emanating from learning theory) were effective and therefore preferred to psychotherapy (Wampold, 2001b). This is an argument not too different from Barlow's (2004) distinction between psychological treatments and generic psychotherapy, discussed earlier.

On the other hand, a model that emphasizes the common factors predicts that, with some qualifications, all cogent treatments, embraced by therapist and client and competently delivered to a client motivated to engage in the process, are equally effective. The logic is simple: It is the common factors discussed in this book that lead to successful outcomes, and as long as those common factors are capably used by therapist and client, the treatment will be beneficial. To those steeped in a medical tradition, as most people are in Western societies, the notion is counterintuitive: The potency of some medications, particularly newly developed, must surely be more effective than the treatments offered to our parents and grandparents. But, as Saul Rosenzweig observed in 1936, counterintuitively, the dodo said, "All have won, and all must have prizes." And it indeed appears that the evidence leads to the conclusion that all treatments intended to be therapeutic are equally effective.

The evidence for the equivalence of all treatments has been accumulating since the time that researchers rigorously examined the outcomes of psychotherapy. When Smith and Glass (1977; Smith et al., 1980) conducted their meta-analyses that showed that psychotherapy was effective, they also examined the relative efficacy of various types of treatments. Although at first it appeared that behavioral treatments were superior, as Eysenck suggested, when confounding variables (such as the reactivity of the measures) were controlled, there were no significant differences among treatments. A number of meta-analyses conducted after Smith and Glass have found a similar result: When differences among studies are controlled, treatments appear to be remarkably equivalent (Robinson, Berman, & Neimeyer, 1990; D. A. Shapiro & Shapiro, 1982; Wampold, Minami, Baskin, & Tierney, 2002).

The effects of confounding variables have been illustrated, for example, by Robinson et al. (1990), who found that for the treatment of adult depression, cognitive–behavioral approaches were superior to behavioral approaches, and both of these treatments as well as cognitive therapies were superior to general verbal therapies. However, the differences were entirely accounted for by the allegiance of the researcher. Allegiance of the researcher is present when the researcher is an advocate for one of the treatments being studied. Often, this occurs when the researcher developed one of the treatments or has argued for the superiority of the treatment; this allegiance is often conveyed to therapists in the study when the researcher trains and supervises the therapists, and the therapists know that there is a belief that one treatment is believed to be superior to the others. In Robinson et al.'s (1990) study, when allegiance of the researcher to a particular treatment was accounted for, the differences among treatments disappeared (see Wampold, 2001b, for a discussion of allegiance effects more generally).

One way to control for many of the confounds among studies is to limit meta-analyses to only those studies that directly compare two or more psychotherapies (Shadish & Sweeney, 1991). This is a strategy used by Gloaguen, Cottraux, Cucherat, and Blackburn (1998), who compared cognitive treatments for adult depression with other treatments and found that cognitive therapies were superior to a class of therapies that were labeled as *other therapies*. Unfortunately, several of the other therapies were not really therapies intended by the researchers to be therapeutic but were rather administered to control for common factors by providing a warm and empathic therapist, but one who delivered no particular treatment. This is particularly problematic because psychotherapy trials are not blinded, and the therapist generally knows that he or she is delivering a treatment the researchers consider to be a sham. It is no wonder that the researchers' favored treatment is superior to these controls, as the comparison treatment is not a treatment at all and certainly not one that a therapist would choose to use. A good example of such a bogus treatment is "supportive counseling" used by Foa, Rothbaum, Riggs, and Murdock (1991) in a clinical trial of cognitive–behavioral therapy (CBT) for women who were sexually assaulted and experiencing posttraumatic stress disorder (PTSD):

> Patients were taught a general problem-solving technique. Therapists played an indirect and unconditionally supportive role. Homework consisted of the patient's keeping a diary of daily problems and her attempts at problem solving. Patients were immediately redirected to focus on current daily problems if discussions of the assault occurred. (p. 718)

Clearly, this "supportive counseling" is not a means that therapists would use to treat recently assaulted women.

Wampold et al. (1997) addressed the issues of confounding and treatments not intended to be therapeutic by examining only studies that directly compared two treatments intended to be therapeutic for adult disorders. They found that the differences among treatments were consistent with a hypothesis that all treatments are equally effective and that the upper bound for the difference among treatments was an effect size of .2, which is an extremely small difference. Moreover, the comparisons of treatments that were very different did not produce larger effects than comparisons of treatments that were similar, another finding consistent with equality of effectiveness.

Wampold et al.'s (1997) meta-analysis was criticized because it asked the general question "Are all psychotherapies equivalent?" rather than the specific question "Are all treatments for a particular disorder equivalent?" or an even the more specific question "Are all treatments for a particular disorder for a particular population equivalent?" The argument can be made that generically all treatments are about equally effective, but for specific disorders, some treatments are more effective because they contain "specific psychological procedures targeted at the psychopathology at hand," which is the argument made by Barlow (2004, p. 873) and Crits-Christoph (1997). This argument is made most perspicuously with regard to anxiety disorders, in which it is claimed that behavioral and cognitive–behavioral treatments are more scientifically justified and more effective. An argument has also been made that the dodo bird conjecture may apply to adults, at least to some adult disorders, but not to children. Nevertheless, recent meta-analyses and primary studies have produced evidence that suggests that these criticisms of the dodo bird conjecture do not threaten the validity of the conclusions that all treatments are equally effective.

First, look at the literature with regard to particular disorders, especially those that are most prevalent. It appears that there are absolutely no differences among treatments intended to be therapeutic for the treatment of adult depression, one of the most prevalent of all mental disorders. Earlier meta-analyses demonstrated that when comparing the effects of treatment versus control groups, the relative advantages of cognitive treatments were due to allegiance of the researcher (e.g., Robinson et al., 1990). Later meta-analyses of direct comparison appeared to demonstrate that cognitive treatments were superior to *verbal therapies* (i.e., noncognitive, nonbehavioral treatments; Gloaguen et al., 1998); however, when treatments that were not intended to be therapeutic (e.g., supportive counseling used as a control for common factors) were omitted, verbal therapies were as effective as cognitive therapies (Wampold et al., 2002). Indeed, it seems that all treatments that have been examined in clinical trials meet the criteria to be classified as an EST; by 1998, the EST list included cognitive therapy, interpersonal therapy, brief dynamic therapy, psychoeducational treatment, self-control therapy, and reminiscence therapy for geriatric clients (Chambless et al., 1998), a list that spans much of the array of psychotherapy orientations. Moreover, process–experiential treatment, a treatment derived from the humanistic tradition, has been found to be as effective as CBT, the gold standard in depression treatment (Watson, Gordon, Stermac, Kalogerakos, & Steckley, 2003). Thus, it appears that for the treatment of adult depression, many treatments from a variety of theoretical orientations are equally effective.

It should be noted that there have been isolated instances in which one treatment for depression has been found to be superior to another treatment; for example, Dimidjian et al. (2006) found that behavioral activation was superior to cognitive–behavioral therapy for severely depressed clients. In these instances, however, no cogent explanation for the differences has been provided, and no systematic pattern of results has suggested any treatment is superior to another for the treatment of depression (Wampold, 2007).

With regard to anxiety, Wampold (2001b, 2006a) reviewed the meta-analyses for various anxiety disorders and found no evidence that one particular treatment for any of the anxiety disorders has been shown to be more effective than any other. Particularly informative is the research on PTSD because PTSD is a disorder that is attributable to a discrete event or series of events and thus it would appear that treatments based on classical conditioning paradigms would be particularly effective. Accordingly, Foa and her colleagues have developed a treatment protocol involving prolonged imaginal exposure and in vivo exposure along with cognitive restructuring. As expected, this treatment has been shown to be quite effective (Foa et al., 1991, 2005). Nevertheless, several treatments with very different treatment rationales have also been shown to be effective, including eye movement desensitization and reprocessing, cognitive therapy without exposure, hypnotherapy, psychodynamic therapy, and present-centered therapy. A recent meta-analysis examining direct comparison among these treatments found all of them to be equally effective (Benish, Imel, & Wampold, 2008). It is interesting that two of the aforementioned treatments—namely cognitive therapy without exposure and present-centered therapy—were designed to exclude any therapeutic actions that might involve exposure, which is actually difficult to accomplish in any psychotherapy (e.g., clients are not allowed to talk about their traumas because that involves imaginal exposure). Nevertheless, the two treatments without exposure were as effective as the treatments in which exposure was incidental (e.g., psychodynamic) or central (CBT including prolonged and in vivo exposure; Benish et al., 2008). As various treatments for anxiety disorders are rigorously tested, they are found to be effective; recently, psychodynamic therapy for panic disorder has been found to be effective (Milrod et al., 2007).

With regard to childhood disorders, it has been claimed that cognitive and behavioral treatments are superior to other treatments (Weiss & Weisz, 1995; Weisz, Weiss, Han, Granger, & Morton, 1995). However, recent meta-analyses have again indicated that all therapies intended to be therapeutic for youth are equally effective. Spielmans, Pasek, and McFall (2007) examined all direct comparisons of CBT for childhood depression and anxiety with other treatments and found that (a) CBT was not superior to non-CBT bona fide treatments and (b) full CBT treatments were not superior to one or more of the components of these treatments. Miller, Wampold, and Varhely (2008) meta-analyzed studies that directly contrasted two or more treatments for youth with diagnoses of depression, anxiety, conduct disorder, and attention deficit disorders (i.e., the most prevalent disorders of youth) and did find small differences among treatments, but these differences were due entirely to allegiance effects. For a more complete summary related to children, see chapter 11 in this volume.

It appears that for the most prevalent disorders of adults and children, all treatments intended to be therapeutic are equally effective. It is important to note that treatments intended to be therapeutic are cogent treatments (a) provided by a clinician who believes in the treatment and (b) accepted by the client. The finding of equivalence of psychotherapy effectiveness is contrary to the medical model that stipulates that some ingredients are more potent than others and suggests that the common factors play a critical role in producing the benefits of psychotherapy. Before taking up the evidence for the common factors, however, the evidence for specific ingredients is considered.

## Is There Evidence for Specificity in Psychotherapy?

As discussed earlier, the hallmark of modern medicine is the notion of specificity, which stipulates that the effectiveness of treatment is due to the specific ingredients in the particular treatments. There are two complementary ways that medicine documents specificity: The first involves showing the superiority of the drug or procedure to a placebo and the second involves a prototypic system-specific sequence (Wampold, 2007). The evidence in each of these two areas is now reviewed.

*Placebo-Controlled (and Related) Research in Psychotherapy*

Placebo-controlled group designs in medicine have three interrelated requirements: blinding, indistinguishability, and randomization. The double-blind requirement in medicine stipulates that neither the patient nor the administrator of the treatment is knowledgeable about whether the specific treatment (e.g., a particular drug) or the placebo is being administered. This is necessary to rule out differential expectations of success by either the administrator of the treatment or the patient. Furthermore, the drug and the placebo must be indistinguishable to accomplish blinding. Finally, to be valid, the experiment needs to assign participants randomly to conditions. The development of the randomized double-blind placebo-controlled design was critical to establishing modern medicine as scientifically based because it ruled out such threats as increased hope and expectations for success of patients and the charisma and personal influence of the physicians. Shortly after medicine adopted this design, Rosenthal and Frank (1956) recommended that it be used in psychotherapy to establish specificity. In psychotherapy, the placebo control is a treatment that involves a therapist and client but contains no specific ingredients; typically, the therapist responds empathically but does not provide a cogent treatment to the client. Such treatments are often called *nonspecific, supportive counseling,* or *common factor controls.*

Several reviews of the placebo literature have shown that treatments intended to be therapeutic are superior to these placebo-type control groups (Lambert & Bergin, 1994; Stevens, Hynan, & Allen, 2000). Many researchers interpret this as evidence for the specific effects of treatment techniques included in bona fide therapies (Stevens et al., 2000). However, three critical issues render this claim for specificity problematic. The first issue is that psychotherapy trials cannot be blinded, and the placebos are not indistinguishable from the treatment, as discussed previously (Baskin, Tierney, Minami, & Wampold, 2003; Imel & Wampold, 2008; Wampold, 2001b; Wampold, Minami, Tierney, Baskin, & Bhati, 2005). Most important, the therapists are necessarily aware of the treatment they are providing and consequently are aware in the placebo condition that they are delivering a treatment that is not intended to be therapeutic and for which the expectation exists that it will not be as effective as the real treatment. Thus, a therapist's belief in the effectiveness of the placebo-type treatment is compromised. Moreover, because the treatment and the placebo are not indistinguishable, the client also likely knows that he or she is receiving the less desirable treatment. Consequently, differences between treatments could be due to a therapist's lack of belief in the treatment or a client's knowledge that he or she is receiving the control treatment, rather than to the specific techniques included in the experimental treatment.

A second issue is that one of the common factors is the delivery of a treatment of some kind: a treatment that has a cogent and convincing rationale (see chap. 5, this volume). Without a treatment, there can be no collaborative effort to establish goals of therapy, and the therapist and client cannot agree on the tasks needed to accomplish the goals, which are two components of the therapeutic alliance, a critical common factor (see chap. 4, this volume). Thus, these placebo-type controls lack two of the most important aspects of common factors models: a treatment intended to be therapeutic and two components of the therapeutic alliance.

A third issue is that in studies comparing a specific treatment with placebo-type controls, the two treatments are not structurally equivalent. *Structural equivalence* refers to the similarity of two treatments in terms of therapist training, number and length of sessions, format (group vs. individual), and the degree to which clients are allowed to discuss topics germane to their treatment (Baskin et al., 2003). Often, the placebo-type control is deficient in one or more of these areas (e.g., fewer sessions), in which case the superiority of the treatment to the control may be due to this deficiency rather than to the potency of the specific ingredients in the treatment. Baskin et al. (2003) evaluated the effect of structural equivalence in a meta-analysis and found that as the structural equivalence of a placebo-type control condition approached that of the bona fide therapy, differences between conditions became quite small (i.e., not statistically different). That is, if the placebo-type control was similar to the bona fide treatment, it was as effective, even though it did not contain all the common factors. Thus, the differential effectiveness of placebo-type controls and bona fide psychotherapies is not likely due to the effects of specific techniques.

A rigorous way to examine specificity that avoids many of the problems associated with placebo-type controls is to either remove a critical ingredient or to add a theoretically important component to an established treatment. These designs, often called *component designs*, are used occasionally to test for specificity. An exemplary component study was conducted by Jacobson et al. (1996), who dismantled CBT for depression by comparing CBT with behavioral treatment (BT). CBT and BT were structurally equivalent except that BT lacked the cognitive components thought to be essential for the effectiveness of CBT. The results, which were surprising to the authors, revealed that the treatments, with and without the cognitive components, were equally effective, calling into question the specificity of CBT for depression. In 2001, Ahn and Wampold meta-analytically examined all component studies in adult psychotherapy and found no evidence to support the claim that removing or adding a specific ingredient to a treatment altered outcomes.

In contrast to medical research, in psychotherapy it is difficult to design trials to establish specificity. Nevertheless, a rigorous examination of placebo-type control research and component studies provides little evidence for specificity.

## The Prototypic System-Specific Sequence in Psychotherapy

Although in medicine placebo-controlled research provides evidence for specific ingredients in a treatment, typically the notion of specificity also requires a theoretical and empirical demonstration of how the ingredient affects the biological system to cure the patient or remediate the symptoms (Wampold, 2007). According to Wampold (2007), in medicine the prototypic sequence is as follows:

> (a) A biological explanation for the illness, based on scientific research, is established, (b) a treatment is designed or a substance is hypothesized to remediate the biological deficit, (c) administration of the substance demonstrably alters the biology of the patient in the expected way and other substances do not, (d) the change in the biology remediates the illness (a cure or management of chronic illness). (p. 867)

It is interesting that when Rosenthal and Frank (1956) suggested psychotherapy researchers use the placebo to establish specificity in psychotherapy, they also indicated that psychotherapy researchers needed to determine a chain of empirical results that would establish the specificity sequence in a manner similar to that used in medicine. However, establishing the specificity in psychology is more difficult than in medicine. Nevertheless, efforts in this regard have not provided evidence that the specific actions prescribed in various psychotherapies are responsible for the benefits of psychotherapy.

As a first example of the difficulties with the specificity sequence, consider the case of systematic desensitization, which was one of the first, if not the first, behavioral "talk" treatments (Fishman & Franks, 1992) and one that has been empirically tested and found to be effective, as evidenced by its designation as an EST (Chambless et al., 1998). The original rationale for systematic desensitization proposed by Wolpe in 1958 was based on classical conditioning (more specifically, reciprocal inhibition), but by the late 1970s it had been shown quite unequivocally that this explanation was flawed (Fishman & Franks, 1992). Several other explanations were offered in its place, including extinction, expectancy effects, cognitive reassessment, and treatment credibility (Kirsch & Henry, 1977; Wampold, 2001b). To date, there have been no conclusive studies demonstrating how systematic desensitization works. Systematic desensitization is a relatively simple psychotherapy that is delivered in a constrained manner, yet the specificity sequence cannot be established because the psychological bases for the benefits cannot be established.

One of the profound difficulties that underlie attempts to determine the specificity sequence for psychological treatments is that it relies on a flawed diagnostic system. In medicine, the biological etiology for many diseases has been established, and if it has not been established, there are empirically based theories that guide treatment development. In the area of mental health disorders, diagnostic nosologies (e.g., the *DSM*) are descriptive rather than etiological (Widiger & Trull, 2007) and often reflect cultural notions of what is dysfunctional (Wakefield, 1992, 1999). Not having a definitive psychological model for dysfunction prevents confirmation of the specificity sequence, as is illustrated by panic disorder, in which the six best psychological explanations provided for this disorder have either been falsified or are not falsifiable (Roth, Wilhelm, & Petit, 2005). It is not surprising, therefore, that a variety of treatments based on a range of explanations for panic have been shown to be effective, including the seemingly theoretically polar opposites CBT (Barlow, Craske, Cerny, & Klosko, 1989) and psychodynamic psychotherapy (Milrod et al., 2007).

One way to avoid the dilemma presented by diagnostic systems is to examine subtypes of disorders, in which the subtypes are based on etiological rather than descriptive factors. This is an argument made by Follette and Houts (1996) with regard to the dodo bird effect in the treatment of depression:

> If one assumed that depressive symptoms were one possible endpoint from a number of etiological pathways and that any group of persons with depression contained a number from each pathway, then comparative outcome studies are forever doomed to get equivalent results because those who might have had a biological cause might respond to medication but not those were interpersonally unskilled, and so on. So far there is little evidence that there are common etiological pathways that describe a uniform course or response to treatment for any reasonable proportion of the *DSM–IV* categories. (p. 1128)

Specificity would be strongly supported if etiological subtypes moderated treatment efficacy, as suggested by Follette and Houts (1996). Nevertheless, the many attempts to establish that etiological subtypes are more effective in one type of treatment (e.g., clients with dysfunctional cognitions receiving CBT) than in another (these clients in non-CBT) have not confirmed the matching hypothesis (Wampold, 2001b). Simply put, there is little evidence that any particular treatment can be matched to any client on the basis of the nature of the disorder (i.e., etiological subtypes). There is some evidence that various types of persons do better with certain types of clients, as suggested by technical eclecticism (Beutler & Clarkin, 1990). For example, there is some evidence to suggest that so-called characterologically resistant clients have better outcomes in structured rather than unstructured treatments (Beutler, Harwood, Alimohamed, & Malik, 2002), but such a finding does not establish the specificity of any particular ingredient of a treatment. Indeed, that some types of clients find some types of treatments more acceptable and useful is consistent with many common factors models (see chap. 3, this volume); corroborative efforts of the therapist and client are critical to the success of therapy, and client acceptance of the explanation of treatment is therefore critical (Baldwin, Wampold, & Imel, 2007; Imel & Wampold, 2008; Wampold, 2007).

There have also been claims made that two treatments could be equally effective because the purported mechanisms of each are equally potent. For example, CBT and response prevention/exposure (RPE) are both treatments with empirical support for the treatment of obsessive–compulsive disorder. It is hypothesized that CBT works by focusing on the cognitive aspects of obsessive–compulsive disorder (i.e., the obsessions), whereas RPE works by focusing on the behavioral aspects (i.e., the compulsions). However, the application of both CBT and RPE first reduces compulsions, which in turn leads to a reduction in obsessions, suggesting that the two treatments work through the same mechanism (Anholt et al., 2008).

There is a final area of psychotherapy research that sheds light on the specificity sequence. If an ingredient is critical to the success of a treatment, then the degree to which the therapy contains the ingredient (i.e., the degree to which the therapist includes the ingredient in his or her delivery of the treatment) should be correlated with outcome. The degree to which the treatment contains these critical ingredients is referred to as *therapist adherence to the treatment protocol*. Although some evidence has suggested that some degree of adherence is important, other findings have indicated that there is either no relationship between adherence and outcome or that high and possibly rigid levels of adherence may even be detrimental (Imel & Wampold, 2008; Wampold, 2001b).

A number of studies have found adherence unrelated to outcome (Imel & Wampold, 2008; Wampold, 2001b). An interesting result in this regard was reported by Shaw et al. (1999) in an analysis of data for the CBT condition from the National Institute of Mental Health Treatment of Depression Collaborative Research Program. After controlling for pretreatment symptoms and the provision of support by the therapist, Shaw et al. found that adherence measures were unrelated to outcome. However, in this study competence was also assessed, and although competence in delivering CBT was unrelated to outcome, including adherence and competence in the model simultaneously revealed a significant correlation between competence and outcome, which is the classical suppression effect. Adherence suppresses the relationship of competence to adherence, suggesting that aspects of competence unrelated to adherence (i.e., general competence in therapy rather than competence in CBT) are important. So, it appears that adherence to the CBT protocol may actually detract from the competence of the therapist.

The suggestion that adherence might exert a negative influence has been shown in several early studies of adherence (Castonguay, Goldfried, Wiser, Raue, & Hayes, 1996; Henry, Schacht, Strupp, Butler, & Binder, 1993; Henry, Strupp, Butler, Schacht, & Binder, 1993). A recent report related to adherence is informative because it occurred in the context of a rigorous clinical trial of an EST. Huppert, Barlow, Gorman, Shear, and Woods (2006) examined client motivation and adherence to CBT in the treatment for panic. Among clients who were less motivated to change, therapist adherence to the treatment protocol resulted in poorer outcomes, whereas for more motivated clients, therapist adherence was unrelated to outcome. This result suggests that for clients who do not seem to believe the treatment will work, the greater the degree to which the therapist continues to deliver the ingredients of the treatment, the less the client will benefit, probably because the agreement on the tasks of therapy is low.

*Conclusions for Specificity*

A thorough review of the literature provides precious little evidence for the specificity of any psychotherapy, thereby suggesting that the common factors are the potent aspects of treatment. However, the absence of research evidence for specificity is not sufficient; there must actually be evidence that supports the common factors. Through the years, this evidence has been accumulating (Norcross, 2002). Unfortunately, the evidence has become quite diffuse because integrated models of the common factors have not been emphasized. That is, evidence for a particular factor has been studied isolated from other factors, creating a potpourri of results that limits the utility of common factor research to improve the quality of psychotherapy (Imel & Wampold, 2008). The purpose of this volume is to examine how the common factors can be integrated in such a way as to lead to improved outcomes.

## COMMON FACTORS

The remainder of this chapter briefly reviews the literature on common factors models and research. This sketch foreshadows the various chapters in this book in that the evidence supporting the importance of various common factors is presented.

### The Nature of the Common Factors

As noted, Rosenzweig in 1936 originated the common factors notion (see Prologue, this volume); he described a number of *implicit common factors* that explain treatment successes, including the following: (a) the inspiring or stimulating aspects of the therapist's personality, (b) the reintegration of personality through the systematic application of some therapeutic ideology, (c) implicit psychological processes such as catharsis or social reconditioning, and (d) the reformulation of psychological events. Although common factors models have never been a predominate force in psychotherapy (Arkowitz, 1992), there has been enough interest that by 1990 Grencavage and Norcross found nearly 90 common factors referenced in the literature. A number of attempts have been made to classify the common factors into categories to make sense of the structure of the common factors (Grencavage & Norcross, 1990; Lambert & Bergin, 1994; Tracey, Lichtenberg, Goodyear, Claiborn, & Wampold, 2003; Weinberger, 2002; Weinberger, Rasco, & Hofmann, 2007).

Missing from these attempts to list and then categorize the common factors is that the common factors are not analogues of specific ingredients that can be added and removed singularly (Imel & Wampold, 2008). One often reads that the most prominent common factor is the relationship with an empathic healer, but quite obviously this ingredient cannot be removed from psychotherapy and still have a practice that would be classified as psychotherapy. Consequently, the common factors cannot be experimentally manipulated in the same manner as specific ingredients, but this does not suggest logically that such factors cannot be responsible for the benefits of psychotherapy.

Another issue with listing and categorizing common factors is that such factors are intertwined with each other and with the specific treatments that are delivered. Over the years, there have been several attempts to develop integrated models involving the common factors. The most notable integrated model has been presented by Frank and Frank, most recently in 1991. Wampold and colleagues (Imel & Wampold, 2008; Wampold, 2001b, 2007; Wampold, Imel, Bhati, & Johnson Jennings, 2007) and Duncan, Miller, and Sparks (2004) have extended this model by emphasizing the contextual nature of psychotherapy. In the remainder of this chapter, the intertwined nature of the common factors is discussed by examining the most prominent common factors, research in support of these common factors, and the ways in which the common factors overlap with each other.

## The Intertwined Common Factors

The intertwined nature of the common factors can be demonstrated by choosing any prominent one and examining the research and theory related to it. In this chapter, the investigation begins with the focus on therapist effects, that is, the professional psychotherapist.

Historically, the development of clinical trials focused on the intervention being studied and ignored the provider of the intervention (Wampold,

2001a; Wampold & Bhati, 2004). For example, an early application (circa 1920s) of randomized designs examined the relative worth of various educational programs and ignored the provider (i.e., the teacher) of the programs. That is, it was assumed that the teachers would deliver the educational programs uniformly so that the outcomes would not be dependent on the teacher. Later, farmers and physicians were ignored, whereas emphasis was placed on farming methods (e.g., crop varieties and fertilizers) and medical interventions, respectively. Psychotherapy followed suit, emphasizing clinical trials of particular forms of psychotherapy (Goldfried & Wolfe, 1998). Indeed, analyses of clinical trials rarely examined the degree to which therapists were responsible for the benefits of the treatment (Wampold, 2006b), leaving unanswered the question of whether some therapists consistently produce better outcomes than other therapists, regardless of the type of psychotherapy.

Essentially, it appears that even in clinical trials in which therapists are selected for their skill, are trained and supervised, and are monitored to maintain adherence to the treatment protocol, a significant proportion of the variability in outcomes is attributable to therapists within treatments, and this therapist effect is at least one order of magnitude greater than any differences among treatments in these trials (Crits-Christoph et al., 1991; Huppert et al., 2001; Kim, Wampold, & Bolt, 2006). Similarly, in naturalistic settings, it is becoming clear that some therapists are more effective than other therapists, regardless of the type of therapy administered (Lutz, Leon, Martinovich, Lyons, & Stiles, 2007; Wampold & Brown, 2005).

The presence of therapist effects raises the critical question, "What are the characteristics and actions of effective therapists?" Although we do not know for certain (Beutler et al., 2004), one good candidate is related to the working alliance, a prominently mentioned common factor. The *working alliance* is defined as the bond between the therapist and client as well as the agreement about the tasks and goals of therapy (Bordin, 1979; Bordin, Horvath, & Greenberg, 1994; Hatcher, Barends, Hansell, & Gutfreund, 1995; Hatcher & Barends, 2006; Horvath & Bedi, 2002; Horvath & Luborsky, 1993). Several meta-analyses have shown that the alliance, measured early in therapy, is strongly associated with outcomes (Horvath & Bedi, 2002; Horvath & Symonds, 1991; Martin, Garske, & Davis, 2000). It is important to note that the alliance–outcome relationship is robust in that it appears across various therapies, including those that do not emphasize this aspect, such as CBT, as well as the more relational therapies, such as psychodynamic and humanistic treatments; indeed, the alliance is related to outcomes in psychopharmacology (Blatt, Zuroff, Quinlan, & Pilkonis, 1996; Klein et al., 2003; Zuroff & Blatt, 2006).

DeRubeis, Brotman, and Gibbons (2005), however, raised the possibility that the alliance is not critical to outcome in therapy because there is ambiguity about cause and effect of the alliance and outcome. First, it may be that the alliance is due to prior gains made in therapy and therefore is the effect of therapeutic progress rather than the cause. That is, the alliance measured, say at Session 3, is a consequence of early symptom reduction, and this reduction is responsible for ultimate improvement of the client, rather than the alliance. Various analyses that have examined the time course of alliance and symptoms have produced convincing evidence that the alliance is not the result of early improvement and that subsequent improvement can be traced to the alliance rather than early improvement (Klein et al., 2003; Zuroff & Blatt, 2006). A second issue raised by DeRubeis et al. (2005) was that the alliance between therapist and client may be due, in fact, to the client; that is, some clients come to therapy with an ability to form an alliance (Mallinckrodt, 1991), and it is these clients who progress in therapy. Baldwin et al. (2007) showed, on the contrary, that client contributions to the alliance were not related to outcome; those clients who formed a better alliance with a particular therapist did not have better outcomes than did clients who formed a poorer alliance with the same therapist. A third possibility is the one that places the emphasis on the therapist: Therapists who get better outcomes generally are the therapists who are better able to form an alliance with a variety of clients. Indeed, it is this possibility that was demonstrated by Baldwin et al. They found that therapists who generally form better alliances also had better outcomes. So, a client who has difficulty forming relationships has a better outcome with a therapist who can form better alliances across clients. This client has a relatively poor alliance with the more effective therapist but that alliance is better than it would have been with a less effective therapist, and the ultimate outcome will also be better. Baldwin et al. showed that much of the variability in therapist effectiveness was due to their variability in forming an alliance.

It appears that the alliance is a robust common factor and that the therapist's contribution to the alliance is important. However, the alliance is dependent on the delivery of a particular treatment. Although it is possible to form a relationship with a healer, there can be no agreement about the tasks and goals of therapy and critical aspects of the alliance without a particular treatment. As Frank and Frank (1991) emphasized, two common factors are the *myth* and *ritual*. The myth is the rationale for the treatment and the explanation for the client's difficulties, which are communicated to the client by the therapist in a convincing way. In the common factors perspective, the rationale and explanation need not be scientific truth; what is important is that the myth be accepted by the client and lead to adaptive responses (Imel & Wampold, 2008; Wampold, 2007; Wampold et al., 2007). The acceptance of an alternative and adaptive explanation for one's problems is insight, according to the common factors model (Wampold et al., 2007). The adaptive client actions are part of the ritual, which is roughly equivalent to the therapeutic actions. Psychological treatments all have in common some rationale and explanation and some therapeutic actions; these are the aspects of treatment that make treatment per se a common factor, as explained in chapter 5 in this volume.

A good working alliance is an indication that the client has accepted the rationale for the treatment, the explanation for the disorder, and is willing to participate in the process of therapy. A critical component of how this leads to change is involved in replacing a maladaptive explanation with an adaptive one. The maladaptive explanation is discouraging because the client cannot see how any action will lead to progress: Put simply, they are stuck. Frank and Frank (1991) would say they are demoralized, whereas Bandura (1997) would say that they have low self-efficacy for change. Acceptance of an alternative explanation changes the client's expectation, which is a critical component of any healing practice (Wampold, 2007). Over the years, modern medicine has discounted the importance of expectations, and indeed medicine is based on the demonstration that medical interventions are more effective than placebos, which are designed to control for expectations. However, research on placebos has demonstrated that expectations themselves result in demonstrable change in the body and account for much of the benefits of many medical procedures (Wampold et al., 2005). It is then not surprising that expectations are critical to the effectiveness of psychotherapy (Greenberg, Constantino, & Bruce, 2006; Kirsch, 2005), as discussed in chapter 5 in this volume.

Another critical component of the alliance involves *agreement* about the tasks and goals of therapy; that is, therapist and client are on the same page with regard to the process of therapy. Research indicates that successful psychotherapy involves collaborative and purposeful work (Hatcher & Barends, 2006), which raises the critical point that psychotherapy is not a treatment administered to a client but a process in which the client is engaged (Wampold, 2007). This leads to the conclusion that critical common factors involve the client (Bohart & Tallman, 1999; Duncan et al., 2004). If one considers that in any study of psychotherapy, the largest amount of variance is what in research design is called *error variability*. In actuality, this is client variability. Although not all of unexplained variance is easily identified as due to clients per se, without a doubt one cannot understand what makes therapy work without understanding the client's contribution, as discussed in chapter 3 in this volume.

## Mobilizing the Common Factors

If the common factors are critical to the success of psychotherapy, how can they be mobilized to increase the benefits that accrue to clients? Of course, education and training in the common factors is important. There is some evidence, for example, that specific manualized training in the alliance leads to better alliances (Crits-Christoph et al., 2006).

Discussion of education and training in an important way begs the question because such efforts are concentrated in the graduate training of therapists. It has become clear that despite the training and despite the fact that practicing therapists are achieving admirable outcomes, there is much variability in outcomes among therapists. How can the quality of outcomes be improved across the board for practicing therapists?

The answer to this question may be quite a simple one and one that applies to learning most any skill: continued practice with feedback. Learning to sail involves practice with feedback from the environment and from experts. Without feedback, learning any skill is almost impossible. Yet the field of psychotherapy has only recently begun to measure the outcomes of clients in practice and use these outcomes as feedback to therapists (Lambert, Hansen, & Finch, 2001; Miller, Duncan, & Hubble, 2005). It is not surprising, perhaps, that feedback has been found to improve the quality of services (Lambert et al., 2001) often dramatically, as discussed in chapter 8 and other chapters in this book. Clearly, feedback is an effective means to mobilize the common factors in psychotherapy.

## IMPLICATIONS

A brief review of the history reveals that psychotherapy and medicine are intertwined. It is not surprising then that psychotherapy has focused on establishing particular treatments for particular disorders. Nevertheless, the research evidence indicates that a variety of treatments, when administered by therapists who believe in the treatment and when accepted by the clients, are equally effective. Indeed, there is little evidence that the specific ingredients of any treatment are responsible for the benefits of therapy. On the other hand, there is a plethora of evidence that suggests that therapists vary in the outcomes that are produced and that these differences are due to common factors, such as the therapist's ability to form an alliance with his or her clients. These results have several implications for research and practice:

- *Clinical trials comparing two treatments should be discontinued.* Much money has been spent on clinical trials, with the same result: "Both treatments were more effective than no treatment, but there were no differences in outcomes between the two treatments." Continued research that looks at new variations of old treatments will yield little that can be transported to systems of care to improve the outcomes of clients.

- *Research should be devoted to understanding the process of therapy and how outcomes can be improved.* Therapy has been shown to work, but it is now time to understand how the common factors can be mobilized to increase the benefits. In many of the chapters that follow, innovative research is reported that is beginning to shed light on what works and what does not. For example, feedback to therapists about their clients' progress has been shown to improve outcomes (see chap. 8 and 12, this volume). Such results have enormous implications for improving mental health services and will lead to a better understanding of the important elements of psychotherapy.
- *Particular treatments should not be mandated.* Because there is absolutely no evidence that one treatment for a particular disorder is more effective than any other, it makes no sense to mandate treatments. The notion of requiring clinicians to use empirically supported treatment or evidence-based treatments simply is not supported by the research evidence.
- *Clinicians should be accountable for the outcomes of their services.* Rather than accountability deriving from documentation that a particular treatment was delivered, accountability should emanate from the therapist (see chap. 9, this volume). Of course, to be accountable, therapists need to have access to information about their outcomes. This information is a critical component of effective services because, as discussed in several chapters, knowing the outcomes of clients results in better outcomes. That is, to a great extent, therapists are self-correcting.

## QUESTIONS FROM THE EDITORS

1. *Given the significant contributions of common factors to outcome, how can the historical and current paucity of research on these factors be explained?*

First, characterizing the amount of research on common factors in terms of paucity is not quite right. There is a great deal of research on the common factors, particularly on the therapeutic alliance. What seems to be lacking, in some contexts, is recognition that the evidence supports the common factors rather than specific ingredients. As discussed in this chapter, clinical science seems focused on identification of the most effective treatment for particular disorders, as in medicine. The research supporting common factors is often ignored.

The focus on treatment is fostered by funding agencies, such as the National Institute of Mental Health, which are partial to RCTs. Research on the common factors typically is not experimental; that is, the presence or absence of a common factor cannot be manipulated. Thus, this research is not privileged by being classified as experimental. However, this should not detract from the fact that common factors may be causal to outcomes in psychotherapy. Indeed, as shown in this chapter and in many of the other chapters in this volume, there is a wealth of evidence supporting the common factors.

*2. What role, if any, does researchers' allegiance play in studies on the common factors?*

As mentioned in this chapter, researcher allegiance in RCTs has been shown to be strong. Researchers who have an allegiance to one treatment in a comparison of treatments typically find that their treatment is more effective. How this works is not quite clear, but it appears that the therapists in the study are influenced by the researcher's allegiance. For example, a researcher who may have developed one of the treatments often trains and supervises therapists, and the therapists are quite aware that this treatment is expected to be better. That is, the researchers have communicated to the therapists the expectation that the favored treatment is superior, and the therapists in turn convey that expectation to the clients.

It also is not clear how allegiance affects studies that investigate the common factors. My own meta-analyses showing that all treatments are equally effective have been criticized as being influenced by my allegiance to the dodo bird conjecture. However, there is a difference between this allegiance and the allegiance of researchers in RCTs of particular treatments. In a meta-analysis, the critics have access to the studies and can expose any research bias by reanalyzing the data. Indeed, Smith and Glass (1977) were roundly criticized when they found that behavioral treatments were not really more effective than other treatments. However, a number of reanalyses, aimed at exposing Smith and Glass's bias, failed to reach a different conclusion.

# REFERENCES

Ahn, H., & Wampold, B. E. (2001). A meta-analysis of component studies: Where is the evidence for the specificity of psychotherapy? *Journal of Counseling Psychology, 48*, 251–257.

Anholt, G. E., Kempe, P., de Haan, E., van Oppen, P., Cath, D. C., Smit, J. H., et al. (2008). Cognitive versus behavior therapy: Processes of change in the treatment of obsessive–compulsive disorder. *Psychotherapy and Psychosomatics, 77*, 38–42.

Arkowitz, H. (1992). Integrative theories of therapy. In D. K. Freedheim (Ed.), *History of psychotherapy: A century of change* (pp. 261–303). Washington, DC: American Psychological Association.

Baldwin, S. A., Wampold, B. E., & Imel, Z. E. (2007). Untangling the alliance–outcome correlation: Exploring the relative importance of therapist and patient variability in the alliance. *Journal of Consulting and Clinical Psychology*, 75, 842–852.

Bandura, A. (1997). *Self-efficacy: The exercise of control*. New York: Freeman.

Barlow, D. H. (2004). Psychological treatments. *American Psychologist*, 59, 869–878.

Barlow, D. H., Craske, M. G., Cerny, J. A., & Klosko, J. S. (1989). Behavioral treatment of panic disorder. *Behavior Therapy*, 20, 261–282.

Barlow, D. H., Gorman, J. M., Shear, M. K., & Woods, S. W. (2000). Cognitive–behavioral therapy, imipramine, or their combination for panic disorder: A randomized controlled trial. *JAMA*, 283, 2529–2536.

Baskin, T. W., Tierney, S. C., Minami, T., & Wampold, B. E. (2003). Establishing specificity in psychotherapy: A meta-analysis of structural equivalence of placebo controls. *Journal of Consulting and Clinical Psychology*, 71, 973–979.

Benish, S., Imel, Z. E., & Wampold, B. E. (2008). The relative efficacy of bona fide psychotherapies of post-traumatic stress disorder: A meta-analysis of direct comparisons. *Clinical Psychology Review*, 28, 746–758.

Beutler, L. E., & Clarkin, J. (1990). *Differential treatment selection: Toward targeted therapeutic interventions*. New York: Brunner/Mazel.

Beutler, L. E., Harwood, T. M., Alimohamed, S., & Malik, M. (2002). Functional impairment and coping style. In J. C. Norcross (Ed.), *Psychotherapy relationships that work: Therapist contributions and responsiveness to patients* (pp. 145–170). New York: Oxford University Press.

Beutler, L. E., Malik, M., Alimohamed, S., Harwood, T. M., Talebi, H., Noble, S., et al. (2004). Therapist variables. In M. J. Lambert (Ed.), *Bergin and Garfield's handbook of psychotherapy and behavior change* (5th ed., pp. 227–306). New York: Wiley.

Blatt, S. J., Zuroff, D. C., Quinlan, D. M., & Pilkonis, P. A. (1996). Interpersonal factors in brief treatment of depression: Further analysis of the National Institute of Mental Health treatment of depression collaborative research program. *Journal of Consulting and Clinical Psychology*, 64, 162–171.

Bohart, A. C., & Tallman, K. (1999). *How clients make therapy work: The process of active self-healing*. Washington, DC: American Psychological Association.

Bordin, E. S. (1979). The generalizability of the psychoanalytic concept of the working alliance. *Psychotherapy: Theory, Research & Practice*, 16, 252–260.

Bordin, E. S., Horvath, A. O., & Greenberg, L. S. (1994). Theory and research on the therapeutic working alliance: New directions. *The working alliance: Theory, research, and practice* (pp. 13–37). Oxford, England: Wiley.

Caplan, E. (1998). *Mind games: American culture and the birth of psychotherapy*. Berkeley: University of California Press.

Castonguay, L. G., Goldfried, M. R., Wiser, S., Raue, P. J., & Hayes, A. M. (1996). Predicting the effect of cognitive therapy for depression: A study of unique and common factors. *Journal of Consulting and Clinical Psychology*, 64, 497–504.

Chambless, D. L., Baker, M. J., Baucom, D. H., Beutler, L. E., Calhoun, K. S., Daiuto, A., et al. (1998). Update on empirically validated therapies, II. *The Clinical Psychologist, 51*, 3–16.

Chambless, D. L., & Hollon, S. D. (1998). Defining empirically supported therapies. *Journal of Consulting and Clinical Psychology, 66*, 7–18.

Crits-Christoph, P. (1997). Limitations of the dodo bird verdict and the role of clinical trials in psychotherapy research: Comment on Wampold et al. (1997). *Psychological Bulletin, 122*, 216–220.

Crits-Christoph, P., Baranackie, K., Kurcias, J. S., Carroll, K., Luborsky, L., McLellan, T., et al. (1991). Meta-analysis of therapist effects in psychotherapy outcome studies. *Psychotherapy Research, 1*, 81–91.

Crits-Christoph, P., Connolly Gibbons, M. B., Crits-Christoph, K., Narducci, J., Schamberger, M., & Gallop, R. (2006). Can therapists be trained to improve their alliances? A preliminary study of alliance-fostering psychotherapy. *Psychotherapy Research, 16*, 268–281.

Cushman, P. (1992). Psychotherapy to 1992: A history situated interpretation. In D. K. Freedheim (Ed.), *History of psychotherapy: A century of change* (pp. 21–64). Washington, DC: American Psychological Association.

DeRubeis, R. J., Brotman, M. A., & Gibbons, C. J. (2005). A conceptual and methodological analysis of the nonspecifics argument. *Clinical Psychology: Science and Practice, 12*, 174–183.

Dimidjian, S., Hollon, S. D., Dobson, K. S., Schmaling, K. B., Kohlenberg, R. J., Addis, M. E., et al. (2006). Randomized trial of behavioral activation, cognitive therapy, and antidepressant medication in the acute treatment of adults with major depression. *Journal of Consulting and Clinical Psychology, 74*, 658–670.

Duncan, B. L., Miller, S. D., & Sparks, J. A. (2004). *The heroic client: A revolutionary way to improve effectiveness through client-directed, outcome-informed therapy* (Rev. ed.). San Francisco: Jossey-Bass.

Eysenck, H. J. (1952). The effects of psychotherapy: An evaluation. *Journal of Consulting Psychology, 16*, 319–324.

Eysenck, H. J. (1961). The effects of psychotherapy. In H. J. Eysenck (Ed.), *Handbook of abnormal psychology* (pp. 697–725). New York: Basic Books.

Eysenck, H. J. (1966). *The effects of psychotherapy*. New York: International Science Press.

Fishman, D. B., & Franks, C. M. (1992). Evolution and differentiation within behavior therapy: A theoretical and epistemological review. In D. K. Freedheim (Ed.), *History of psychotherapy: A century of change* (pp. 159–196). Washington, DC: American Psychological Association.

Foa, E. B., Hembree, E. A., Cahill, S. P., Rauch, S. A. M., Riggs, D. S., Feeny, N. C., et al. (2005). Randomized trial of prolonged exposure for posttraumatic stress disorder with and without cognitive restructuring: Outcome at academic and community clinics. *Journal of Consulting and Clinical Psychology, 73*, 953–964.

Foa, E. B., Rothbaum, B. O., Riggs, D. S., & Murdock, T. B. (1991). Treatment of post-traumatic stress disorder in rape victims: A comparison between cognitive–behavioral procedures and counseling. *Journal of Consulting and Clinical Psychology, 59,* 715–723.

Follette, W. C., & Houts, A. C. (1996). Models of scientific progress and the role of theory in taxonomy development: A case study of the DSM. *Journal of Consulting and Clinical Psychology, 64,* 1120–1132.

Frank, J. D. (1992). Historical developments in research centers: The Johns Hopkins Psychotherapy Research Project. In D. K. Freedheim (Ed.), *History of psychotherapy: A century of change* (pp. 392–396). Washington, DC: American Psychological Association.

Frank, J. D., & Frank, J. B. (1991). *Persuasion and healing: A comparative study of psychotherapy* (3rd ed.). Baltimore: Johns Hopkins University Press.

Garfield, S. L. (1995). *Psychotherapy: An eclectic–integrative approach.* New York: Wiley.

Gloaguen, V., Cottraux, J., Cucherat, M., & Blackburn, I. (1998). A meta-analysis of the effects of cognitive therapy in depressed patients. *Journal of Affective Disorders, 49,* 59–72.

Goldfried, M. R., & Wolfe, B. E. (1998). Toward a more clinically valid approach to therapy research. *Journal of Consulting and Clinical Psychology, 66,* 143–150.

Greenberg, R. P., Constantino, M. J., & Bruce, N. (2006). Are patient expectations still relevant for psychotherapy process and outcome? *Clinical Psychology Review, 26,* 657–678.

Grencavage, L. M., & Norcross, J. C. (1990). Where are the commonalities among the therapeutic common factors? *Professional Psychology: Research and Practice, 21,* 372–378.

Harrington, A. (2008). *The cure within: A history of mind–body medicine.* New York: Norton.

Hatcher, R. L., Barends, A., Hansell, J., & Gutfreund, M. J. (1995). Patients' and therapists' shared and unique views of the therapeutic alliance: An investigation using confirmatory factor analysis in a nested design. *Journal of Consulting and Clinical Psychology, 63,* 636–643.

Hatcher, R. L., & Barends, A. W. (2006). How a return to theory could help alliance research. *Psychotherapy: Theory, Research, Practice, Training, 43,* 292–299.

Henry, W. P., Schacht, T. E., Strupp, H. H., Butler, S. F., & Binder, J. (1993). Effects of training in time-limited dynamic psychotherapy: Mediators of therapists' responses to training. *Journal of Consulting and Clinical Psychology, 61,* 441–447.

Henry, W. P., Strupp, H. H., Butler, S. F., Schacht, T. E., & Binder, J. (1993). Effects of training in time-limited psychotherapy: Changes in therapist behavior. *Journal of Consulting and Clinical Psychology, 61,* 434–440.

Hollon, S. D., Stewart, M. O., & Strunk, D. (2006). Enduring effects for cognitive behavior therapy in the treatment of depression and anxiety. *Annual Review of Psychology, 57,* 285–315.

Horvath, A. O., & Bedi, R. P. (2002). The alliance. In J. C. Norcross (Ed.), *Psychotherapy relationships that work: Therapist contributions and responsiveness to patients* (pp. 37–70). New York: Oxford University Press.

Horvath, A. O., & Luborsky, L. (1993). The role of the therapeutic alliance in psychotherapy. *Journal of Consulting and Clinical Psychology, 61*, 561–573.

Horvath, A. O., & Symonds, B. D. (1991). Relation between working alliance and outcome in psychotherapy: A meta-analysis. *Journal of Counseling Psychology, 38*, 139–149.

Huppert, J. D., Barlow, D. H., Gorman, J. M., Shear, M. K., & Woods, S. W. (2006). The interaction of motivation and therapist adherence predicts outcome in cognitive behavioral therapy for panic disorder: Preliminary findings. *Cognitive and Behavioral Practice, 13*, 198–204.

Huppert, J. D., Bufka, L. F., Barlow, D. H., Gorman, J. M., Shear, M. K., & Woods, S. W. (2001). Therapists, therapists variables, and cognitive behavioral therapy outcomes in a multicenter trial for panic disorder. *Journal of Consulting and Clinical Psychology, 69*, 747–755.

Imel, Z. E., Malterer, M. B., McKay, K. M., & Wampold, B. E. (2008). A meta-analysis of psychotherapy and medication in unipolar depression and dysthymia. *Journal of Affective Disorders , 110*, 197–206.

Imel, Z. E., & Wampold, B. E. (2008). The common factors of psychotherapy. In S. D. Brown & R. W. Lent (Eds.), *Handbook of counseling psychology* (4th ed., pp. 249–266). New York: Wiley.

Jacobson, N. S., Dobson, K. S., Truax, P. A., Addis, M. E., Koerner, K., Gollan, J. K., et al. (1996). A component analysis of cognitive–behavioral treatment for depression. *Journal of Consulting and Clinical Psychology, 64*, 295–304.

Kim, D. M., Wampold, B. E., & Bolt, D. M. (2006). Therapist effects in psychotherapy: A random effects modeling of the NIMH TDCRP data. *Psychotherapy Research, 16*, 161–172.

Kirsch, I. (2005). Placebo psychotherapy: Synonym or oxymoron? *Journal of Clinical Psychology, 61*, 791–803.

Kirsch, I., & Henry, D. (1977). Extinction versus credibility in the desensitization of speech anxiety. *Journal of Consulting and Clinical Psychology, 45*, 1052–1059.

Klein, D. N., Schwartz, J. E., Santiago, N. J., Vivian, D., Vocisano, C., Castonguay, L. G., et al. (2003). Therapeutic alliance in depression treatment: Controlling for prior change and patient characteristics. *Journal of Consulting and Clinical Psychology, 71*, 997–1006.

Kraemer, H. C., & Kupfer, D. J. (2006). Size of treatment effects and their importance to clinical research and practice. *Biological Psychiatry, 2005*, 990–996.

Lambert, M. J., & Bergin, A. E. (1994). The effectiveness of psychotherapy. In A. E. Bergin & S. L. Garfield (Eds.), *Handbook of psychotherapy and behavior change* (4th ed., pp. 143–189). New York: Wiley.

Lambert, M. J., Hansen, N. B., & Finch, A. E. (2001). Patient-focused research: Using patient outcome data to enhance treatment effects. *Journal of Consulting and Clinical Psychology, 69*, 159–172.

Leykin, Y., Amsterdam, J. D., DeRubeis, R. J., Gallop, R., Shelton, R. C., & Hollon, S. D. (2007). Progressive resistance to a selective serotonin reuptake inhibitor but not to cognitive therapy in the treatment of major depression. *Journal of Consulting and Clinical Psychology, 75*, 267–276.

Lutz, W., Leon, S. C., Martinovich, Z., Lyons, J. S., & Stiles, W. B. (2007). Therapist effects in outpatient psychotherapy: A three-level growth curve approach. *Journal of Counseling Psychology, 54*, 32–39.

Mallinckrodt, B. (1991). Clients' representations of childhood emotional bonds with parents, social support, and formation of the working alliance. *Journal of Counseling Psychology, 38*, 401–409.

Marmor, J. (1962). Psychoanalytic therapy as an educational process. In J. H. Masserman (Ed.), *Science and psychoanalysis* (Vol. 5, pp. 286–299). New York: Grune & Stratton.

Martin, D. J., Garske, J. P., & Davis, M. K. (2000). Relation of the therapeutic alliance with outcome and other variables: A meta-analytic review. *Journal of Consulting and Clinical Psychology, 68*, 438–450.

Miller, S. D., Duncan, B. L., & Hubble, M. A. (2005). Outcome-informed clinical work. In J. C. Norcross & M. R. Goldfried (Eds.), *Handbook of psychotherapy integration* (2nd ed., pp. 84–102). New York: Oxford University Press.

Miller, S. D., Wampold, B. E., & Varhely, K. (2008). Direct comparisons of treatment modalities for youth disorders: A meta-analysis. *Psychotherapy Research, 18*, 5–14.

Milrod, B., Leon, A. C., Busch, F., Rudden, M., Schwalberg, M., Clarkin, J., et al. (2007). A randomized controlled clinical trial of psychoanalytic psychotherapy for panic disorder. *American Journal of Psychiatry, 164*, 265–272.

Minami, T., Wampold, B. E., Serlin, R. C., Hamilton, E., Brown, G. S., & Kircher, J. (2008). Benchmarking the effectiveness of psychotherapy treatment for adult depression in a managed care environment: A preliminary study. *Journal of Consulting and Clinical Psychology, 76*, 116–124.

Norcross, J. C. (Ed.). (2002). *Psychotherapy relationships that work: Therapist contributions and responsiveness to patients.* New York: Oxford University Press.

Robinson, L. A., Berman, J. S., & Neimeyer, R. A. (1990). Psychotherapy for the treatment of depression: A comprehensive review of controlled outcome research. *Psychological Bulletin, 108*, 30–49.

Rosenthal, D., & Frank, J. D. (1956). Psychotherapy and the placebo effect. *Psychological Bulletin, 53*, 294–302.

Rosenzweig, S. (1936). Some implicit common factors in diverse methods of psychotherapy: "At last the Dodo said, 'Everybody has won and all must have prizes'". *American Journal of Orthopsychiatry, 6*, 412–415.

Roth, W. T., Wilhelm, F. H., & Petit, D. (2005). Are current theories of panic falsifiable? *Psychological Bulletin, 131,* 171–192.

Shadish, W. R., & Sweeney, R. B. (1991). Mediators and moderators in meta-analysis: There's a reason we don't let dodo birds tell us which psychotherapies should have prizes. *Journal of Consulting and Clinical Psychology, 59,* 883–893.

Shapiro, A. K., & Shapiro, E. S. (1997). *The powerful placebo: From ancient priest to modern medicine.* Baltimore: Johns Hopkins University Press.

Shapiro, D. A., & Shapiro, D. (1982). Meta-analysis of comparative therapy outcome research: A critical appraisal. *Behavioural Psychotherapy, 10,* 4–25.

Shaw, B. F., Elkin, I., Yamaguchi, J., Olmsted, M., Vallis, T. M., Dobson, K. S., et al. (1999). Therapist competence ratings in relation to clinical outcome in cognitive therapy of depression. *Journal of Consulting and Clinical Psychology, 67,* 837–846.

Smith, M. L., & Glass, G. V. (1977). Meta-analysis of psychotherapy outcome studies. *American Psychologist, 32,* 752–760.

Smith, M. L., Glass, G. V., & Miller, T. I. (1980). *The benefits of psychotherapy.* Baltimore: Johns Hopkins University Press.

Spielmans, G. I., Pasek, L. F., & McFall, J. P. (2007). What are the active ingredients in cognitive and behavioral psychotherapy for anxious and depressed children? A meta-analytic review. *Clinical Psychology Review, 27,* 642–654.

Stevens, S. E., Hynan, M. T., & Allen, M. (2000). A meta-analysis of common factor and specific treatment effects across domains of the phase model of psychotherapy. *Clinical Psychology: Science and Practice, 7,* 273–290.

Task Force on Promotion and Dissemination of Psychological Procedures. (1995). Training in and dissemination of empirically-validated psychological treatment: Report and recommendations. *The Clinical Psychologist, 48,* 2–23.

Taylor, E. (1999). *Shadow culture: Psychology and spirituality in America.* Washington, DC: Counterpoint.

Tracey, T. J. G., Lichtenberg, J. W., Goodyear, R. K., Claiborn, C. D., & Wampold, B. E. (2003). Concept mapping of therapeutic common factors. *Journal of Counseling Psychology, 13,* 401–413.

VandenBos, G. R., Cummings, N. A., & DeLeon, P. H. (1992). A century of psychotherapy: Economic and environmental influences. In D. K. Freedheim (Ed.), *A history of psychotherapy: A century of change.* Washington DC: American Psychological Association.

Wakefield, J. C. (1992). The concept of mental disorder: On the boundary between biological facts and social values. *American Psychologist, 47,* 373–388.

Wakefield, J. C. (1999). Evolutionary versus protype analyses of the concept of disorder. *Journal of Abnormal Psychchology, 108,* 374–399.

Wampold, B. E. (2001a). Contextualizing psychotherapy as a healing practice: Culture, history, and methods. *Applied and Preventive Psychology, 10,* 69–86.

Wampold, B. E. (2001b). *The great psychotherapy debate: Model, methods, and findings.* Mahwah, NJ: Erlbaum.

Wampold, B. E. (2006a). Do therapies designated as empirically supported treatments for specific disorders produce outcomes superior to non-empirically supported treatment therapies? In J. C. Norcross, L. E. Beutler, & R. F. Levant (Eds.), *Evidence-based practices in mental health: Debate and dialogue on the fundamental questions* (pp. 299–308). Washington, DC: American Psychological Association.

Wampold, B. E. (2006b). The psychotherapist. In J. C. Norcross, L. E. Beutler, & R. F. Levant (Eds.), *Evidence-based pratices in mental health: Debate and dialogues on the fundamental questions* (pp. 200–208). Washington, DC: American Psychological Association.

Wampold, B. E. (2007). Psychotherapy: The humanistic (and effective) treatment. *American Psychologist, 62,* 857–873.

Wampold, B. E., & Bhati, K. S. (2004). Attending to the omissions: A historical examination of the evidenced-based practice movement. *Professional Psychology: Research and Practice, 35,* 563–570.

Wampold, B. E., & Brown, G. S. (2005). Estimating therapist variability: A naturalistic study of outcomes in managed care. *Journal of Consulting and Clinical Psychology, 73,* 914–923.

Wampold, B. E., Imel, Z. E., Bhati, K. S., & Johnson Jennings, M. D. (2007). Insight as a common factor. In L. G. Castonguay & C. E. Hill (Eds.), *Insight in psychotherapy* (pp. 119–139). Washington, DC: American Psychological Association.

Wampold, B. E., Minami, T., Baskin, T. W., & Tierney, S. C. (2002). A meta-(re)analysis of the effects of cognitive therapy versus "other therapies" for depression. *Journal of Affective Disorders, 68,* 159–165.

Wampold, B. E., Minami, T., Tierney, S. C., Baskin, T. W., & Bhati, K. S. (2005). The placebo is powerful: Estimating placebo effects in medicine and psychotherapy from clinical trials. *Journal of Clinical Psychology, 61,* 835–854.

Wampold, B. E., Mondin, G. W., Moody, M., Stich, F., Benson, K., & Ahn, H. (1997). A meta-analysis of outcome studies comparing bona fide psychotherapies: Empirically, "All must have prizes." *Psychological Bulletin, 122,* 203–215.

Watson, J. C., Gordon, L. B., Stermac, L., Kalogerakos, F., & Steckley, P. (2003). Comparing the effectiveness of process-experiential with cognitive-behavioral psychotherapy in the treatment of depression. *Journal of Consulting and Clinical Psychology, 71,* 773–781.

Weinberger, J. (2002). Short paper, large impact: Rosenweig's influence on the common factors movement. *Journal of Psychotherapy Integration, 12,* 67–76.

Weinberger, J., Rasco, C., & Hofmann, S. G. (2007). Empirically supported common factors. *The art and science of psychotherapy* (pp. 103–129). New York: Routledge/Taylor & Francis.

Weiss, B., & Weisz, J. R. (1995). Relative effectiveness of behavioral versus nonbehavioral child psychotherapy. *Journal of Consulting and Clinical Psychology, 63,* 317–320.

Weisz, J. R., Weiss, B., Han, S. S., Granger, D. A., & Morton, T. (1995). Effects of psychotherapy with children and adolescents revisited: A meta-analysis of treatment outcome studies. *Psychological Bulletin, 117,* 450–468.

Widiger, T. A., & Trull, T. J. (2007). Plate tectonics in the classification of personality disorders: Shifting to a dimensional model. *American Psychologist, 2007,* 71–83.

Wolpe, J. (1958). *Psychotherapy by reciprocal inhibition.* Palo Alto, CA: Stanford University.

Zuroff, D. C., & Blatt, S. J. (2006). The therapeutic relationship in brief treatment of depression: Contributions to clinical improvement and enhanced adaptive capacities. *Journal of Consulting and Clinical Psychology, 74,* 130–140.

# 3

# CLIENTS: THE NEGLECTED COMMON FACTOR IN PSYCHOTHERAPY

ARTHUR C. BOHART AND KAREN TALLMAN

Facts don't cease to exist because they are ignored.
—Robert Louis Stevenson

Professional discourse and practice have long privileged the position and point of view of the therapist. In the "drama" of therapy, clinicians restructure clients' cognitions, extinguish fears, bring forth insight, unlock repressed affects, help restore brain functioning, and loosen the bonds of familial terror. Clients, in contrast, have nearly always played Nell Fenwick to the field's Dudley Do-Rights, bound to the tracks of destruction by weak ego structures, regressive potential, borderline defenses, lack of skills, and other presumed deficits. Thus, therapists "intervene," whereas clients "respond," or worse, "resist" the heroic efforts of the helper (cf. Angus, 1992). Told in this way, it is hard if not impossible to imagine a counternarrative, one in which the consumer of therapeutic services is more protagonist than prop, managing at least some workable accommodations no matter how debilitating his or her problems (Rosenbaum, 1996).

Yet the fact is that clients' active involvement in the therapeutic process is critical to success. Indeed, in a comprehensive review of 50 years of literature on the subject for the fifth edition of the *Handbook of Psychotherapy and Behavior Change*, Orlinsky, Rønnestad, and Willutzki (2004) stated, "the quality of the patient's participation . . . [emerges] as the *most* [italics added] important

83

determinant of outcome" (p. 324)—more so than therapist attitudes, behaviors, or techniques. The authors identified 11 additional variables linked to outcome. These included the following 10: client suitability, client cooperation versus resistance, client experience of the therapeutic bond, client contribution to the bond, client interactive collaboration, client expressiveness, client affirmation of the therapist, client openness versus defensiveness, therapeutic realizations (clients' in-session impacts of therapy events), and treatment duration. Note the number of factors that are directly related to the client.

Furthermore, the client and factors in the client's life account for more variance in therapeutic outcome than any other factor. Asay and Lambert (1999), on the basis of their assessment of the literature, portioned 40% of variance of outcome to the client and to factors in his or her life. Wampold's (2001) meta-analysis suggests that about 13% of total outcome variance is explained by treatment (therapist, alliance, model or technique, allegiance, and placebo), leaving 87% of the variance attributed to client or extratherapeutic factors as well as unexplained and error variance. It is not unreasonable to suppose that a substantial portion of the unexplained variance is due to the client.

Years ago, researchers Bergin and Garfield (1994) called for a reformation in psychotherapy. After reviewing the evidence, they challenged practitioners and theoreticians to think anew:

> Clients are not inert objects upon which techniques are administered. . . . [Therefore] it is important to rethink the terminology that assumes that "effects" are like Aristotelian impetus causality. *As therapists have depended more upon the client's resources, more change seems to occur* [italics added]. (pp. 825–826)

Although this call is finally beginning to be heeded, client contributions to therapy continue to be neglected in most theoretical models of change, with a few exceptions (cf. Bohart & Tallman, 1999; Duncan, Miller, & Sparks, 2004; Duncan & Moynihan, 1994). The therapist and his or her techniques are still seen as the primary curative factors. This emphasis on the primacy of techniques has unfortunately intensified as the proposition of evidence-based practice has risen in popularity.

Once more, the time has come to set the story straight, to spotlight the largest yet most neglected factor in treatment outcome: the client. Although experimental studies of client factors are few and far between and most research favors correlational, qualitative, and retrospective designs, a strong case emerges for the potency of the human client in successful psychotherapy. This chapter begins with a short survey of the potential for self-righting and self-healing. We then consider research regarding the client's role as an active contributor to the therapy process. We review data regarding the factors traditionally thought to account for the effectiveness of psychotherapy and offer an alternative account highlighting the importance of the client. The chapter concludes with the assertion that the client offers the best explanation for the dodo verdict as well as a discussion of the implications of a client-centered paradigm for psychotherapy practice, training, and the broader field of mental health.

## HUMAN POTENTIAL FOR CHANGE

Research on the human potential for self-healing is considerable. It comes from several sources, including the following: (a) self-generated change and spontaneous recovery, (b) placebo effects, (c) resilience and posttraumatic growth, and (d) the corrective effects of self-expression or disclosure.

### Self-Generated Change and Spontaneous Recovery

Studies have repeatedly demonstrated that people overcome significant problems without the benefit of professional intervention. When asked, 90% of individuals polled report having overcome a significant health, emotional, addiction, or lifestyle problem in the prior year (Gurin, 1990). Data provide support for such self-reports, even for problems most view as extreme. For instance, many individuals overcome problems considered chronic, such as antisocial behavior (J. T. Tedeschi & Felson, 1994) and substance abuse. About the latter, researchers Miller and Carroll (2006) noted, "Most people who recover from drug problems do so on their own, without formal treatment" (p. 295). Even the course for people who receive personality diagnoses is more benign than commonly believed. Most individuals diagnosed with personality disorders improve over time (Perry, 1993; Skodol et al., 2007). Zanarini, Frankenburg, Hennen, Reich, and Silk (2006) found that over a 10-year period, 88% of those diagnosed with borderline personality disorder achieved remission. These studies are confounded because in many cases the individuals studied had received some kind of treatment. Nonetheless, given that personality disorders are conceived of as engrained, difficult to change personality characteristics, this is encouraging. In this regard, Fonagy and Bateman (2006) pointed out that the natural course of borderline personality disorder is more benign than previously believed and that the treatment resistance of people with this diagnosis may have more to do with the iatrogenic effects of therapy than with the condition itself.

Prochaska (1999) studied how individuals overcome problems without the aid of psychotherapy. People use the same methods and processes used in therapy. As an illustration, though exposure is a common procedure used for treating phobias and trauma, the field of psychotherapy cannot lay exclusive claim to it. The popularity of the old saying "If you are thrown off a horse, get back on" indicates that people have long understood the beneficial effects of the method. Prochaska, Norcross, and DiClemente (1994) have made a compelling case that all change is self-change: Therapy is simply self-change that is professionally coached.

Additional support for the role of the client in the change process is provided by data on spontaneous recovery. Lambert, Shapiro, and Bergin (1986) estimated that about 40% of people recover without professional intervention. Moreover, a strong endorsement of the impact of client resources is found in the pretreatment change literature. Several studies have shown that 60% or more of clients reported the occurrence of improvement in the period between scheduling and attending their first session (Lawson, 1994; Weiner-Davis, de Shazer, & Gingerich, 1987). Finally, Miller and C'de Baca (2001) reported a phenomenon they termed *quantum change*. This refers to the experience of a sudden, significant personal transformation. Interviews with 55 individuals in the Albuquerque, New Mexico, area led the authors to conclude that such experiences were common—further testament to the human capacity for self-change.

## Placebo Effects

*Placebo effects,* or the benefits resulting from the client's expectation that treatment will help, offer more evidence of the significant role that clients play. In a review of 46 meta-analytic studies, for example, Grissom (1996) found that the effect size (ES) of placebo conditions was 0.44 compared with no-treatment control groups. In two of the largest randomized clinical trials ever conducted—the Treatment of Depression Collaborative Research Project (Elkin, 1994) and the Collaborative Cocaine Treatment Study (Crits-Christoph et al., 1999)—participants in the placebo and minimal clinical management conditions achieved outcomes roughly equivalent to those in psychotherapy. The strength of such findings led Honos-Webb (2005) to conclude that placebo control and minimal clinical management meet the criteria for classification as an empirically supported treatment.

Similarly, Kirsch et al.'s (2008) massive review of all studies about selective serotonin reuptake inhibitors (SSRIs) submitted to the Federal Drug Administration reported comparable results of SSRIs and placebos, with differences found between SSRIs and placebos only for the most severely depressed clients, and even these differences were small (Kirsch et al., 2008). The similarity of results between sugar pills and SSRIs suggests that change is far more about the individual and his or her expectations regarding change than the treatment provided. One way of understanding the placebo phenomena is that the client's expectation for change stimulates innate self-healing capabilities; in other words, the placebo effect represents the client's personal agency in action. Consider also that when active placebos, which mimic the side effects of the experimental drug, are used, no differences between drug and placebo conditions emerge (see chap. 7, this volume). It is thought that side effects signal that a powerful drug has been ingested, heightening expectations and releasing client's regenerative processes. Going one step further, techniques in psychotherapy may be also viewed as active placebos that similarly initiate client self-healing. The consistency of the placebo effect demands that it should no longer be denigrated. More attention might be paid to understanding its potency in mobilizing and supporting clients' innate, self-curative processes.

## Resilience and Posttraumatic Growth

Evidence regarding human resilience provides extra support for the human potential for self-healing (Bonanno, 2004). For instance, being exposed to trauma does not necessarily cause posttraumatic stress disorder. Ozer, Best, Lipsey, and Weiss (2003) noted that "roughly 50%–60% of the U.S. population is exposed to traumatic stress but only 5%–10% develop PTSD [posttraumatic stress disorder]" (p. 54). In their literature review, Masten, Best, and Garmazy (1990) concluded, "studies of psychosocial resilience support the view that human psychological development is highly buffered and self-righting" (p. 438). A good example is found in a longitudinal study conducted by Vaillant (1993) of 456 men. Though all were regarded as broken beyond repair at age 25, most self-righted. Approximately 64% were rated in the top 25% of mental health by the time they had entered their 60s. So compelling are the data that Masten (2001) posited that resilience is "a common phenomenon . . . development is robust even in the face of severe adversity" (p. 227).

Personal factors do play a role, such as the person's temperament and disposition, intelligence quotient, and level of self-esteem. Environmental factors such as the presence of a good social support network, a mentor, a role model, or even a therapist are also important. Yet, even children without good environmental buffering often show some resilience (Masten, 2001). Similar results are found in the literature on recovery from traumatic life events. R. G. Tedeschi, Park, and Calhoun (1998) reported, for instance, that 40%–60% of people who suffer a trauma recover on their own or report personal growth following the experience. Such changes include positive self-perception, improved sense of personal strengths, and better interpersonal relationships (Calhoun & Tedeschi, 2006).

## Corrective Effects of Self-Expression or Disclosure

Added support for human resilience comes from research on the beneficial effects of both self-expression and disclosure. Several studies have shown that writing or discussing a troubling or traumatic event facilitates healing (Harvey, Orbuch, Chwalisz, & Garwood, 1991; Hemenover, 2003; Pennebaker, 1997). In one, Segal and Murray (1994) wrote that giving individuals an opportunity to talk into a tape recorder worked about as well as cognitive therapy in managing traumatic experiences.

In sum, as this brief survey shows—encompassing spontaneous recovery, self-generated change, placebo effects, resilience, posttraumatic growth, and the corrective effects of self-expression and disclosure—humans have a good deal of potential for righting themselves when struck by adversity.

## THE CLIENT'S CONTRIBUTION TO THE EFFICACY OF PSYCHOTHERAPY

Additional substantiation of the defining role that clients play in therapy is found in research supporting client (a) involvement and participation; (b) perceptions of psychotherapy; (c) agency, activity, reflexivity, and creativity; (d) integration of therapy experiences into everyday life; and (e) early change.

### Client Involvement and Participation

Recall Orlinsky et al.'s (2004) review of therapeutic process and treatment outcome. They concluded that the quality of the client's participation is "most determinant of outcome" (p. 324). Client participation encompasses openness and willingness to engage in the tasks of psychotherapy, cooperative involvement, and a collaborative versus dependent disposition. In each case, the majority of studies show a positive relationship with success in therapy.

### Client Perception of Psychotherapy

Historically, client perceptions of the therapist and therapy were considered suspect, distorted by psychopathology. The data show otherwise. As an example, the client's perception of the therapeutic relationship has been consistently found to correlate more highly with outcome than the therapist's (Busseri & Tyler, 2004; Zuroff et al., 2000). On a related note, research has shown that client ratings of therapist empathy and the collaborative nature of the relationship correlate as, or more highly, with outcome than ratings by therapists and objective observers (Bohart, Elliott, Greenberg, & Watson, 2002).

Similarly, Levitt and Rennie (2004) reported that when therapists and clients looked at tapes of their interactions, the perspectives of the therapists and clients only partially overlapped. They noted, "Three stories may be occurring at once: the story of the dialogue between the client and the therapist, the client's inner story, and the therapist's inner story" (p. 308). Others have also reported only a modest relationship between the clients' and therapists' views of the therapy process (Elliott et al., 1994; Rosenbaum & Talmon, 2006).

Combine these two findings—that clients perception of the therapy relationship predicts outcome and that clients perceive therapy differently than do therapists—and the implication emerges that clients select from therapy what they need to get better. For instance, Mackrill (2008) had clients keep diaries on their experiences both inside and outside of therapy. He found that clients were highly active in integrating their therapy experiences in their own ways into their everyday lives. As an example, one client focused on the importance of positive thinking before starting therapy. Later in therapy, the client interpreted what was happening in terms of learning to use positive thinking. Positive thinking was not one of the therapist's goals. Clients, apparently, enter therapy with their own ideas about what they need (Philips, Werbart, Wennberg, & Schubert, 2007), and these ideas influence how they construe and use what therapists offer (Hubble, Duncan, & Miller, 1999). Similarly, Bohart and Boyd (1997) established that clients perceived empathic responses from therapists as supportive, if they felt in need of support, and as insightful, when insight was needed.

### Client Agency, Activity, Reflexivity, and Creativity

Clients, therefore, are anything but passive recipients of therapeutic wisdom. On the contrary, they continuously evaluate what is happening in therapy and then actively work to arrange events to suit their purposes. Hoerner (2007) found that clients perceive themselves as agentic, valued their own contributions to the process, and attributed the results to their efforts. Consider a classic study conducted by Garfinkel (1967). Participants posed problems to a therapist whose responses were limited to a simple yes or no answer. In a wrinkle sure to be rejected by any modern institutional review board, the therapists' answers to the queries were entirely random. Despite this less than helpful experimental condition, participants pieced together coherent accounts of their experience and derived solutions to their presenting problems.

Since Garfinkel's research, qualitative studies (Levitt, 2004; Levitt & Rennie, 2004; Rennie, 2000) have shown that clients are highly active, albeit often at a covert level, during sessions. This literature indicates that clients often enter therapy with a plan and work to steer sessions in directions that they perceive will be beneficial. They even redirect their therapist if he or she is off course. Greaves (2006) found in her study of 13 clients, that

> the clients exhibited initiative and engaged in meaning-making processes
> to make sense of their difficulties, redefine and remoralize themselves, and

try out new ways of being. Not only did they act in planning and management capacities, they also played the role of truth-seeker, motivator, advo-
cator, and negotiator to further the pursuit and attainment of their goals.
They blended their own wisdom with their therapist's expertise in idiosyncratic ways, after having prepared their therapist to potentially offer
the most appropriate assistance. These clients also nurtured a strong therapeutic relationship and utilized learning and healing opportunities within
the context of that relationship. (p. xii)

Research shows, too, that clients rework therapeutic blunders in ways that
enhance therapeutic success (Levitt, 2004; Levitt & Rennie, 2004; Tallman,
Robinson, Kay, Harvey, & Bohart, 1994).

Closely related to agency, activity, and reflexivity is client creativity.
Although rarely examined, much of the evidence cited previously supports
the role that client creativity plays in successful outcome. How else can one
explain clients using therapeutic errors to positive effect? It is as though clients
give their therapists the benefit of the doubt. In short, they want their therapists to be successful; the therapists' success means their success. Most practicing clinicians have also experienced what Talmon (1990) found in interviews
with former clients. He noted that many "reported following suggestions that
I could not remember having made. They created their own interpretations,
which were sometimes quite different from what I recollected and sometimes
more creative and suitable versions of my suggestions" (p. 60). More directly,
Selby's (2004) qualitative analysis showed that half of clients exhibited
creativity or inventiveness that both altered the direction and facilitated
the success of therapy.

## How Clients Relate Therapy to Their Everyday Lives

As Mackrill (2008) observed, we do not know much about how clients
actually integrate their therapy experiences with everyday life. Dreier (2000),
on the basis of his studies of family therapy, concluded that therapy does not
take place primarily in the therapist's office. Clients actively transform what
they have learned in therapy and apply it to their life situations. "Clients con-
figure the meaning of therapy within the structure of their ongoing social practice" (Dreier, 2000, p. 253).

For example, Moertl (2007) found that clients talked over their day treatment experiences with friends and family and reflected on these clinic experiences while at home. Clients also participate in activities such as reading
self-help books, reflecting and self-questioning, thinking about dialogues with
the therapist, or allowing time before or after the session to prepare (Levitt,
Butler, & Hill, 2006). Conversely, Moertl (2007) found that clients also trans-
ferred experiences from everyday life into the day clinic. For instance, they

compared their relationships at home with relationships at the clinic, using strategies at the clinic that were effective at home. Mackrill (2008) had clients keep diaries and found that they actively learned through their own efforts of integrating information gleaned from their own experiments, friends, movies, clairvoyants, television, and other outside sources of ideas with what they were learning in therapy. Finally, Kühnlein (1999) interviewed 49 clients who had received cognitive–behavior therapy and found that participants did not blindly adopt what was presented in therapy. Instead, they took what they found useful and combined it with their own previously existing schemas.

## Early Change

One significant bit of evidence for the importance of the client's contribution and resources to success in psychotherapy can be found in the emerging evidence for early change (e.g., Brown, Burlingame, Lamberg, Jones, & Vaccaro, 2001; Howard, Kopta, Krause, & Orlinsky, 1986). Consider the classic Howard et al. (1986) article on the dose–effect relationship: First, 30% of clients, now called *early responders,* improved by the second session; 60% to 65% of people experienced significant symptomatic relief within one to seven visits, which increased to 70% to 75% after 6 months and to 85% at 1 year. Now consider, as an example, that in 1986, one of the most prevalent orientations of therapists was psychodynamic, which traditionally views change in terms of years rather than weeks. The majority of clients in Howard et al.'s study achieved change during the very preliminary stages of therapy, perhaps even before, according to the model, the transference relationship was set and therapy had really begun. The point, that these early changes occurred before the major mechanisms of a theoretical approach had time to become operative, can also be made about other orientations (Snyder, Michael, & Cheavens, 1999).

Not all clients are early responders. In fact, different clients follow different change trajectories (Stulz, Lutz, Leach, Lucock, & Barkham, 2007). However, the fact that early change is so common reinforces the idea that clients and their resources frequently are more responsible for change in therapy than therapists' models, techniques, and theories. Why not all clients are early responders and what to do about that is an important issue and awaits further investigation.

In a related finding, the best predictor of change appears to be higher levels of distress at the start of therapy, more so than the client's diagnosis, chronicity of the problem, or the treatment population (Brown et al., 2001). On the other hand, others have reported that clients who are rated as more functionally impaired, who are diagnosed with personality disorders, or who have had poor early relationships with caregivers do more poorly in therapy than those without these histories (Castonguay & Beutler, 2006).

It is not clear what these findings mean or how to reconcile them. Do diagnoses of functional impairment, personality disorder, and early relationship issues imply that clients are so impaired that they are robbed of a capacity to engage in proactive self-healing efforts? Are there clients who lack the capacity for self-healing? Not necessarily. The fact that higher levels of distress are the best predictor of outcome suggests that being motivated to get involved in therapy may be more important than hypothesized personal deficits. At the same time, it may be that long-engrained patterns of behavior may make change more difficult. It may also be that therapy administered in the studies of client impairment was not what was needed to support these clients' self-healing efforts. Finally, it may also be that some clients elicit negative therapist relationship behaviors that in turn interfere with their ability to make use of the therapy environment (see chap. 4, this volume). Further research and analysis is needed. The fact remains that many clients respond positively very quickly in therapy, before most models of psychotherapy would predict. This only makes sense if it is the client who is driving the bus and the therapist and treatment approach are but passengers on the ride to change.

In sum, available evidence shows that clients are not dependent variables on which the independent variable of therapy operates. Far from it; they are active, generative agents, working to get what they want and need, protecting themselves when needed, and even supporting the therapist when they deem it necessary. Clients modify old concepts and use their revisions, create new concepts, think of alternatives, and integrate what they learn.

## EVALUATION OF THE TRADITIONAL MODEL OF PSYCHOTHERAPY

The traditional model, patterned after physicians' treatment of physical diseases, holds that specific interventions are needed for the treatment of specific disorders. In this worldview, the therapist, an expert, diagnoses the client's problem and then chooses and delivers the appropriate intervention. In combination, therapist expertise and the technique itself are considered the forces behind successful psychotherapy.

Traditional beliefs notwithstanding, the empirical evidence does not support this view of the factors responsible for the efficacy of psychotherapy. First, as Wampold argues in chapter 2 of this volume, all bona fide therapeutic approaches work about equally well, regardless of diagnosis. Second, research also challenges the importance of technique. Indeed, estimates based on meta-analytic studies have shown that specific techniques or models of therapy contribute little to therapeutic success. For instance, Wampold (2001) attributed 13% of variance in outcome to treatment, and of that, only about 8% is due to techniques; in other words, of the total variance of change, model differences account for but 1% of the variance (or an ES of 0.20). In a review for the fifth edition of the *Handbook of Psychotherapy and Behavior Change,* Beutler et al. (2004) reported correlations ranging from 0 to .11 between specific techniques and outcome.

These data fit with what clients say about therapy. Even when prompted, clients rarely mention particular techniques when asked to reflect on the helpful aspects of psychotherapy. In an analysis of client interviews, for example, Levitt (2004) found that clients did not focus on or even recall specific interventions. They did attend to the tenor of the therapeutic relationship and new insights they achieved. Instead of procedures, studies have consistently shown that clients emphasize (a) feeling understood, accepted, and being heard; (b) having a safe space to explore feelings, thoughts, behaviors, and experiences; (c) support for dealing with crises; (d) support for trying out new behaviors; and (e) advice (e.g., Cullari, 2000; Elliott & James, 1989; Kagan, Angus, & Pos, 2007; Levitt et al., 2006; Rodgers, 2003; Timulak, 2007; Westra, Angus, & Stala, 2007). Specific activities such as therapist confrontation of the client (Moertl, 2007; Werbart & Johannson, 2007), doing practical exercises (Levitt et al., 2006; Von Below & Werbart, 2007), and getting tools and strategies from their therapists (Carey et al., 2007; Timulak, 2007) are sometimes mentioned, but they are not emphasized as often as factors such as feeling understood.

Two additional sources of evidence undermine conventional beliefs regarding the importance of the therapist's expertise and technique. First, although therapists have been shown to exert significant effects on success, the field has struggled to provide any consistent evidence that professional training, experience, discipline, licensure, or certification impacts outcome (Beutler et al., 2004; Christensen & Jacobson, 1994; Horvath & Bedi, 2002; Najavits & Strupp, 1994; Wampold, 2006). Second, although considerable research has supported the contribution of the therapeutic relationship to improvement, there is evidence that neither a therapist nor therapeutic relationship are necessary for change to occur.

On this score, Norcross (2006) reviewed research on self-help books and programs, and reported effects as strong as, or almost as strong as, those delivered by a therapist. These results have been supported by meta-analyses (Gould & Clum, 1993; Gregory, Canning, Lee, & Wise, 2004). For instance, Gregory et al. (2004) found an ES of 0.77 for bibliotherapy and concluded that that "compares favorably with data from studies of individual psychotherapy" (p. 277). In one representative study, Jacobs et al. (2001) found that a simple form of computer-assisted therapy produced overall outcomes equivalent to those provided by a therapist, although there was more clinically significant change in the group of clients who saw therapists. The computer program prompted clients to think about what they wanted and how to obtain it. Clients in these studies presented with a wide range of problems, including depression, anxiety, and substance abuse.

However, a recent meta-analysis of studies for depression and anxiety suggested that therapy with professional therapists does better than self-help. Menchola, Arkowitz, and Burke (2007) found that compared with control groups, self-help had an ES of 1.0. This is a large ES and comparable with those found for psychotherapy in other research reports (e.g., Wampold, 2001). However, the ES for professionally provided psychotherapy compared with self-help was 0.31. This suggests that therapy does provide something over and above self-help. It is important to note, though, that although the 0.31 difference between the self-help and psychotherapy ES was statistically significant, it is small compared with the large effect of self-help. Furthermore, the 0.31 difference is less than the difference of 0.4 considered necessary to be of clinical significance (e.g., Elliott, Greenberg, & Lietaer, 2004). Overall, the data support the conclusion that self-help is as effective or almost as effective as psychotherapy for many disorders, again supporting the significant role of the client in therapeutic change.

THE CLIENT AS ACTIVE SELF-HEALER: CONCLUSIONS

Although the research may appear at times to be a potpourri of findings from unrelated research areas, it is important to recognize that investigating client factors is not easy and is hampered by largely ex post facto analysis and nonexperimental designs. Nevertheless, evidence from multiple sources converges to make a convincing case for client centrality in clinical change, providing a parsimonious explanation of why all bona fide approaches to therapy work about equally well and self-help procedures nearly as well as professional-provided therapy.

In short, it is the client, more so than the therapist or technique, who makes therapy work. The client's abilities to use whatever is offered surpass any differences that might exist in techniques or approaches. Clients use and tailor what each approach provides to address their problems. Thus, for example, a client can use cognitive, interpersonal, or antidepressant therapies (Elkin, 1994); emotional exploration procedures; or empathically based client-centered therapy (Greenberg & Watson, 1998) to move him- or herself out of depression.

We have argued (Bohart, 2000; Bohart & Tallman, 1999; Tallman & Bohart, 1999; cf. also Duncan et al., 2004) that these findings call for a new paradigm, one that takes as its central assumption that it is clients who make therapy work. Clients are not submissive recipients of an intervention. They actively operate on therapists' inputs, transforming bits and pieces of the process into information and experiences which, in turn, are used to make change occur. Their effort, involvement, intelligence, and creativity enable them to accommodate and metabolize different therapeutic approaches and achieve positive outcomes. In other words, clients are the common factor across varying forms of psychotherapy. Such a view is not meant to minimize the importance of therapists. Clearly, clients come to therapy because they have not been successful resolving problems with the resources available to them. Clients need support and, often, some kind of useful structure that they can use to resolve their problems (see chap. 5, this volume). Instead of technical know-how, the therapist helps primarily by supporting, nurturing, or guiding and structuring the client's self-change efforts. This may include the suggestion of techniques.

## IMPLICATIONS

Viewing the client as the common factor has immediate implications for clinical practice, training, and the field at large.

### Implications for Clinical Practice

*Therapists should enlist and promote client strengths, resources, and personal agency.*

Perhaps the single largest implication of the view of the client as the active self-healer is that therapists should rely more heavily on client resources and strengths. Consider a study by Gassman and Grawe (2006). They conducted minute-by-minute analyses of 120 sessions involving 30 clients treated for a range of psychological problems. They found that unsuccessful therapists focused on problems but neglected client strengths. When the unsuccessful therapists did focus on clients' strengths, they did so more at the end of a therapy session. Successful therapists focused on their clients' strengths from the very start of an appointment. Gassman and Grawe (2006) concluded that successful therapists "created an environment in which the patient felt he was perceived as a well functioning person. As soon as this was established, productive work on the patient's problems was more likely" (p. 10).

Strength-based approaches are increasingly becoming a part of many psychotherapies. It has always been a part of some, such as Duncan, Solovey, and Rusk's (1992) client-directed approach, the solution-focused approach (e.g., Berg & Miller, 1992), narrative therapies (e.g., Anderson & Gehart, 2006), and person-centered therapy (Bohart, 2007). No matter the therapy, recruiting and promoting client strengths means, at times, tapping into resources and abilities of which clients may not be aware. Therapists can note and then share such discoveries with clients. An aspect of this work is finding strength in seemingly dysfunctional behaviors (Honos-Webb, 2005, 2006; Mosher, Hendrix, & Fort, 2004) and recognizing that clients' identities and innate abilities transcend descriptions of pathology (Duncan et al., 2004).

*Therapists should believe that clients are motivated and capable of proactive change.*

There is no such thing as an unmotivated client. His or her motivations might not match the therapist's, but clients are indeed driven by personal desires. Understanding and honoring those motivations is critical to client-centered clinical work. Several authors have suggested that there is even some underlying sense or positive rationale underlying negative, self-defeating, or dysfunctional patterns of behavior (Linehan, 1997; Miller & Rollnick, 2002). This underlying sense or rationale is often implicit. Recognizing that this sense exists and then helping clients access and unpack the implicit meanings involved can help them mobilize positive motivation for change. As Cantor (2003) noted,

> What observers of human behavior often lose sight of are the alternative routes that different individuals take toward personally fulfilling ends. By focusing on the process of working on goals, how individuals see their tasks, what they are trying to do, what kinds of social supports they mobilize in the process—it is often possible to see meaning and positive purpose in what may appear to an observer to be at best unnecessary or at worst self-defeating behavior. (p. 52)

Moreover, and in concert with embracing the client's motivations for change, therapists should also believe in the client's innate ability to change. Too many pathology-based prognostications about clients pervade the field. It would seem that a field dedicated to helping people change would believe that change is not only possible but probable. Believing in the client's propensities for change seems to follow the data presented in this chapter. Given the amount of variance accounted for by the client relative to models, allegiance to this belief is perhaps more important that any commitment to a given approach.

*Therapists should promote client involvement: Psychotherapy is a collaborative endeavor.*

As Orlinsky et al.'s (2004) review makes clear, psychotherapy is most effective when it nurtures and supports maximum client involvement and participation. Therapists facilitate client involvement by providing an atmosphere in which clients can be open, participate, test ideas, and make mistakes. Bachelor, Laverdière, Gamache, and Bordeleau (2007) found that the majority of clients (76%) could be classified as either *active* or *mutual collaborators*, placing the primary emphasis in treatment on their own efforts or on joint involvement with the therapist. Thus, therapists are in line with the empirical evidence when they listen to clients, establish common ground, and work together to forge solutions. Although some therapeutic models are more didactic in nature than others, all can be pursued collaboratively.

*Therapists should listen to clients and privilege their experience and ideas.*

Therapists must listen in a different way to clients. Instead of hearing pathology, they must also hear strengths; instead of deficits, they need to listen to clients' experience; instead of seeing what they know, they must know (i.e., be aware of) what they see. Additionally, therapists must show clients that they not only understand their experience, view of the problem, and potential solutions, but that they will also privilege those perspectives. Easier said than done; therapists can demonstrate their privilege of clients through careful listening, attending to feedback (see chap. 8, this volume), and being willing to adjust services to better fit clients' sensibilities. This includes identifying what clients value and incorporating it into how they proceed.

Listening to clients also entails paying attention to research about what clients say is important. For example, although insight is often maligned as an insufficient condition for change, clients, the evidence indicates, value attaining it (Levitt, 2004; Timulak, 2007; Westra et al., 2007). Werbart and Johansson (2007) found that people in therapy viewed increased self-knowledge as a positive change. Learning about patterns of behavior has also been shown to be valued by clients (Moertl, 2007).

As for emotions, research has found that clients value being able to access, accept, understand, experience, and express painful feelings (Kagan et al., 2007; Werbart & Johansson, 2007; Westra et al., 2007), although this may be culture-specific to Euro-American cultures. Conversely, clients consider being unable to "reach" their feelings or having trouble expressing them significant hindrances (Von Below & Werbart, 2007). Other helpful aspects of therapeutic process reported by clients include the following: taking risks and trying out new behaviors, sharing with others (Moertl, 2007; Werbart & Johannson, 2007), gaining a sense of empowerment (Timulak, 2007), and developing new strategies for attaining goals (Moertl, 2007; Timulak, 2007; Werbart & Johannson, 2007).

Regarding helpful therapist behaviors, research yet again points in the direction of nonspecific factors. Clients have emphasized being understood, accepted, and actively supported. These findings were corroborated in a study (conducted and published by *Psychology Today*) of more than 2,200 clients (Harris Interactive, 2004). Using data gathered online and via telephonic survey, researchers found that clients considered listening skills (63%), personality (52%), personal connection (45%), and activity level (38%) as the most essential qualities of a good clinician. Other studies have found that clients' progress in treatment is hindered when therapists (a) make hurtful remarks; (b) are authoritarian; (c) do not listen; (d) remain silent, distant, or unresponsive; (e) refuse to give advice, ideas, or practical exercises; (f) differ significantly from the client in personality; and (g) are distant and untrustworthy (Conrad & Auckenthaler, 2007; Von Below & Werbart, 2007). In all, research about client preferences suggests that clients want a safe space to talk with someone who will listen and appreciate what they think is important. Is that too much to ask?

## Implications for Training

*Train therapists to value clients: their strengths, resources, ideas, and propensity for self-healing.*
Therapists in training should be encouraged to do the following:

- Begin with the assumption that clients make therapy work— that clients are both resilient and reasonable, but stuck in a difficult situation.
- Take seriously the client's perspective on the problem and honor that perspective. Encourage clients to understand that there are multiply correct points of view. Certainly no one point of view offered by approaches to psychotherapy can be said to be "the" correct one.
- Expect clients will get better, and believe that therapy works and that the person sitting across from them will change. Trainees can gain confidence in knowing this by tracking client progress via outcome measures and making notes of the new skills, ideas, goals, and insights clients mention each week.
- Support the clients' efforts so they can leave therapy and be effective problem solvers on their own. Allow clients to originate some of the solutions.

*Train therapists to listen; listening is an art.*
Therapists in training should be taught the following:

- Be effective, supportive listeners instead of being diagnosticians or interventionists. Diagnosis encourages an external perspective on the client as well as a view of the client as broken or damaged. The introduction to pathology and diagnosis should be delayed until the therapist gains skills in relating to clients. Instruction in the art of dialogue and the study of communication should be included before the introduction of models and techniques. Put models and techniques in their place—not discounting them, but understanding their relative importance in psychotherapeutic change. Use a collaboration metaphor for therapy rather than the widely accepted adversarial, often combative, metaphor. It is not "us" against "them" or even "us" against the problem or pathology. It is both the therapist and client in partnership against the obstacles the client views in his or her life.

- Value the power of listening. Beginning therapists should practice their listening skills in triads, acting as the therapist, the client, and the observer. As conversation unfolds and methods of exploration are tried, trainees learn to evaluate any given position or technique from multiple points of view. Firsthand experience of varied perspectives encourages flexibility and an ongoing appreciation of diversity of views.

- Be comfortable with silence. Silence is critical when the client is thinking effectively, engaging in self-reflection, imagining new possibilities, and considering changes.

- Include client feedback in their understanding of their listening and relational skills. It is the client's perceptions that make the difference: You are not listening until the client says you are.

## Implications for the Field

*Abandon empirically supported treatments: Embrace the American Psychological Association's evidence-based practice.*

The evidence-based practice (EBP) movement has become a central component of health care policy and research over the past decade. In 1995, Division 12 (Society of Clinical Psychology) within the American Psychological Association (APA) formed the Task Force on the Promotion and Dissemination of Psychological Procedures, with the stated objective of identifying treatment approaches for which empirical evidence existed (Chambless & Hollon, 1998; Task Force on the Promotion and Dissemination of Psychological Procedures, 1995). The criteria used by the committee to evaluate existing research were based on customary ideas about how psychotherapy works. Thus, all the approaches designated as empirically validated in the committee's original report had been tested in a randomized clinical trial using a treatment manual and had focused on specific treatments for specific disorders.

However, if it is the client who ultimately (in collaboration with the therapist) makes therapy work by how he or she uses the procedures and experiences offered, then the empirically supported treatments approach is misguided (Bohart, 2006). The emphasis should be more on helping individual clients use their own resources to change rather than on applying standardized treatment packages. There is some movement in this direction.

In May 2006, the APA Presidential Task Force on EBP published a revised definition of EBP in psychology. Recognizing that the report of the prior Task Force had been used by various government and commercial entities to mandate the use of the approaches labeled as *empirically supported*, the committee moved beyond a simplistic "specific treatments for specific disorders" paradigm, to defining EBP as "the integration of the best available research with clinical expertise in the context of patient characteristics, culture, and preferences" (p. 273). The role of clients as an important factor in clinical decision making was recognized. This definition merits celebration, acknowledging as it does the central role that clients play in the execution, efficacy, and evaluation of psychotherapy. EBP is not synonymous with a list of empirically supported treatments (Norcross, Levant, & Beutler, 2006), although under the APA Task Force statement, empirically supported treatments are to be included as one thing for the clinician to consider. However, in addition, other empirically sound methods exist for ensuring that practice is informed by the best evidence (Bohart & Tallman, 1999; Duncan et al., 2004; Hubble et al., 1999; Orlinsky et al., 2004).

*Renew interest in person-centered care.*

The data reviewed in this chapter, and elsewhere in this volume, provide strong support for a person-centered orientation to clinical practice. Currently popular in medicine, this way of working calls for a collaborative, patient-involved model of service delivery. It is an approach in which listening to the patients' stories becomes an integral part of what physicians do (Charon, 2006; Tallman, Janisse, Frankel, Sung, Krupat, & Hsu, 2007).

In mental health care, clients not only desire but also demand that treatment be more person centered. Variously called *survivors* or *consumers*, people, particularly those who have at some time been diagnosed with schizophrenia or bipolar disorder, want to take an active role in directing services they receive. In several states, members of the recovery movement or their advocates sit on various mental health commissions and have a major say in policy. Cohen (2005) pointed out those groups often explicitly reject the traditional medical view of emotional suffering and treatment, choosing instead to embrace a paradigm that emphasizes client resources and community activism. An emphasis on creating or using real-life support networks and opportunities both in work and in relationships is also seen. Briefly, Cohen's study of 36 survivors, most diagnosed with schizophrenia, showed that the majority cited self-help, support of family and friends, social activism, exercise, as well as one-on-one psychotherapy as the most common and helpful methods for facilitating recovery. Only 25% reported the use of drugs as helpful. It is unfortunate that the one movement that explicitly recognizes clients as active, empowered agents in their own right has been met with mixed feelings by the mental health establishment.

The person-centered orientation also dovetails with the field's increasing awareness regarding cultural diversity. As APA's revised definition of EBP indicates, therapy needs to be informed by the client's culture and personal preferences. Obviously, solutions developed collaboratively, in the context of clients' cultural experiences, are likely to be more meaningful to the individual, hence successful. Here again, utilization and mobilization of client resources trump the application of a specific technique to a specific problem. Finally, the person-centered perspective fits perfectly with the current zeitgeist (see chap. 8, this volume) toward client-based outcome feedback and the privileging of the client's voice achieved by routine assessment and use of the client's perceptions of the benefit of services. Using client feedback to tailor mental health services finally makes clients true partners in the therapeutic endeavor.

Changing the governing paradigm by taking seriously the active, generative nature of clients leads to fundamental changes in how the process of therapy is viewed and conducted. This process at once becomes collaborative in theory and practice, not merely collaborative in the sense that the client complies with and participates in a predetermined treatment plan. From such a vantage point, each person in the process is an expert in his or her own right. Together, practitioners, researchers, and clients combine their efforts to ensure that the client is no longer the most neglected common factor in psychotherapy.

## QUESTIONS FROM THE EDITORS

1. *What has been the most important finding about the client's role in psychotherapy since the first edition? What research needs to be conducted to establish further the client's pivotal role?*

We would say that the most important finding is that the client is important. In recent years there has been a significant increase in studies on the client's role in therapy. Writers are now mentioning clients as a critical factor in how therapy works. As mentioned previously, the recent APA Task Force on EBP included the client as one of the three major factors to be taken into account in deciding how best to proceed in therapy.

In terms of research, there really is not one particular finding but rather a convergence of results. Findings continue to accumulate showing that clients are active interpreters of the therapy environment and that the nature of the outcomes clients achieve depend in part on their active (and creative) integration of what therapy has to offer with their own plans, goals, and agendas.

Research has also found that focusing on clients' strengths and resources is important to make therapy work across different approaches.

Concerning future research, there has been almost no work done on client expertise, although therapists of many different persuasions pay lip service to the idea that the client is the expert on his or her own life. That clients apply such expertise to help solve their own problems in therapy is a major thesis of this chapter. Yet, there is virtually no research on this subject. Much more also needs to be done to learn how clients actively engage in the therapeutic process on a session by session basis and how they integrate what they experience into their lives outside therapy. More research needs to be done to identify why some clients benefit from care whereas others do not. What are the causes from the client's point of view? Is it really due to a deficit in the client? Or is it possible that there is a mismatch between the therapy provided and the client? Or, finally, is it that the therapy does not sufficiently address itself to client concerns and perspectives in such a way as to best involve them? Perhaps the recent efforts, highlighted in this volume, to integrate client feedback and tailor services to client preferences will shed more light on the issue.

*2. How do you reconcile evidence suggesting that certain clients do less well in therapy (e.g., clients rated as more functionally impaired, diagnosed with personality disorders, and assessed as having relationship problems from childhood) with other data showing that client ratings of distress are better predictors of change than diagnosis or client functional impairment?*

These findings on distress suggest that the most important factor in how well therapy works is, once again, client involvement and participation. Presumably, more highly distressed clients are more motivated to participate. That this dwarfs diagnosis, functional impairment, and so forth is significant. It suggests that the motivated participation of the client is the most important factor.

The data suggesting that clients who are more functionally impaired do less well in therapy are part of a larger picture that shows that different clients have different healing trajectories in therapy. The traditional interpretation is to blame the client: It is his or her psychological impairment that impedes therapy. An alternative possibility is that the typical therapy environment, typical therapy behavior, and typical therapy solutions do not work equally well in mobilizing the self-healing capacities of all clients. The traditional model of therapy—in which the expert therapist is the one who decides what the client's problem is, diagnoses it, and then chooses and prescribes the treatment—may get in the way of listening to the client to find out what works best for him or her. This may be particularly important with clients who might not adapt well to the traditional therapy environment. Or, the failed therapy itself creates the noted impairment: Client dysfunction is an iatrogenic effect of ineffective therapy. In an interesting project, Duncan, Hubble, and Miller (1997) deliberately tried to work with clients other therapists had found intractable. By working in a more collaborative way with these clients than they had been worked with in the past, these clients were able to be successful. More research to understand how clients approach and work with what is offered in therapy is needed before we conclude that their relative lack of success is due to their defects.

3. *You talk about the client as active self-healer. We (the editors) have talked about "heroic clients." Is it possible that such talk could stigmatize individuals who do not self-right in everyday life and instead need psychotherapy and individuals who do not get better in therapy?*

First, one must keep in mind that the literature on resilience shows that not everyone is equally resilient. Resilience is a complex product of individual personality factors interacting with life historical events and the facilitating or nonfacilitating aspects of one's current environment. Although 40% to 60% of individuals who experience traumatic events show signs of posttraumatic growth, conversely, 40% to 60%—a substantial number—do not.

Therefore, there is nothing unusual about needing help to self-right. Indeed, even those who exhibit resilience or posttraumatic growth have usually had the aid of other people, perhaps a mentor, teacher, or supportive family member. We believe the evidence supports humans' considerable potential to self-right. They may need a therapist to help them mobilize it. The evidence regarding the importance of listening to clients as proactive agents and finding ways to mobilize client's generative capacities is compelling. Unfortunately, we have both experienced too many cases of therapists who "know what's best for you" and impose their view on clients, which often implies that the client is damaged in some way and not capable of self-healing. The case of Molly, presented in Duncan et al. (1997), is a classic example of how therapists repeatedly imposed their perspectives on the client and ignored her voice. When a therapist finally listened, Molly was able to figure out a solution for herself. Why she had not done that in everyday life is another question, but it shows that clients have this potential, and it is not uncommon for them to need the aid of a professional to mobilize it.

Therapy offers at least two things people may not have in their everyday lives. First, it offers a supportive interpersonal relationship in which one can think together with another human being. A supportive other can help mobilize hope and renewed effort. In everyday life, many people do not have the kind of relationship that would help them work through their difficulties. Secondly, it provides a good workspace. Clients in everyday life may not have the time, place, or emotionally safe space to focus productively on their problems.

Although we believe it is ultimately clients' own generative capacities that lead them to productively use whatever they experience in therapy, it does not mean those who do not improve should be blamed. As we have previously stated, it could be that the therapy did not mobilize their self-healing capacities. Additionally, our therapy models underestimate the importance of clients' ecological circumstances. Therapy models focus on fixing factors inside clients, which presumably allows them to successfully cope with their life spaces. However, the therapist is never just working with the client but with their life circumstances, as well. Robert Elliott's (2002) work with his hermeneutic single case efficacy design for studying psychotherapy outcome has shown how complex change is and how much it is influenced by clients' circumstances. Without stigmatizing clients, therapists need to understand how circumstances both inside and outside of therapy may be making it difficult for clients to achieve positive outcomes in therapy.

## REFERENCES

American Psychological Association Presidential Task Force on Evidence-Based Practice. (2006). Evidence-based practice in psychology. *American Psychologist, 61,* 271–285.

Anderson, H., & Gehart, D. (2006). *Collaborative therapy: Relationships and conversations that make a difference.* New York: Routledge.

Angus, L. E. (1992). Metaphor and the communication interaction in psychotherapy: A multimethodological approach. In S. G. Toukmanian & D. L. Rennie (Eds.), *Psychotherapy process research: Paradigmatic and narrative approaches* (pp. 187–210). Newbury Park, CA: Sage.

Asay, T. P., & Lambert, M. J. (1999). The empirical case for the common factors in therapy: Quantitative findings. In M. A. Hubble, B. L. Duncan, & S. D. Miller (Eds.), *The heart and soul of change: What works in therapy* (pp. 33–56). Washington, DC: American Psychological Association.

Bachelor, A., Laverdière, O., Gamache, D., & Bordeleau, V. (2007). Clients' collaboration in therapy: Self-perceptions and relationships with client psychological functioning, interpersonal relations, and motivation. *Psychotherapy: Theory, Research, Practice, Training, 44,* 175–192.

Berg, I. K., & Miller, S.D. (1992). *Working with the problem drinker: A solution-focused approach.* New York: Norton.

Bergin, A. E., & Garfield, S. L. (1994). Overview, trends, and future issues. In A. E. Bergin & S. L. Garfield (Eds.), *Handbook of psychotherapy and behavior change* (4th ed., pp. 821–830). New York: Wiley.

Beutler, L. E. Malik, M., Alimohamed, S., Harwood, T. M., Talebi, H., Noble, S., et al. (2004). Therapist variables. In M. J. Lambert (Ed.), *Bergin and Garfield's handbook of psychotherapy and behavior change* (5th ed., pp. 227–306). New York: Wiley.

Bohart, A. C. (2000). The client is the most important common factor: Clients' self-healing capacities and psychotherapy. *Journal of Psychotherapy Integration, 10,* 127–150.

Bohart, A. C. (2006). The active client. In J. C. Norcross, L. E. Beutler, & R. F. Levant (Eds.), *Evidence-based practices in mental health: Debate and dialogue on the fundamental questions* (pp. 218–225). Washington, DC: American Psychological Association.

Bohart, A. C. (2007). The actualizing person. In M. Cooper, M. O'Hara, P. F. Schmid, & G. Wyatt (Eds.), *The handbook of person-centred psychotherapy and counselling* (pp. 47–63). Hampshire, England: Palgrave Macmillan.

Bohart, A. C., & Boyd, G. (1997, December). *Clients' construction of the therapy process: A qualitative analysis.* Paper presented at the meeting of the North American Association of the Society for Psychotherapy Research, Tucson, AZ.

Bohart, A. C., Elliott, R., Greenberg, L. S., & Watson, J. C. (2002). Empathy. In J. C. Norcross (Ed.), *Psychotherapy relationships that work* (pp. 89–108). New York: Oxford University Press.

Bohart, A. C., & Tallman, K. (1999). *How clients make therapy work: The process of active self-healing.* Washington, DC: American Psychological Association.

Bonanno, G. A. (2004). Loss, trauma, and human resilience: Have we underestimated the human capacity to thrive after extremely aversive events? *American Psychologist, 59,* 20–28.

Brown, G. S., Burlingame, G. M., Lambert, M. J., Jones, E., & Vaccaro, J. (2001). Pushing the quality envelope: A new outcomes management system. *Psychiatric Services, 52,* 925–934.

Busseri, M. A., & Tyler, J. D. (2004). Client–therapist agreement on target problems, working alliance, and counseling outcome. *Psychotherapy Research, 14,* 77–88.

Calhoun, L. G., & Tedeschi, R. G. (2006). The foundations of posttraumatic growth: An expanded framework. In L. G. Calhoun & R. G. Tedeschi (Eds.), *Handbook of posttraumatic growth: Research and practice* (pp. 1–23). Mahwah, NJ: Erlbaum.

Cantor, N. (2003). Constructive cognition, personal goals, and the social embedding of personality. In L. G. Aspinwall & U. M. Staudinger (Eds.), *A psychology of human strengths* (pp. 49–60). Washington, DC: American Psychological Association.

Carey, T. A., Carey, M., Stalker, K., Mullan, R. J., Murray, L. K., & Spratt, M. B. (2007). Psychological change from the inside looking out: A qualitative investigation. *Counselling & Psychotherapy Research, 7,* 178–187.

Castonguay, L. G., & Beutler, L. F. (2006). Common and unique principles of therapeutic change: What do we know and what do we need to know? In L. G. Castonguay & L. E. Beutler (Eds.), *Principles of therapeutic change that work* (pp. 353–370). New York: Oxford University Press.

Chambless, D. L., & Hollon, S. D. (1998). Defining empirically supported therapies. *Journal of Consulting and Clinical Psychology, 66,* 7–18.

Charon, R. (2006). *Narrative medicine: Honoring the stories of illness.* New York: Oxford University Press.

Christensen, A., & Jacobson, N. S. (1994). Who (or what) can do psychotherapy: The status and challenge of nonprofessional therapies. *Psychological Science, 5,* 8–14.

Cohen, O. (2005). How do we recover? An analysis of psychiatric survivor oral histories. *Journal of Humanistic Psychology, 45*, 333–354.

Conrad, A., & Auckenthaler, A. (2007, June). *Client reports on failure in psychotherapy—Further support for the contextual model of psychotherapy?* Paper presented at the conference of the Society for Psychotherapy Research, Madison, WI.

Crits-Christoph, P., Siqueland, L., Blaine, J., Frank, A., Luborsky, L., Onken, L. S., et al. (1999). Psychosocial treatments for cocaine dependence: National Institute on Drug Abuse Collaborative Cocaine Treatment Study. *Archives of General Psychiatry, 56*, 493–502.

Cullari, S. (2000). *Counseling and psychotherapy.* New York: Allyn & Bacon.

Dreier, O. (2000). Psychotherapy in clients' trajectories across contexts. In C. Mattingly & L. Garro (Eds.), *Narrative and the cultural construction of illness and healing* (pp. 237–258). Berkeley: University of California Press.

Duncan, B. L., Hubble, M. A., & Miller, S. D. (1997). *Psychotherapy with "impossible" cases: Efficient treatment of therapy veterans.* New York: Norton.

Duncan, B. L., Miller, S. D., & Sparks, J. A. (2004). *The heroic client: A revolutionary way to improve effectiveness through client-directed, outcome-informed therapy.* San Francisco: Jossey-Bass.

Duncan, B. L., & Moynihan, D. (1994). Applying outcome research: Intentional utilization of the client's frame of reference. *Psychotherapy, 31*, 294–301.

Duncan, B. L., Solovey, A., & Rusk, G. (1992). *Changing the rules: A client-directed approach.* New York: Guilford Press.

Elkin, I. (1994). The NIMH treatment of depression collaborative research program: Where we began and where we are. In A. E. Bergin & S. L. Garfield (Eds.), *Handbook of psychotherapy and behavior change* (4th ed., pp. 114–142). New York: Wiley.

Elliott, R. (2002). Hermeneutic single-case efficacy design. *Psychotherapy Research, 12*, 1–21.

Elliott, R., & James, E. (1989). Varieties of client experience in psychotherapy: An analysis of the literature. *Clinical Psychology Review, 9*, 443–467.

Elliott, R., Greenberg, L. S., & Lietaer, G. (2004). Research on experiential psychotherapies. In M. J. Lambert (Ed.), *Bergin and Garfield's handbook of psychotherapy and behavior change* (5th ed., pp. 493–540). New York: Wiley.

Elliott, R., Shapiro, D. A., Firth-Cozens, J., Stiles, W. B., Hardy, G. E., Llewelyn, S. P., & Margison, F. R. (1994). Comprehensive process analysis of insight events in cognitive–behavioral and psychodynamic–interpersonal psychotherapies. *Journal of Counseling Psychology, 41*, 449–463.

Fonagy, P., & Bateman, M. (2006). Progress in the treatment of borderline personality disorder. *British Journal of Psychiatry, 188*, 1–3.

Garfinkel, H. (1967). *Studies in ethnomethodology.* New York: Prentice-Hall.

Gassman, D. & Grawe, K. (2006). General change mechanisms: The relation between problem activation and resource activation in successful and unsuccessful therapeutic interactions. *Clinical Psychology and Psychotherapy, 13*, 1–11.

Gould, R. A., & Clum, G. A. (1993). A meta-analysis of self-help treatment approaches. *Clinical Psychology Review, 13,* 169–186.

Greaves, A. L. (2006). *The active client: A qualitative analysis of thirteen clients' contribution to the psychotherapeutic process.* Unpublished doctoral dissertation, University of Southern California, Los Angeles.

Greenberg, L. S., & Watson, J. E. (1998). Experiential therapy of depression: Differential effects of client-centered relationship conditions and process experiential interventions. *Psychotherapy Research, 8,* 210–224.

Gregory, R. J., Canning, S. S., Lee, T. W., & Wise, J. C. (2004). Cognitive bibliotherapy for depression: A meta-analysis. *Professional Psychology: Research and Practice, 35,* 275–280.

Grissom, R. J. (1996). The magical number .7 ± .2: Meta-meta-analysis of the probability of superior outcome in comparisons involving therapy, placebo, and control. *Journal of Consulting and Clinical Psychology, 64,* 973–982.

Gurin, J. (1990, March). Remaking our lives. *American Health,* pp. 50–52.

Harris Interactive. (2004, April). *Therapy in America: A poll sponsored by Psychology Today and PacifiCare..* Retrieved December 8, 2007, from http://www.psychologytoday.com/pto/topline_report_042904.pdf

Harvey, J. H., Orbuch, T. L., Chwalisz, K. D., & Garwood, G. (1991). Coping with sexual assault: The roles of account-making and confiding. *Journal of Traumatic Stress, 4,* 515–531.

Hemenover, S. H. (2003). The good, the bad, and the healthy: Impacts of emotional disclosure of trauma on resilient self-concept and psychological distress. *Personality and Social Psychology Bulletin, 29,* 1236–1244.

Hoerner, C. (2007, June). *Client experiences in psychotherapy: The importance of being active.* Paper presented at the conference of the Society for Psychotherapy Research, Madison, WI.

Honos-Webb, L. (2005). The meaning vs. the medical model in the empirically supported treatments program: A consideration of the empirical evidence. *Journal of Contemporary Psychotherapy, 35,* 55–66.

Honos-Webb, L. (2006). *Listening to depression: How understanding your pain can heal your life.* Oakland, CA: New Harbinger.

Horvath, A. O., & Bedi, B. P. (2002). The alliance. In J. C. Norcross (Ed.), *Psychotherapy relationships that work* (pp. 37–70). New York: Oxford University Press.

Howard, K. I., Kopta, S. M., Krause, M. S., & Orlinsky, D. E. (1986). The dose–effect relationship in psychotherapy. *American Psychologist, 41,* 159–164.

Jacobs, M. K., Christensen, A., Snibbe, J. R., Dolezal-Wood, S., Huber, A., & Polterok, A. (2001). A comparison of computer-based versus traditional individual psychotherapy. *Professional Psychology: Research and Practice, 32,* 92–96.

Kagan, F., Angus, L., & Pos, A. (2007, June). *Client experiences in emotion-focused and client-centered brief therapy for depression: A qualitative analysis.* Paper presented at the conference of the Society for Psychotherapy Research, Madison, WI.

Kirsch, I., Deacon, B. J., Huedo-Medina, T. B., Scoboria, A., Moore, T. J., & Johnson, B. T. (2008). Initial severity and antidepressant benefits: A meta-analysis of data submitted to the Food and Drug Administration. *PLoS Medicine, 5*(2), e45.

Kühnlein, I. (1999). Psychotherapy as a process of transformation: Analysis of post-therapeutic autobiographical narrations. *Psychotherapy Research, 9,* 274–288.

Lambert, M. J., Shapiro, D. A., & Bergin, A. E. (1986). The effectiveness of psychotherapy. In S. L. Garfield & A. E. Bergin (Eds.), *Handbook of psychotherapy and behavior change* (3rd ed., pp. 157–212). New York: Wiley.

Lawson, D. (1994). Identifying pretreatment change. *Journal of Counseling and Development, 72,* 244–248.

Levitt, H. M. (2004, November). *What client interviews reveal about psychotherapy process: Principles for the facilitation of change in psychotherapy.* Paper presented at the meeting of the North American Society for Psychotherapy Research, Springdale, UT.

Levitt, H., Butler, M., & Hill, T. (2006). What clients find helpful in psychotherapy: Developing principles for facilitating moment-to-moment change. *Journal of Counseling Psychology, 53,* 314–324.

Levitt, H. M., & Rennie, D. L. (2004). Narrative activity: Clients' and therapists' intentions in the process of narration. In L. E. Angus & J. McLeod (Eds.), *The handbook of narrative and psychotherapy* (pp. 299–314). Thousand Oaks, CA: Sage.

Linehan, M. (1997). Validation and psychotherapy. In A. C. Bohart & L. S. Greenberg (Eds.), *Empathy reconsidered* (pp. 353–392). Washington, DC: American Psychological Association.

Mackrill, T. (2008). *The therapy journal project: A cross-contextual qualitative diary study of psychotherapy with adult children of alcoholics.* Unpublished doctoral dissertation, Copenhagen University, Copenhagen, Denmark.

Masten, A. S. (2001). Ordinary magic: Resilience processes in development. *American Psychologist, 56,* 227–238.

Masten, A. S., Best, K. M., & Garmazy, N. (1990). Resilience and development: Contributions from the study of children who overcome adversity. *Development and Psychopathology, 2,* 425–444.

Menchola, M., Arkowitz, H. S., & Burke, B. L. (2007). Efficacy of self-administered treatments for depression and anxiety. *Professional Psychology: Research and Practice, 38,* 421–429.

Miller, W. R., & C'de Baca, J. (2001). *Quantum change.* New York: Guilford Press.

Miller, W. R., & Carroll, K. M. (2006). Drawing the scene together: Ten principles, ten recommendations. In W. R. Miller & K. M. Carroll (Eds.), *Rethinking substance abuse: What the science shows, and what we should do about it* (pp. 293–312). New York: Guilford Press.

Miller, W. R., & Rollnick, S. (2002). *Motivational interviewing: Preparing people for change* (2nd ed.). New York: Guilford Press.

Moertl, K. (2007, June). *Patients' narratives about their process of change in a partial hospitalization program*. Paper presented at the conference of the Society for Psychotherapy Research, Madison, WI.

Mosher, L. R., Hendrix, V., & Fort, D. C. (2004). *Soteria*. Philadelphia: Xlibris.

Najavits, L. M., & Strupp, H. (1994). Differences in the effectiveness of psychodynamic therapists: A process–outcome study. *Psychotherapy, 31*, 114–123.

Norcross, J. C. (2006). Integrating self-help into psychotherapy: 16 practical suggestions. *Professional Psychology: Research and Practice, 37*, 683–693.

Norcross, J. C., Beutler, L. E., & Levant, R.F. (Eds.). (2006). *Evidence-based practices in mental health: Debate and dialogue on the fundamental questions* (pp. 200–207). Washington, DC: American Psychological Association.

Orlinsky, D. E., Rønnestad, M. H., & Willutzki, U. (2004). Fifty years of psychotherapy process–outcome research: Continuity and change. In M. J. Lambert (Ed.), *Bergin and Garfield's handbook of psychotherapy and behavior change* (5th ed., pp. 307–390). New York: Wiley.

Ozer, E. J., Best, S. R., Lipsey, T. L., & Weiss, D. S. (2003). Predictors of posttraumatic stress disorder and symptoms in adults: A meta- analysis. *Psychological Bulletin, 129*, 52–71.

Pennebaker, J. W. (1997). Writing about emotional experiences as a therapeutic process. *Psychological Science, 8*, 162–166.

Perry, J. C. (1993, Spring). Longitudinal studies of personality disorders. *Journal of Personality Disorders, 1*(Suppl. 1), 63–85.

Philips, B., Werbart, A., Wennberg, P., & Schubert, J. (2007). *Journal of Clinical Psychology, 63*, 213–232.

Prochaska, J. O. (1999). How do people change, and how can we change to help many more people? In M. A. Hubble, B. L. Duncan, & S. D. Miller (Eds.), *The heart and soul of change: What works in therapy* (pp. 227–258). Washington, DC: American Psychological Association.

Prochaska, J. O., Norcross, J. C., & DiClemente, C. C. (1994). *Changing for good*. New York: Morrow.

Rennie, D. L. (2000). Aspects of the client's conscious control of the psychotherapeutic process. *Journal of Psychotherapy Integration, 10*, 151–168.

Rodgers, B. (2003). An exploration into the client at the heart of therapy: A qualitative perspective. *Person-Centered & Experiential Psychotherapies, 2*, 19–30.

Rosenbaum, R. (1996). Form, formlessness, and formulation. *Journal of Psychotherapy Integration, 6*, 107–117.

Rosenbaum, R., & Talmon, M. (2006, September). *Implementing single-session approaches in community clinics*. One-day workshop for Mental Health Association, State of Victoria, Australia, Bendigo, Australia.

Segal, D. L., & Murray, E. J. (1994). Emotional processing in cognitive therapy and vocal expression of feeling. *Journal of Social and Clinical Psychology, 13*, 189–206.

Selby, C. E. (2004). *Psychotherapy as creative process: A grounded theory exploration.* Unpublished doctoral dissertation, Saybrook Graduate School, San Francisco.

Skodol, A. E., Bender, D. S., Pagano, M. E., Shea, M. T., Yen, S., Sanislow, C. A., et al. (2007). Positive childhood experiences: Resilience and recovery from personality disorder in early adulthood. *Journal of Clinical Psychiatry, 68,* 1102–1108.

Snyder, C. R., Michael, S. T., & Cheavens, J. S. (1999). Hope as a psychotherapeutic foundation of common factors, placebos, and expectancies. In M. A. Hubble, B. L. Duncan, & S. Miller (Eds.), *The heart and soul of change: What works in therapy* (pp. 179–200). Washington, DC: American Psychological Association.

Stulz, N., Lutz, W., Leach, C., Lucock, M., & Barkham, M. (2007). Shapes of early change in psychotherapy under routine outpatient conditions. *Journal of Consulting and Clinical Psychology, 75,* 864–874.

Tallman, K., & Bohart, A. C. (1999). The client as a common factor: Clients as self-healers. In M. A. Hubble, B. L. Duncan, & S. D. Miller (Eds.), *The heart and soul of change: What works in therapy* (pp. 91–132). Washington, DC: American Psychological Association.

Tallman, K., Janisse, T., Frankel, R. M., Sung, S. H., Krupat, E., & Hsu, J. T. (2007). Communication practices of physicians with high patient-satisfaction ratings. *The Permanente Journal, 11,* 19–29.

Tallman, K., Robinson, E., Kay, D., Harvey, S., & Bohart, A. (1994, August). *Experiential and non-experiential Rogerian therapy: An analogue study.* Paper presented at the 102nd Annual Convention of the American Psychological Association, Los Angeles, CA.

Talmon, M. (1990). *Single session therapy.* San Francisco: Jossey-Bass.

Task Force on Promotion and Dissemination of Psychological Procedures, Division of Clinical Psychology of the American Psychological Association. (1995). Training and dissemination of empirically-validated psychological treatments: Report and recommendations. *The Clinical Psychologist, 48,* 3–23.

Tedeschi, J. T., & Felson, R. B. (1994). *Violence, aggression, and coercive actions.* Washington, DC: American Psychological Association.

Tedeschi, R. G., Park, C. L., & Calhoun, L. G. (Eds.). (1998). *Posttraumatic growth.* Mahwah, NJ: Erlbaum.

Timulak, L. (2007). Identifying core categories of client-identified impact of helpful events in psychotherapy: A qualitative meta-analysis. *Psychotherapy Research, 17,* 305–314.

Vaillant, G. E. (1993). *The wisdom of the ego.* Cambridge, MA: Harvard University Press.

Von Below, C., & Werbart, A. (2007, June). *Dissatisfied psychotherapy patients—What went wrong?* Paper presented at the conference of the Society for Psychotherapy Research, Madison, WI.

Wampold, B. E. (2001). *The great psychotherapy debate: Models, methods, and findings.* Mahwah, NJ: Erlbaum.

Wampold, B. E. (2006). The therapist. In J. C. Norcross, L. E. Beutler, & R. F. Levant (Eds.), *Evidence-based practices in mental health: Debate and dialogue on the fundamental questions* (pp. 200–207). Washington, DC: American Psychological Association.

Weiner-Davis, M., de Shazer, S., & Gingerich, W. (1987). Building on pretreatment change to construct the therapeutic solution: An exploratory study. *Journal of Marital and Family Therapy, 13*, 359–364.

Werbart, A., & Johansson, L. (2007, June). *Patients' view of therapeutic action in group psychotherapy*. Paper presented at the conference of the Society for Psychotherapy Research, Madison, WI.

Westra, H., Angus, L., & Stala, D. (2007, June). *Client experiences of motivational interviewing for generalized anxiety disorder: A qualitative analysis*. Paper presented at the conference of the Society for Psychotherapy Research, Madison, WI.

Zanarini, M. C., Frankenburg, F. R., Hennen, J., Reich, D. B., & Silk, K. (2006). Prediction of the ten year course of borderline personality disorder. *American Journal of Psychiatry, 163*, 827–832.

Zuroff, D. C., Blatt, S. J., Sotsky, S. M., Krupnick, J. L., Martin, D. J., Sanislow, C. A., & Simmens, S. (2000). Relation of therapeutic alliance and perfectionism to outcome in brief outpatient treatment of depression. *Journal of Consulting and Clinical Psychology, 68*, 114–124.

# 4

# THE THERAPEUTIC RELATIONSHIP

JOHN C. NORCROSS

Listening creates a holy silence. When you listen generously to people, they can hear the truth in themselves, often for the first time. And when you listen deeply, you can know yourself in everyone.
—Rachel Remen, *Kitchen Table Wisdom*

Let us act like Einstein and begin our journey into the therapeutic relationship with a thought experiment (*Gedankenexperiment*). Like Einstein riding a beam of light into the universe, ask yourself: What accounts for the success of psychotherapy? Ponder it quietly for a moment.

Now, consider a more personal question: What accounted for the success of your own personal therapy? More than 75% of mental health professionals have undergone personal psychotherapy, typically on more than one occasion (Geller, Norcross, & Orlinsky, 2005). What made it effective? Give that some thought.

Your probable answer is that many factors account for the success of psychotherapy, including the client, the therapist, their relationship, the treatment method, and the context. Yet, when pressed for a single response, in my experience, about 80% of psychotherapists will answer: "the relationship." As every human knows intuitively in his or her bones, it is the nurture and comfort of the other human. Your probable answer matches the cumulative findings of psychotherapy research.

Suppose we asked a neutral scientific panel from outside the field to review the corpus of psychotherapy research to determine what is the most powerful phenomenon we should be studying, practicing, and teaching. Henry (1998) concluded that the panel

> would find the answer obvious, and *empirically validated*. Across studies, the largest portion of outcome variance not attributable to preexisting client characteristics involves individual therapist differences and the emergent therapeutic relationship between client and therapist, regardless of technique or school of therapy. (p. 128)

That is the main thrust of 4 decades of empirical research. In more strident moments, one could adapt Bill Clinton's unofficial campaign slogan: "It's the relationship, stupid!"

Indeed, of the multitude of factors that account for success in psychotherapy, clinicians of different orientations converge on this point: The therapeutic relationship is the cornerstone. To be sure, some clinicians conceptualize the relationship as a precondition of change, others as the fertile soil that permits change, and still others as the central mechanism of change itself. Nonetheless, the most common of common factors, the most convergence amongst the professional divergence, is the therapeutic relationship (Grencavage & Norcross, 1990; Weinberger, 1995).

Highlighting the therapeutic relationship as a mechanism of change raises the proverbial temptation to devalue other change mechanisms, such as the client's contribution and the treatment method. This chapter, as does the present volume, avoids such simple dichotomies and archaic polarizations. Focusing on one area—the psychotherapy relationship—should not convey the impression that it is the only area of importance nor should it trivialize or degrade the others. I argue for the centrality, not the exclusivity, of the therapeutic relationship. The treatment method, the individual therapist, the therapy relationship, the client, and their optimal combinations are all vital contributors to the success of psychotherapy. All must be studied.

We can operationally define the *client–therapist relationship* as the feelings and attitudes that therapist and client have toward one another and how these are expressed (Gelso & Carter, 1994; also see Gelso & Hayes, 1998). This definition is general but concise, reasonably consensual, and theoretically neutral.

My aim in this chapter is to traverse the empirical research on what works in the therapeutic relationship and to translate that research into clinical practices. Decades of research can guide therapists in what to do, what not to do, and how to adapt to individual clients and contexts. The chapter begins with clients' voices: what research into their experiences reveals about the therapeutic relationship. Then, I review the research on what works in the therapeutic relationship in general. The ensuing section covers the research on what works for particular clients, that is, how to responsively tailor the therapeutic relationship to enhance the efficacy of treatment. The chapter concludes with a brief, practice-friendly review of what does *not* work in the therapeutic relationship and offers final thoughts on integrating the relationship into the larger treatment context.

## WHAT WORKS ACCORDING TO CLIENTS

Before turning to sophisticated empirical research on the robust association between the therapy relationship and treatment outcomes, let us consider a large body of clinical experience and client reports attesting to the powerful, if not curative, nature of the therapy relationship (Norcross & Lambert, 2005). When clinicians ask clients what was helpful in their psychotherapy, clients routinely identify the therapeutic relationship (Sloane, Staples, Cristol, Yorkston, & Whipple, 1975). At least 100 such studies have appeared in the literature with similar conclusions. Clients do not emphasize the effectiveness of particular techniques or methods. Instead, they primarily attribute the effectiveness of their treatment to the relationship with their therapists (Elliott & James, 1989; Strupp, Fox, & Lessler, 1969).

**Representative Studies**

In an illustrative study, researchers asked outpatients to list curative factors that they believed to be associated with their successful cognitive–behavioral therapy (Murphy, Cramer, & Lillie, 1984). The factors endorsed by the majority of clients were advice (79%), talking to someone interested in my problems (75%), encouragement and reassurance (67%), talking to someone who understands (58%), and instillation of hope (58%). The clients in the study were mainly from the lower socioeconomic class, whom past research has suggested expect more expert advice in therapy (Goin, Yamamoto, & Silverman, 1965).

In an investigation of psychodynamic therapy (Najavits & Strupp, 1994), 16 therapists were assigned clients with similar difficulty levels. After 25 sessions, therapists were evaluated according to outcome, length of treatment, and therapist in-session behavior. Therapists whose clients evidenced better outcomes used more positive and fewer negative behaviors than the less effective therapists, with the largest differences occurring in relationship behaviors rather than technical skills. Warmth, understanding, and affirmation were considered positive, whereas subtle forms of belittling, blaming, ignoring, neglecting, attacking, and rejecting were considered negative. From these results, the authors concluded that "basic capacities of human relating—warmth, affirmation, and a minimum of attack and blame—may be at the center of effective psychotherapeutic intervention. Theoretically based technical interventions were not nearly as often significant in this study" (Najavits & Strupp, 1994, p. 121).

The massive National Institute of Mental Health (NIMH) Treatment of Depression Collaborative Research Program evaluated the effectiveness of interpersonal therapy, cognitive therapy, antidepressant medication plus clinical management, and a placebo plus clinical management (Elkin et al., 1989). Clients' experiences on the helpful aspects of their psychotherapy experiences were examined as part of the research program. Their most frequent responses fell into the categories of "my therapist helped" (41%) and "learned something new" (36%). In fact, at posttreatment fully 32% of the clients receiving placebo plus clinical management wrote their therapists were the most helpful part of their "treatment" (Gershefski, Arnkoff, Glass, & Elkin, 1996).

As a final illustration, consider the studies on the most informed consumers of psychotherapy: psychotherapists themselves. In two studies, American (N = 727) and British (N = 710) psychologists were asked to reflect on their psychotherapy experiences and to nominate any lasting lessons acquired concerning the practice of psychotherapy (Bike, Norcross, & Schatz, 2009: Norcross, Dryden, & DeMichele, 1992). The most frequent responses all involved the interpersonal relationships and dynamics of psychotherapy: the centrality of warmth, empathy, and the personal relationship; the importance of transference and countertransference; the inevitable humanness of the therapist; and the need for therapist reliability and commitment. Conversely, a review of five published studies that identified covariates of harmful therapies received by mental health professionals concluded that the harm was typically attributed to distant and rigid therapists, emotionally seductive therapists, and poor client–therapist matches (Orlinsky & Norcross, 2005).

The tendency in psychotherapy research is to look past clients' narrative reports of successful psychotherapy because they lack the precision and causation afforded by quantitative analysis. Although quantitative analysis surely provides an invaluable perspective, it often looks past the interpersonal experiences of our clients. Psychotherapy is an intensely relational and affective pursuit—that is what our clients tell us time and again.

## Practice Implications

- *Listen to clients*. What is missing in most psychotherapy journals and textbooks is the client's voice (Gabbard & Freeman, 2006). The consumer movement in health care forcibly reminds therapists to listen to the client's experiences, preferences, and realities. Their voices consistently, eloquently tell us to cultivate and customize the therapeutic relationship (Duncan, Miller, & Sparks, 2004).

- *Privilege the client's experience.* The empirical research on therapist empathy and the therapeutic alliance (to be reviewed shortly) repeatedly informs us that it is the client's experience of empathy and collaboration that best predicts treatment success (e.g., Bohart & Greenberg, 1997; Bedi, Davis, & Williams, 2005; Horvath & Bedi, 2002): the client's experience, not the therapist's experience. The practice imperative is to privilege the client's theory and experience of change, not the therapist's (Duncan & Miller, 2000).
- *Request feedback on the therapy relationship.* Psychotherapists are comparatively poor at gauging their client's experiences of their empathy and the alliance, although therapists frequently believe they are accurate (Hannan et al., 2005). A meta-analysis found that client and therapist alliance ratings only correlated an average of .33 (Tryon, Collins, & Felleman, 2006). The clinical upshot is to request real-time feedback from clients on their response to the therapy relationship. The benefits of doing so include empowering clients, promoting explicit collaboration, making mid-therapy adjustments as needed, and enhancing treatment success (Lambert, 2005). (Several methods of systematically gathering client feedback are provided in chap. 8, this volume.)
- *Avoid critical or pejorative comments.* Client reports and the empirical research converge in warning therapists to avoid negative communication patterns that detract from outcome, especially in treating more difficult clients (Lambert & Barley, 2002). These patterns include comments or behaviors that are critical, attacking, rejecting, blaming, or neglectful (Najavits & Strupp, 1994). Although this sounds like elementary advice, difficult clients who themselves attack, reject, and blame are likely to provoke negative communications from their therapists over time.
- *Ask what has been most helpful in this therapy.* If you have not yet tried it, ask your clients toward the conclusion of a successful course of therapy what has been most helpful to them. They are likely to be amazed by the ubiquity and centrality of the therapy relationship: "you listened carefully," "you respected and liked me," "I could tell you anything," "you believed in me," "we worked well together." You are also likely to receive responses that are representations or transitional objects for respect, listening, and support. In my practice, for example, many clients recall fondly my offering them a bottle of water, juice, or soda at the beginning of our sessions. The Diet Pepsi, a returned phone call,

or a sliding fee scale served as concrete symbols of the amorphous but genuine relationship.

## WHAT WORKS IN GENERAL

Hundreds upon hundreds of research studies convincingly demonstrate that the therapeutic relationship makes substantial and consistent contributions to psychotherapy outcome. These studies were efficiently summarized in a series of meta-analyses commissioned and published by an American Psychological Association Division 29 (Division of Psychotherapy) task force (Norcross, 2001, 2002) on empirically supported (therapy) relationships.

Two specific objectives informed the work of the task force: first, to identify elements of effective therapy relationships; second, to identify effective methods of tailoring therapy to the individual client on the basis of his or her (nondiagnostic) characteristics. Thus, we sought to answer the dual pressing questions of What works in general in the therapy relationship? and What works best for particular clients?

The task force reviewed the extensive body of empirical research and generated a list of effective relationship elements and effective means for customizing therapy to the individual client. The evidentiary criteria for making these judgments entailed number of supportive studies, consistency of the research results, magnitude of the positive relationship between the element and outcome, directness of the link between the element and outcome, experimental rigor of the studies, and external validity of the research base.

For each relationship element judged to be effective by that task force, I define the relationship element, describe the findings of an illustrative study, present the meta-analytic results, and most important, offer clinical practices predicated on that research.

### Empathy

Carl Rogers's (1957) definition of *empathy* has guided most of the research: "Empathy is the therapist's sensitive ability and willingness to understand clients' thoughts, feelings, and struggles from their point of view" (p. 98). Empathy involves entering the private, perceptual world of the other and, in therapeutic contexts, communicating that understanding back to the client in ways that can be received and appreciated.

A meta-analysis of 47 studies (encompassing 190 tests) revealed a median $r$ of .26 between therapist empathy and psychotherapy outcome (Bohart, Elliott, Greenberg, & Watson, 2002). This translates into a conventional effect size (ES) of 0.32. Empathy is linked to outcome because it serves a positive relationship function, facilitates a corrective emotional experience, promotes exploration and meaning creation, and supports clients' active self-healing.

In a classic study, W. R. Miller, Taylor, and West (1980) examined the comparative effectiveness of several behavioral approaches in reducing alcohol consumption. The authors also collected data on the contribution of therapist empathy to treatment outcome. At the 6- to 8-month follow-up interviews, client ratings of therapist empathy correlated significantly ($r = .82$) with client outcome, thus accounting for 67% of the variance. Although there were methodological limitations to this early study, the results demonstrated that the importance of empathy was not restricted to person-centered or insight-oriented therapies. Moreover, this study provided impetus for W. R. Miller's development of *motivational interviewing,* a person-centered directive therapy that relies on expressing empathy and rolling with the resistance to help clients explore and resolve their ambivalence about change (W. R. Miller & Rollnick, 2002).

Of course, individual clients experience and interpret therapist behavior quite differently. In one interesting study of perceptions of empathy (Bachelor, 1988), 44% of clients valued a cognitive form of empathic response, 30% an affective form of empathy, and the remainder a nurturing and disclosing empathic response. These results lead to the following conclusions: No single, invariably facilitative empathic response exists, and clients respond according to their own unique needs (Bachelor & Horvath, 1999).

The most obvious practice implication is to convey empathy to all clients in all forms of psychotherapy. Therapists must make efforts to understand their clients, and this understanding must be communicated through responses that the client perceives as empathic. This stance contrasts with therapists responding primarily out of their own needs or agendas. Nor do empathic therapists parrot client's words or simply reflect the content of words. On the contrary, they understand and communicate the clients' moment-to-moment experiences and their implications. In helping clients access as much internal information as possible, empathic therapists attend to what is not said and is at the periphery of awareness as well as what is said and is in focal awareness (Bohart et al., 2002).

To highlight an earlier point, the primary means of ascertaining whether the psychotherapist is indeed empathic is to secure feedback from the client. Clinicians are inadequate judges of clients' experience of empathy (Batchelor & Horvath, 1999). Clinicians' intentions or efforts to be emphatic are insufficient; client reception of empathy is necessary.

## Alliance

The *alliance* refers to the quality and strength of the collaborative relationship between client and therapist. It is typically measured as agreement on the therapeutic goals, consensus on treatment tasks, and a relationship bond (Bordin, 1976; Horvath & Greenberg, 1994). This construct and its multiple measures go by several names: *working alliance, therapeutic alliance*, or simply, the *alliance*. And this construct is incontrovertibly the most popular researched element of the therapeutic relationship today. In fact, some people erroneously have begun to equate the alliance with the entire therapeutic relationship. Remember: The relationship is far broader and inclusive than the alliance alone.

Across 89 studies, the median correlation of the relation between the alliance and therapy outcome among adults was .21, a modest but very robust association (Horvath & Bedi, 2002). Across 23 studies of child and adolescent therapy, the weighted mean correlation between alliance and outcome was .20 (Shirk & Karver, 2003; see also chap. 11, this volume). A weighted mean correlation of .20 and .21 corresponds to an ES (*d*) of 0.45, a medium-sized effect. Nevertheless, this effect is large when one considers that the average ES for psychotherapy versus no treatment is 0.80, and the average ES for differences among treatments, when there are differences among bona fide treatments, is 0.20 (Wampold, 2001). Accordingly, the alliance is potent and amazingly consistent, certainly more than differences among treatments.

Individual studies provide clearer illustrations of the connection between the alliance and client outcome. Effect sizes and probability values, one must remember, translate into vital human statistics: happier and healthier people.

One early study (Gaston, Marmar, Gallagher, & Thompson, 1991) used hierarchical regression analysis to examine the alliance in older depressed clients who participated in behavioral, cognitive, or brief psychodynamic therapy. Clients completed the California Psychotherapy Alliance Scales after the 5th, 10th, and 15th sessions. The alliance uniquely contributed to outcome with increasing variance as therapy progressed. The alliance assessed at the 5th session accounted for 19% to 32% of treatment outcome and for 36% to 57% of outcome at the 15th session.

The salutary impact of the alliance is not restricted to psychotherapy. Several studies have examined the impact of the therapeutic alliance in pharmacotherapy. In the NIMH Collaborative Study, the therapeutic alliance in pharmacotherapy emerged as the leading force in reducing a client's depression (Krupnick et al., 1996). A perceived positive therapeutic alliance early in treatment predicted more rapid and better improvement in all four pharmacotherapy and psychotherapy conditions (Zuroff & Blatt, 2006). In a study of pharmacotherapy for bipolar disorder, the alliance (as rated by the client) with the prescribing physician predicted long-term mood outcomes ($r = .37$) and medication compliance ($r = .48$) for up to 28 months following an acute episode (Gaudiano & Miller, 2006; see also chap. 7, this volume).

The meta-analytic results, combined with individual studies, point to a host of recommended clinical practices. First, develop a strong alliance early in treatment, probably within three to five sessions. If the alliance has not solidified by the fifth session, then the probability for success is jeopardized (Horvath & Bedi, 2002). Second, construct a thoughtful systemic plan for cultivating and maintaining the multiple alliances inherent in multiperson therapies (Kazdin, Marciano, & Whitley, 2005; Shelef, Diamond, Diamond, & Liddle, 2005). Third, recognize that an alliance is harder to establish with clients who are more disturbed, delinquent, homeless, drug abusing, fearful, anxious, dismissive, and preoccupied (Horvath & Bedi, 2002). Fourth, on the therapist side, foster a stronger alliance by using communication skills, empathy, openness, and a paucity of hostile interactions. Fifth, as noted in the following sections, strive to reach consensus on goals and respective tasks, which contributes to alliance formation and then to treatment success. The early sessions should always entail soliciting the client's goals and specifying the respective contributions of client and therapist alike. Sixth and finally, emphasize, particularly in the initial sessions, the relational bond, the special sense of understanding, safety, and trust.

## Cohesion

Cohesion in group therapy—a parallel of the therapeutic alliance in individual therapy—also demonstrates consistent associations to client benefit. *Cohesion* refers to the forces that cause members to remain in the group, a "sticking togetherness." Approximately 80% of the studies support positive relationships between cohesion (mostly member-to-member) and therapy outcome (Burlingame, Fuhriman, & Johnson, 2002; Tschuschke & Dies, 1994).

From this empirical research come a set of treatment principles for fostering cohesion and group outcomes (Burlingame et al., 2002). In particular, the leader or leaders of group therapy can

- Conduct pregroup preparation that sets treatment expectations, defines group rules, and instructs members in rules and skills needed for effective group participation.
- Establish clarity regarding group processes in early sessions (as higher levels of structure usually lead to higher levels of disclosure and cohesion).
- Model real-time observations, guide effective interpersonal feedback, and maintain a moderate level of control and affiliation.

- Time and deliver feedback to group members carefully so feedback is largely positive early on, feedback is balanced between positive and negative in later sessions, and the receiver is ready and open.
- Manage one's own emotional presence in the group because the leader not only affects the relationship with individual members but also all group members as they vicariously experience the leader's manner of relating.
- Facilitate group members' emotional expression, responsiveness of others to that expression, and shared meaning from such expression.

## Goal Consensus and Collaboration

*Goal consensus* refers to therapist–client agreement on treatment goals and expectations. *Collaboration* is the mutual involvement of the participants in the helping relationship. Although goal consensus and collaboration are frequently measured as part of the alliance, for clinical, research, and training purposes, they must be separated. We need to know, specifically, what in the therapy relationship (and the alliance) is effective. Fully 68% (17 of 25) of the studies found a positive association between goal consensus and outcome, and 89% (32 of 36) of the studies reported the same for collaboration and outcome (Tryon & Winograd, 2002).

In an interesting study, investigators explored the specific behavior of therapists contributing to a client's perception of a facilitative alliance (Creed & Kendall, 2005). Collaboration behaviors included the therapist presenting treatment as a team effort, helping set goals for therapy, encouraging specific feedback from the client, and building a sense of togetherness by using words like *we, us,"* and *let's*. These collaborative behaviors predicted early client ratings of the alliance and therapist-rated alliances by the seventh session.

To promote treatment success, research and experience suggest that clinicians should begin to develop consensus at intake. In later sessions with their clients, they should encourage a process of shared decision making in which goals are frequently discussed, reevaluated, and agreed on. Collaborative therapists attend verbally to client problems, address topics of importance to them, and resonate to client attributions of blame regarding their problems. Collaboration involves the behaviors identified and validated in the Creed and Kendall (2005) study cited earlier. Therapists who mutually create homework assignments with clients achieve better therapy outcomes, particularly if they check on these assignments in the next session (Kazantzis, Deane, & Ronan, 2000). In short, the therapist and client journey together toward a mutual destination.

Therapist empathy, the alliance, cohesion in group therapy, goal consensus, and collaboration are demonstrably effective elements of the therapy relationship. The task force designated another set of seven relational elements as probably effective because of a less compelling body of extant research. These are summarized in less detail in the sections that follow.

## Positive Regard

This therapist quality is characterized as warm acceptance of the client's experience without conditions. It is understood as a prizing, an affirmation, and a deep nonpossessive caring. The early research reviews (e.g., Truax & Carkhuff, 1967; Orlinsky & Howard, 1978) were very supportive of the association between positive regard and therapy outcome, with approximately two thirds of the studies in the positive direction. Recent reviews of more rigorous studies published since 1990 found that 49% (27 of 55) of all associations were significantly positive and 51% (28 of 55) did not achieve significance. No studies reported negative associations between positive regard and outcome (Farber & Lane, 2002). When treatment outcome and therapist positive regard were both rated by clients, the percentage of positive findings jumped to 88% (Farber & Lane, 2002).

Clinically, the research results indicate, first, that the provision of positive regard or validation is strongly indicated in practice. Second, similar to empathy and the alliance, it is the client's perception of the therapist's positive regard that has the strongest association with outcome. At the risk of redundancy, supportive therapists should privilege their client's experience. Third, therapists cannot be merely content with feeling good about their clients but should ensure that their positive feelings are communicated to them. This does not require a stream of compliments or an outpouring of love. Rather, it speaks to the need for therapists to communicate a caring, respectful attitude that affirms a client's basic sense of worth (Duncan & Moynihan, 1994; Farber & Lane, 2002). Fourth, when working with challenging clients who tend to devalue others, therapists need to demarcate their support for the person of the client from their distaste of particular behaviors. Put differently, therapists can separate the "sinner from the sin" and thereby prize the client as whole.

## Congruence/Genuineness

The two facets here are the therapist's personal integration in the relationship and the therapist's capacity to communicate his or her personhood to the client as appropriate. Across 20 studies (and 77 separate results), 34% found a positive relation between therapist congruence and treatment outcome, and 66% found no significant associations (M. G. Klein, Kolden, Michels, &

Chisholm-Stockard, 2002). The percentage of positive studies increased to 68% when congruence was tested in concert with empathy and positive regard, supporting Roger's original conviction that the facilitative conditions (empathy, positive regard, congruence) work together and cannot be easily distinguished. Therapist congruence is higher when therapists have more self-confidence, good mood, increased involvement or activity, responsiveness, smoothness of speaking exchanges, and when clients have high levels of self-exploration/experiencing.

### Feedback

*Feedback* is defined as descriptive and evaluative information provided to clients from therapists about the client's behavior or the effects of that behavior. Across 11 studies empirically investigating the feedback–outcome connection, 73% were positive and 27% were nonsignificant (Claiborn, Goodyear, & Horner, 2002). Note that this research concerns therapist feedback to clients, not client feedback to therapists (for the latter, see chap. 8, this volume).

To enhance the clinical effectiveness of feedback, therapists can take the following steps (Claiborn et al., 2002):

- increase their credibility, which makes acceptance of feedback more positive;
- prepare the client to receive and make use of the feedback;
- structure the feedback and explain its goals in a clear way;
- give positive feedback, especially early to establish the relationship;
- precede or sandwich negative feedback with positive comments; and
- proceed cautiously with clients suffering from low self-esteem and negative mood, who are apt to bias processing of feedback in a negative direction.

### Repair of Alliance Ruptures

A *rupture* in the therapeutic alliance is a tension or breakdown in the collaborative relationship. Therapists should be aware that clients often have negative feelings about the treatment or the relationship. Additionally, they may be reluctant to broach their concerns for fear of the therapist's reactions. Many clients do not tell us about ruptures; they often "vote with their feet" and do not return. As such, therapists must be attuned to subtle indications of alliance ruptures and take the initiative in exploring their client's reactions (Safran, Muran, Samstag, & Stevens, 2002). Once more, here is where direct monitoring of the client's experience of the treatment and the relationship pays dividends. Proactive monitoring can detect ruptures and improve the chances for therapy success. The small body of research indicates that the frequency and severity of ruptures are increased by rigid adherence to a treatment manual and an excessive number of transference interpretations. By contrast, the research suggests that repairs of ruptures can be facilitated by the therapist responding nondefensively, attending directly to the alliance, and adjusting his or her behavior (Safran et al., 2002).

### Self-Disclosure

*Therapist self-disclosure* refers to therapist statements and behaviors that reveal something personal about the practitioner. Analogue research suggests that nonclients commonly have positive perceptions of therapist self-disclosure. In actual therapy, disclosures are perceived as helpful for enhanced empathy and immediate outcomes, although the effect on the ultimate outcome of therapy is unclear (Hill & Knox, 2002). The research suggests that therapists should disclose infrequently and, when they do disclose, do so to validate reality, normalize experiences, strengthen the alliance, or offer alternative ways to think or act. Therapists should avoid self-disclosures that are for their own needs, remove the focus from the client, or blur the treatment boundaries.

### Management of Countertransference

Although variously defined, *countertransference* refers to reactions in which the unresolved conflicts of the psychotherapist, usually but not always unconscious, are involved. The limited research supports the interrelated conclusions that therapists acting out countertransference hinders psychotherapy. On the other hand, effectively managing countertransference aids the process and probably the outcome of therapy (Gelso & Hayes, 2002). In managing countertransference, five central therapist skills have been implicated: self-insight, self-integration, anxiety management, empathy, and conceptualizing ability.

### Quality of Relational Interpretations

In the clinical literature, *interpretations* are therapist interventions that attempt to bring material to consciousness that was previously out of awareness. In the research literature, interpretations are behaviorally coded as making connections, going beyond what the client has overtly recognized, and pointing out themes or patterns in the client's behavior. The research correlating frequency of interpretations and outcome has yielded mixed findings. However, the evidence suggests that high rates of transference interpretations lead to poorer outcomes, especially for clients with low quality of object relations (Crits-Christoph & Gibbons, 2002). In contrast, other research has highlighted the importance of the quality of interpretations. Better outcomes are achieved when the therapist addresses central aspects of client interpersonal dynamics (Crits-Christoph & Gibbons, 2002; Luborsky & Crits-Christoph, 1998). The resulting practice implications are to avoid high levels of transference interpretations, particularly for interpersonally challenged clients, and to focus interpretations on the central interpersonal themes for each client.

Taken together, this mass of empirical findings provides reliable evidence that therapists' relational contributions to outcome are identifiable and teachable. We do know what works! Further, these relational behaviors or qualities significantly and causally relate to psychotherapy success at a magnitude as high (or higher) than the particular treatment method (Norcross, 2002; Wampold, 2001).

## WHAT WORKS FOR PARTICULAR CLIENTS

The preceding section addressed relationship behaviors, primarily provided by the psychotherapist, that are effective: what works in general. This section addresses those client behaviors or qualities that may serve as reliable markers for customizing the therapy relationship: what works for particular clients.

The essential truth of behavioral science is that people differ. What works relationally for one person—say, a playful, good-natured tease for an adolescent boy—might be experienced as disrespectful or insensitive by another person. Person-centered therapists characterize these individual differences as idiosyncratic empathy modes.

Clinicians strive to offer or select a therapy that is responsive to the client's condition, characteristics, proclivities, and world views. This process goes by different names—responsiveness, customizing, attunement, tailoring, matchmaking, aptitude by treatment interaction—but the objective is to create a new therapy for each client. The saying "different strokes for different folks" aptly applies.

This position can be easily misunderstood as an authority figure therapist prescribing a specific form of psychotherapy for a passive client. Far from it, the goal is for an empathic therapist to arrange for an optimal relationship collaboratively with an active client on the basis of the client's personality and preferences. If a client frequently resists, for example, then the therapist considers whether she is pushing something that the client finds incompatible (preferences), or the client is not ready to make changes (stage of change), or the client is uncomfortable with a directive style (reactance). Good clinicians pay attention to such matters.

The volume and precision of empirical research on what works best for particular clients pale in comparison with research on what works in general. The empirical research in this area, moreover, tends more toward the correlational and less toward the causal. Consequently, I tentatively summarize below the research on adapting the therapy relationship on just a few such client characteristics that, in the judgment of the Task Force, are demonstrably effective. When we say effective, we mean effective for customizing therapy to the individual client. Here then are three client dimensions—reactance, functional impairment, and stages of change—that may systematically guide therapists in adjusting the relationship to individual differences.

## Reactance

*Reactance* (or *resistance*) refers to being easily provoked and responding oppositionally to external demands. In session, reactance manifests itself in the client's clinical history of high defensiveness, his or her interpersonal style during the interview, response to early interpretations or homework assignments, psychological tests (such as the Minnesota Multiphasic Personality Inventory Paranoid, Defensive, and Hostility scales, for instance), and receptivity to early interpretations or homework assignments. Seasoned clinicians can typically spot highly reactant clients easily, as they can those with low reactance.

Of course, in an interpersonal perspective, we must acknowledge that the therapist's behavior itself may precipitate client reactance! A therapist's authoritarian behaviors, empathic failures, repeated confrontations, or pejorative interpretations may be the culprit for iatrogenic resistance. Let us be careful not to label and blame clients for responding in a reactant manner to resistance-causing therapists.

Varying therapist directiveness to the client's level of reactance improved therapy efficiency and outcome in 80% (16 of 20) of studies (Beutler, Moleiro, & Talebi, 2002). Specifically, clients presenting with high reactance benefit more from self-control methods, minimal therapist directiveness, and paradoxical interventions. By contrast, clients with low reactance benefit more from therapist directiveness and explicit guidance. Listening to the client and attending to his or her progress naturally lead experienced clinicians to similar conclusions. Direct guidance and confrontation with clients who dislike those styles are apt to fail.

In an illustrative study, researchers examined the impact of the interaction between 141 clients' reactance level and their therapists' directiveness on the effectiveness of psychotherapy (Karno & Longabaugh, 2005). Ratings of videotaped treatment sessions were used to measure client reactance and therapist directiveness. The results indicated that therapist directiveness had a negative impact on drinking outcomes for clients high in reactance, but not among clients low in reactance. The more therapists used interpretation and confrontation, the more the high reactant clients drank.

The practice implications entail attending to client interpersonal preferences, considering that stalled progress might result from a therapist pushing too fast or too directly for clients, and adjusting the therapist's level of directiveness to individual client differences. In the main, highly reactant clients do better with low directiveness and more self-control, whereas low reactant clients do better with high directiveness.

## Functional Impairment

This complex dimension reflects the severity of the client's subjective distress as well as reduced behavioral functioning. On the low end of the continuum are clients in little distress and functioning well. On the high end are those in severe and chronic distress, impaired in most areas of functioning (family, social, intimate, occupational). The client's Global Assessment of Functioning (GAF) score and the sheer number and complexity of the client's presenting problems provide a good estimate of functional impairment.

The majority of available studies (74%; 31 of 42) found a significant, inverse relation between level of impairment and treatment outcome. More functionally impaired clients have poorer outcomes (Beutler, Harwood, Alimohamed, & Malik, 2002). At the same time, the research also indicates that clients who manifest impairment in two or more areas of functioning are more likely to benefit from intensive therapy. Such treatment has five characteristics: It is lengthier, more intense, includes psychoactive medication, entails multiple formats (individual couple, family, group), and targets the creation of social support in the natural environment (Beutler, Harwood, et al., 2002; for another interpretation of this research, see chap. 3, this volume).

The research literature corresponds with client voices and preferences. Clients suffering high or chronic distress frequently request that they would profit from "more": more therapy, the addition of group or family therapy, the introduction of psychotropic medication, and greater support in their lives.

## Stages of Change

People progress through a series of stages—precontemplation, contemplation, preparation, action, and maintenance—in both psychotherapy and self-change. More formally, the stages of change can be assessed via a dozen inventories and algorithms (see http://www.uri.edu/research/cprc/measures.

htm). In session, I recommend asking clients a series of quick, discrete questions for each problem behavior:

Do you currently have a problem with_____? (If yes, then in contemplation, preparation, or action stage. If no, then in pre-contemplation or maintenance stage.)

If yes, when will you change it? (Someday: contemplation stage. In the next few weeks: preparation stage. Right now: action stage.)

If no, what leads you to say that? (Because it's not a problem for me: precontemplation stage. Because I have already changed it: maintenance stage.)

A meta-analysis of 47 studies found ESs of 0.70 and 0.80 for the use of different treatment processes in the stages of change (Rosen, 2000). Specifically, cognitive–affective processes are used most by clients in the precontemplation and contemplation stages. Behavioral processes are used most frequently and effectively by those in the action and maintenance stages. Those change processes and treatment methods effective for clients in one stage tend not to be as effective for clients in different stages. For instance, an empathic therapist would probably not request that a client tentatively contemplating ending a relationship do so immediately; the client is simply "not ready yet" to take that step.

The therapist's optimal stance also varies depending on the client's stage of change. Namely, the therapist assumes the position of a nurturing parent with clients in the precontemplation stage, a Socratic teacher with clients in the contemplation stage, an experienced coach with those in the action stage, and a consultant during the maintenance stage (Prochaska & Norcross, 2002). The practice implications encompass assessing the client's stage of change, aligning the therapeutic relationship to that stage, and adjusting tactics as the client moves through the stages. In short, the therapist leads by following the client.

## Additional Characteristics

Researchers are investigating several other, nondiagnostic client dimensions that may call for tailoring the therapy relationship to individual client differences. Among these are clients' preferences (Arnkoff, Glass, & Shapiro, 2002), coping style (Beutler, Harwood, et al., 2002), attachment style (Meyer & Pilkonis, 2002), religious commitment (Worthington & Sandage, 2002), and cultural identification (Sue & Lam, 2002). However, the results of the outcome research on these factors are not yet robust or reliable enough to recommend that therapists routinely use them to tailor the therapeutic relationship.

The overarching lesson of this body of research is to be responsive to clients' requests and needs. This ethical and practical imperative translates into meeting the individual where he or she is, whether that be defined by stage of change, preference, functional impairment, or reactance level. A client who does poorly in one type of relationship (e.g., directive) may do quite well with another. George Eliot (a pseudonym for Mary Ann Evans) wrote in her 1860 novel, *The Mill on the Floss*, "We have no master-key that will fit all cases." Clinical decisions, like Eliot's moral decisions, must be informed by "exerting patience, discrimination, and impartiality" and an insight earned "from a life vivid and intense enough to have created a wide, fellow feeling with all that is human."

## WHAT DOES NOT WORK

Translational research is both prescriptive and proscriptive. It tells us what works and what does not. Seven caveats from the research literature now follow on what should be avoided.

### Confrontations

Controlled research trials, particularly in the addictions field, consistently find a confrontational style to be ineffective. In one review (W. R. Miller, Wilbourne, & Hettema, 2003), confrontation was ineffective in all 12 identified trials. By contrast, expressing empathy, rolling with resistance, developing discrepancy, and supporting self-efficacy—all characteristic of motivational interviewing—have demonstrated large effects with a small number of sessions (Burke, Arkowitz, & Dunn, 2002).

### Negative Processes

Client reports and research studies converge in warning therapists to avoid comments or behaviors that are hostile, pejorative, critical, rejecting, or blaming (Binder & Strupp, 1997; Lambert & Barley, 2002). Therapists who attack a client's dysfunctional thoughts or relational patterns need, repeatedly, to distinguish between attacking the person versus his or her behavior. And, all therapists are advised to manage negative process by learning relational and self-soothing skills.

### Assumptions

Psychotherapists who assume or intuit their client's perceptions of the alliance, empathy, relationship satisfaction, and treatment success are frequently inaccurate. Psychotherapists who specifically and respectfully inquire about their client's perceptions frequently enhance the alliance and prevent premature termination (Lambert, 2005; S. D. Miller, Duncan, Sorrell, & Brown, 2005).

## Therapist Centricity

A recurrent lesson from process–outcome research is that the client's observational perspective on the therapy relationship best predicts outcome (Orlinsky, Rønnestad, & Willutzki, 2004). Psychotherapy practice and research that relies on the therapist's observational perspective, although valuable, simply does not predict outcome as well. Therefore, privilege the client's experiences.

## Rigidity

By inflexibly and excessively structuring treatment, the therapist risks empathic failures and inattentiveness to clients' experiences. Such a therapist is then likely to overlook a breach in the relationship and mistakenly assume she has not contributed to that breach. Dogmatic reliance on particular relational or therapy methods, incompatible with the client, imperils treatment (Ackerman & Hilsenroth, 2001).

## Ostrich Behavior

The nascent research on alliance ruptures in psychotherapy indicate they are common, rarely addressed, and predict premature termination and poor outcomes. Many psychotherapists apparently prefer what we call *ostrich behavior*: burying their heads in the sand and hoping (against hope) that early signs of a rupture do not materialize into a negative outcome. Addressing ruptures in the working alliance is understandably challenging, especially for trainees, but is effective on many fronts.

## Procrustean Bed

As the field of psychotherapy has matured, using an identical therapy relationship (and treatment method) for all clients is now recognized as inappropriate and, in selected cases, even unethical. The efficacy and applicability of psychotherapy are enhanced by tailoring it to the unique needs of the client, not by imposing a *Procrustean bed* onto unwitting consumers of psychological services. (Procrustes, in Greek mythology, was the legendary giant and brigand of Attica, said to be the son of Poseidon. With hospitality, he lured strangers to his inn, and then tied his victims to an iron bed. If their limbs were too long, he would cut them to fit. If too short, he stretched them to the right size.)

Psychotherapists can optimize therapy relationships by simultaneously using what works *and* studiously avoiding what does not work (see Norcross, Koocher, & Garofalo, 2006, for a consensual list of what does not work).

## INTEGRATING RESEARCH AND PRACTICE, INTEGRATING THE RELATIONAL AND TECHNICAL

The research on the therapy relationship is vast, robust, and instructive. As in all pursuits, it is also evolving and not beyond cavil. Before closing, and without resorting to a hackneyed call for more research, allow me a few remarks of caution and constraint. First, current conclusions represent initial steps in aggregating and codifying available research. We all eagerly await updates. My own best guess is that client preferences and attachment styles will soon emerge in research as key guides to how therapists might construct a facilitative therapy relationship.

Second, all findings need to be interpreted within context, such as the modest causal connection between the relationship elements and treatment outcome. Because many facets of the relationship are not subject to randomization and experimental control, it is more difficult to determine a strong, causal relationship between relational elements and treatment outcomes. Nonetheless, dozens of lagged correlational, unconfounded regression, structural equation, and growth curve studies persuasively demonstrate that the therapy relationship causally contributes to outcome (e.g., Barber, Connolly, Crits-Christoph, Gladis, & Siqueland, 2000). For example, using growth-curve analyses (and after controlling for prior improvement and eight prognostically relevant client characteristics), D. N. Klein et al. (2003) found that the early alliance significantly predicted later improvement in 367 chronically depressed clients. Although researchers need to continue to parse out the causal linkages, the therapy relationship has already been shown to exercise causal association to outcome.

For historical and research convenience, we have made distinctions between relationships and techniques. Terms such as *relating* and *interpersonal behavior* are used to describe how therapists and clients behave toward each other. In contrast, terms such as *technique* or *intervention* are used to describe what is done by the therapist. In research and theory, we often treat the how and the what—the relationship and the intervention, the interpersonal and the instrumental—as separate categories. In reality, of course, what one does and how one does it are complementary and inseparable. To remove the interpersonal from the instrumental may be acceptable in research, but it is a fatal flaw when the aim is to extrapolate research results to clinical practice. Although this chapter has focused on key associations between outcome and qualities of the therapeutic relationship, one must always remember that what the therapist does is also influential and inseparable (Orlinsky, 2000). (See also a 2005 special issue of *Psychotherapy* on the interplay of techniques and therapeutic relationship.)

In other words, the value of a treatment method is inextricably bound to the relational context in which it is applied. Hans Strupp, one of my first research mentors, offered an analogy to illustrate the inseparability of these constituent elements. Suppose a parent wants a teenager to clean his or her room. Two methods for achieving this are to establish clear standards and to impose consequences. It's a reasonable approach, but the effectiveness of these two evidence-based methods will vary on whether the relationship between the parent and the teenager is characterized by warmth and mutual respect or anger and mistrust. This is not to say that the methods are useless, but how well they work depends on the context in which they are used.

When all is said and done, when the thousands of empirical studies bearing on the therapeutic relationship are analyzed, here is what can be reliably stated about practice (Norcross, 2001, 2002):

- The therapy relationship makes significant and consistent contributions to psychotherapy outcome for all types of psychological treatments. Thus, practitioners should make the creation and cultivation of a facilitative therapy relationship a primary aim.
- Adapting or tailoring the therapy relationship to specific client needs and characteristics may enhance the effectiveness of treatment. Hence, practitioners are encouraged to adapt the therapy relationship to client characteristics in those ways shown to enhance therapeutic outcome.
- Actively monitoring the quality of the therapeutic relationship improves alliances and reduces negative outcomes. Practitioners should routinely monitor clients' responses to the therapy relationship and treatment.
- The therapy relationship acts in concert with treatment method, client characteristics, and clinician qualities in determining treatment effectiveness. Thus, a comprehensive understanding of effective (and ineffective) psychotherapy considers all of these determinants and their optimal combinations.
- In an era preoccupied with technology and materialism, mental health practitioners should advocate for the research-substantiated benefits of a facilitative and responsive human relationship in psychotherapy.

Coming full circle, if we are to be like Einstein—or at least an interpersonally talented Einstein—what might we do? Cultivate the therapy relationship. Customize the relationship (and treatment) to the particular client and context. Simultaneously use what works. Avoid what does not. Capitalize on what decades of research and millions of clients have told us: Nurture the therapeutic relationship.

## QUESTIONS FROM THE EDITORS

1. *Mindful of the consequence of a sound alliance to outcome and retention (some calling it the* flagship*) and the recent call by many to monitor/measure the alliance, what do you think it will take for the field to embrace alliance assessment as a necessary component of service delivery?*

Beats me. The extant body of research is robust and convincing to most practitioners (including me), and many of my colleagues have incorporated into their sessions various means of directly assessing their clients' experience of the relationship. However, others do not find the research sufficiently compelling or theoretically compatible to implement a formal assessment of alliance.

All psychotherapy innovations take many years to make it from science to service. Recent efforts to accelerate the translation of research into practice might help (Norcross, Hogan, & Koocher, 2008), as long as they do not focus exclusively on specific treatment methods for particular *DSM* categories. Other than that, I am at a loss to explain why more practitioners are not systematically monitoring the therapy relationship and soliciting feedback from their clients. It strikes me as bad science and as bad practice not to do so.

2. *Given the import of a strong therapy relationship to treatment outcome, what implications do you see in the training of graduate students?*

Three immediate implications spring to mind: graduate admissions, curriculum requirements, and competency training. First, we must select students for graduate training who are both academically qualified and interpersonally skilled. We have lost our collective way of late. On the one hand, PhD and MD/DOs programs are very competitive in admissions, but favor entrance examination scores, undergraduate grades, and research experiences over interpersonal skills. On the other hand, many master's programs do emphasize interpersonal skills in admissions decisions, yet are forced to accept the vast majority of applicants for economic survival. For this reason, some students with questionable preparation and mental health are admitted. We need to find a middle way, a way that commits us to selecting rigorously prepared and interpersonally adept people.

Second, every graduate program in mental health should provide explicit training in the effective elements of the therapy relationship and in adapting the relationship to the individual client. To do so will probably require some accountability and accreditation "teeth." Accreditation and certification bodies should develop criteria for assessing, in their evaluation process, the adequacy of training in the therapy relationship.

Third, we need to progress in graduate training from mere exposure to knowledge to demonstrated competence in skills. To know that the therapy relationship is a reliable contributor to outcome is far different from being skilled in creating and cultivating that relationship. I am a strong advocate of competency-based training.

3. *You discuss the important interplay of relationship and technique. It has been suggested that technique represents an instance of the alliance in action. How does such an interdependence of these factors, and the inevitable improvisations and ebb and flow of clinical interaction, help or hinder research about the relationship?*

Research on the effectiveness of the psychotherapy relationship is constrained by therapist responsiveness—the ebb and flow of clinical interaction, as you put it. *Responsiveness* refers to behavior that is affected by emerging context and occurs on many levels—including choice of an overall treatment, case formulation, strategic use of the self and method—and then adjusting those to meet the emerging, evolving needs of the client in any given moment (Stiles, Honos-Webb, & Surko, 1998). Effective psychotherapists are responsive to the different needs of their clients, providing varying levels of relationship elements in different cases and, within the same case, at different moments.

When this occurs, highly effective relational ingredients may have null (or even negative) correlations with outcomes in the cumulative research. Successful responsiveness can confound attempts to find naturalistically observed linear relations of outcome with therapist behaviors (e.g., self-disclosures, positive regard). Because of such problems, the statistical relations between the relationship and outcome cannot always be trusted. By being clinically attuned and flexible, as they should, psychotherapists make it more difficult in research studies to discern what works.

## REFERENCES

Ackerman, S. J., & Hilsenroth, M. J. (2001). A review of therapist characteristics and techniques negatively impacting the therapeutic alliance. *Psychotherapy*, 38, 171–185.

Arnkoff, D. B., Glass, C. R., & Shapiro, S. J. (2002). Expectations and preferences. In J. C. Norcross (Ed.), *Psychotherapy relationships that work: Therapist contributions and responsiveness to patients* (pp. 335–356). New York: Oxford University Press.

Barber, J. P., Connolly, M. B., Crits-Christoph, P., Gladis, L., & Siqueland, L. (2000). Alliance predicts patients' outcomes beyond in-treatment change in symptoms. *Journal of Consulting and Clinical Psychology*, 68, 1027–1032.

Bachelor, A. (1988). How clients perceive therapist empathy: A content analysis of received empathy. *Psychotherapy, 25,* 227–240.

Bachelor, A., & Horvath, A. (1999). The therapeutic relationship. In M. A. Hubble, B. L. Duncan, & S. D. Miller (Eds.), *The heart and soul of change: What works in therapy* (pp. 133–178). Washington DC: American Psychological Association.

Bedi, R. P., Davis, M. D., & Williams, M. (2005). Critical incidents in the formation of the therapeutic alliance from the clients' perspective. *Psychotherapy: Theory, Research, Practice, Training, 42,* 311–323.

Beutler, L. E., Harwood, T. M., Alimohamed, S., & Malik, M. (2002). Functional impairment and coping style. In J. C. Norcross (Ed.), *Psychotherapy relationships that work* (pp. 145–170). New York: Oxford University Press.

Beutler, L. E., Moleiro, C. M., & Talebi, H. (2002). Resistance. In J. C. Norcross (Ed.), *Psychotherapy relationships that work* (pp. 129–143). New York: Oxford University Press.

Bike, D. H., Norcross, J. C., & Schatz, D. M. (2009). Processes and outcomes of psychotherapists' personal therapy: Replication and extension 20 years later. *Psychotherapy, 46,* 19–31.

Binder, J. L., & Strupp, H. H. (1997). "Negative process": A recurrently discovered and underestimated facet of therapeutic process and outcome in the individual psychotherapy of adults. *Clinical Psychology: Science and Practice, 4,* 121–139.

Bohart, A. C., Elliot, R., Greenberg, L. S., & Watson, J. C. (2002). Empathy. In J. C. Norcross (Ed.), *Psychotherapy relationships that work* (pp. 89–107). New York: Oxford University Press.

Bohart, A. C., & Greenberg, L. S. (Eds.). (1997). *Empathy reconsidered: New directions in psychotherapy.* Washington, DC: American Psychological Association.

Bordin, E. S. (1976). The generalizability of the psychoanalytic concept of the working alliance. *Psychotherapy: Theory, Research and Practice, 16,* 252–260.

Burke, B. L., Arkowitz, H., & Dunn, C. (2002). The efficacy of motivational interviewing and its adaptations: What we know so far. In W. R. Miller & S. Rollnick (Eds.), *Motivational interviewing: Preparing people for change* (2nd ed.). New York: Guilford Press.

Burlingame, G. M., Fuhriman, A., & Johnson, J. E. (2002). Cohesion in group psychotherapy. In J. C. Norcross (Ed.), *Psychotherapy relationships that work* (pp. 71–87). New York: Oxford University Press.

Claiborn, C. D., Goodyear, R. K., & Horner, P. A. (2002). Feedback. In J. C. Norcross (Ed.), *Psychotherapy relationships that work* (pp. 217–233). New York: Oxford University Press.

Creed, T. A., & Kendall, P. C. (2005). Therapist alliance-building behavior within a cognitive–behavioral treatment for anxiety in youth. *Journal of Consulting and Clinical Psychology, 73,* 498–505.

Crits-Christoph, P., & Gibbons, M. C. (2002). Relational interpretation. In J. C. Norcross (Ed.), *Psychotherapy relationships that work* (pp. 285–300). New York: Oxford University Press.

Duncan, B. L. & Miller, S. D. (2000). The client's theory of change. *Journal of Psychotherapy Integration, 10,* 169–188.

Duncan, B. L., Miller, S. D., & Sparks, J. A. (2004). *The heroic client: A revolutionary way to improve effectiveness through client-directed, outcome-informed therapy.* San Francisco: Jossey-Bass.

Duncan, B. L., & Moynihan, D. W. (1994). Applying outcome research: Intentional utilization of the client's frame of reference. *Psychotherapy, 31,* 294–301.

Eliot, G. (1860). *The mill on the floss.* London: Blackwood & Sons.

Elkin, I., Shea, T., Watkins, J. T., Imber, S. D., Sotsky, S. M., Collins, I. F., & Glass, D. R. (1989). National Institute of Mental Health treatment of depression collaborative research program: General effectiveness of treatments. *Archives General Psychiatry, 46,* 971–982.

Elliott, R., & James, E. (1989). Varieties of client experience in psychotherapy: An analysis of the literature. *Clinical Psychology Review, 9,* 443–467.

Farber, B. A., & Lane, J. S. (2002). Positive regard. In J. C. Norcross (Ed.), *Psychotherapy relationships that work* (pp. 175–193). New York: Oxford University Press.

Gabbard, G. O., & Freedman, R. (2006). Psychotherapy in the *Journal:* What is missing? *American Journal of Psychiatry, 163,* 182–184.

Gaston, L., Marmar, C. R., Gallagher, D., & Thompson, L. W. (1991). Alliance prediction of outcome beyond in-treatment symptomatic change as psychotherapy processes. *Psychotherapy Research, 1,* 104–112.

Gaudiano, B. A., & Miller, I. W. (2006). Patients' expectancies, the alliance in pharmacotherapy, and treatment outcomes in bipolar disorder. *Journal of Consulting and Clinical Psychology, 74,* 61–676.

Geller, J. D., Norcross, J. C., & Orlinsky, D. E. (Eds.). (2005). *The psychotherapist's own psychotherapy: Patient and clinician perspectives.* New York: Oxford University Press.

Gelso, C. J., & Carter, J. A. (1994). Components of the psychotherapy relationship: Their interaction and unfolding during treatment. *Journal of Counseling Psychology, 41,* 296–306.

Gelso, C. J., & Hayes, J. A. (1998). *The psychotherapy relationship: Theory, research, and practice.* New York: Wiley.

Gelso, C. J., & Hayes, J. A. (2002). The management of countertransference. In J. C. Norcross (Ed.), *Psychotherapy relationships that work* (pp. 267–283). New York: Oxford University Press.

Gershefski, J. J., Arnkoff, D. B., Glass, C. R., & Elkin, I. (1996). Clients' perceptions of their treatment for depression: I. Helpful aspects. *Psychotherapy Research, 6,* 245–259.

Goin, M. K., Yamamoto J., & Silverman, J. (1965). Therapy congruent with class-linked expectations. *Archives of General Psychiatry, 38,* 335–339.

Grencavage, L. M., & Norcross, J. C. (1990). Where are the commonalities among the therapeutic common factors? *Professional Psychology: Research and Practice, 21,* 372–378.

Hannan, C., Lambert, M. J., Harmon, C., Nielsen, S. L., Smart, D. W., Shimokawa, K., & Sutton, S. W. (2005). A lab test and algorithms for identifying clients at risk for treatment failure. *Journal of Clinical Psychology: In Session, 61,* 155–164.

Hill, C. E., & Knox, S. (2002). Self-disclosure. In J. C. Norcross (Ed.), *Psychotherapy relationships that work* (pp. 255–265). New York: Oxford University Press.

Horvath, A. O., & Bedi, R. P. (2002). The alliance. In J. C. Norcross (Ed.), *Psychotherapy relationships that work* (pp. 37–69). New York: Oxford University Press.

Horvath, A. O., & Greenberg, L. S. (Eds.). (1994). *The working alliance: Theory, research, practice.* New York: John Wiley.

Karno, M. P. & Longabaugh, R. (2005). Less directiveness by therapists improves drinking outcomes of reactant clients in alcoholism treatment. *Journal of Consulting and Clinical Psychology, 72,* 262–267.

Kazantzis, N., Deane, F. P., & Ronan, K. R. (2000). Homework assignments in cognitive and behavioral therapy: A meta-analysis. *Clinical Psychology: Science and Practice, 7,* 189–202.

Kazdin, A. E., Marciano, P. L., & Whitley, M. K. (2005). The therapeutic alliance in cognitive–behavioral treatment of children referred for oppositional, aggressive, and antisocial behavior. *Journal of Consulting and Clinical Psychology, 73,* 726–730.

Klein, D. N., Schwartz, J. E., Santiago, N. J., Vivian, D., Vocisano, C., Castonguay, L. G., et al. (2003). Therapeutic alliance in depression treatment: Controlling for prior change and patient characteristics. *Journal of Consulting and Clinical Psychology, 71,* 997–1006.

Klein, M. G., Kolden, G. G., Michels, J. L., & Chisholm-Stockard, S. (2002). Congruence. In J. C. Norcross (Ed.), *Psychotherapy relationships that work* (pp. 195–215). New York: Oxford University Press.

Krupnick, J. L., Stotsky, S. M., Simmons, S., Moyer, J., Watkins, J., Elkin, I., & Pilkonis, P. A. (1996). The role of the therapeutic alliance in psychotherapy and pharmacotherapy outcome: Findings in the National Institute of Mental Health Treatment of Depression Collaborative Research Program. *Journal of Consulting and Clinical Psychology, 64,* 532–539.

Lambert, M. J. (Ed.). (2005) Enhancing psychotherapy outcome through feedback. *Journal of Clinical Psychology: In Session, 61,* 141–217.

Lambert, M. J., & Barley, D. E. (2002). Research summary on the therapeutic relationship and psychotherapy outcome. In J. C. Norcross (Ed.), *Psychotherapy relationships that work* (pp. 17–32). New York: Oxford University Press.

Luborsky, L., & Crits-Christoph, P. (Eds.). (1998). *Understanding transference: The core conflictual relationship theme method* (2nd ed.). Washington, DC: American Psychological Association.

Meyer, B., & Pilkonis, P. A. (2002). Attachment style. In J. C. Norcross (Ed.), *Psychotherapy relationships that work* (pp. 367–382). New York: Oxford University Press.

Miller, S. D., Duncan, B. L., Sorrell, R., & Brown, G. S. (2005). The partners for change outcome management system. *Journal of Clinical Psychology: In Session, 61*, 199–208.

Miller, W. R., & Rollnick, S. (2002). *Motivational interviewing: Preparing people for change* (2nd ed.). New York: Guilford Press.

Miller, W. R., Taylor, C. A., & West J. C. (1980). Focused versus broad-spectrum behavior therapy for problem drinkers. *Journal of Consulting and Clinical Psychology, 48*, 590–601.

Miller, W. R., Wilbourne, P. L., & Hettema, J. E. (2003). What works? A summary of alcohol treatment outcome research. In R. K. Hester & W. R. Miller (Eds.), *Handbook of alcoholism treatment approaches: Effective alternatives* (3rd ed., pp. 13–63). Boston: Allyn & Bacon.

Murphy, P. M., Cramer, D., & Lillie, F. J. (1984). The relationship between curative factors perceived by patients in their psychotherapy and treatment outcome: An exploratory study. *British Journal of Medical Psychology, 57*, 187–192.

Najavits, L. M., & Strupp, H. (1994). Differences in the effectiveness of psychodynamic therapists: A process-outcome study. *Psychotherapy, 31*, 114–123.

Norcross, J. C. (Ed.). (2001). Empirically supported therapy relationships: Summary of the Division 29 Task Force [Special issue]. *Psychotherapy, 38*(4).

Norcross, J. C. (Ed.). (2002). *Psychotherapy relationships that work: Therapist contributions and responsiveness to patient needs*. New York: Oxford University Press.

Norcross, J. C., Dryden, W., & DeMichele J. T. (1992). British clinical psychologists and personal therapy: III. What's good for the goose? *Clinical Psychology Forum, 44*, 29–33.

Norcross, J. C., Hogan, T. P., & Koocher, G. P. (2008). *Clinician's guide to evidence-based practices: Mental health and the addictions*. New York: Oxford University Press.

Norcross, J. C., Koocher, G. P., & Garofalo, A. (2006). Discredited psychological treatments and tests: A Delphi poll. *Professional Psychology: Research & Practice, 37*, 515–522.

Norcross, J .C., & Lambert, M. J. (2005). The therapy relationship. In J. C. Norcross, L. E. Beutler, & R. F. Levant (Eds.), *Evidence-based practices in mental health: Debate and dialogue on the fundamental questions*. Washington, DC: American Psychological Association.

Orlinsky, D. E. (2000, August). *Therapist interpersonal behaviors that have consistently shown positive correlations with outcome*. Paper presented in the symposium "Empirically Supported Therapy Relationships: Task Force of APA's Psychotherapy Division" at the 108th Annual Convention of the American Psychological Association, Washington, DC.

Orlinsky, D. E., & Howard, K. (1978). The relation of process to outcome in psychotherapy. In S. L. Garfield & A. E. Bergin (Eds.), *Handbook of psychotherapy and behavior change* (2nd ed.). New York: Wiley.

Orlinsky, D. E., & Norcross, J. C. (2005). Outcomes and impacts of psychotherapists' personal therapy: A research review. In J. D. Geller, J. C. Norcross, & D. E. Orlinsky (Eds.), *The psychotherapist's personal therapy*. New York: Oxford University Press.

Orlinsky, D. E., Ronnestad, M. H., & Willutzki, U. (2004). Fifty years of psychotherapy process–outcome research: Continuity and change. In M. J. Lambert (Ed.), *Handbook of psychotherapy and behavior change* (5th ed.). New York: Wiley.

Prochaska, J. O., & Norcross, J. C. (2002). Stages of change. In J. C. Norcross (Ed.), *Psychotherapy relationships that work* (pp. 303–313). New York: Oxford University Press.

Rogers, C. R. (1957). The necessary and sufficient conditions of therapeutic personality change. *Journal of Consulting Psychology, 22,* 95–103.

Rosen, C. S. (2000). Is the sequencing of change processes by stage consistent across health problems? A meta-analysis. *Health Psychology, 19,* 593–604.

Safran, J. D., Muran, J. C., Samstag, L. W., & Stevens, C. (2002). Repairing alliance ruptures. In J. C. Norcross (Ed.), *Psychotherapy relationships that work* (pp. 235–253). New York: Oxford University Press.

Shelef, K., Diamond, G. M., Diamond, G. S., & Liddle, H. A. (2005). Adolescent and parent alliance and treatment outcome in multidimensional family therapy. *Journal of Consulting and Clinical Psychology, 73,* 689–698.

Shirk, S. R., & Karver, M. (2003). Prediction of treatment outcome from relationship variables in child and adolescent therapy: A meta-analytic review. *Journal of Consulting and Clinical Psychology, 71,* 452–464.

Sloane, R. B., Staples, F. R., Cristol, A. H., Yorkston, N. J. I., & Whipple, K. (1975). *Short-term analytically oriented psychotherapy vs. behavior therapy.* Cambridge, MA: Harvard University Press.

Stiles, W. B., Honos-Webb, L., & Surko, M. (1998). Responsiveness in psychotherapy. *Clinical Psychology: Science and Practice, 5,* 439–458.

Strupp, H. H., Fox, R. E., & Lessler, K. (1969). *Patients view their psychotherapy.* Baltimore: Johns Hopkins University Press.

Sue, S., & Lam, A. G. (2002). Cultural and demographic diversity. In J. C. Norcross (Ed.), *Psychotherapy relationships that work* (pp. 401–421). New York: Oxford University Press.

Truax, C. B., & Carkhuff, R. R. (1967). *Toward effective counseling and psychotherapy.* Chicago: Aldine.

Tryon, G. S., Collins, S., & Felleman, E. (2006, August). *Meta-analysis of the third session client–therapist working alliance.* Paper presented at the 112th Annual Convention of the American Psychological Association, New Orleans, LA.

Tryon, G. S., & Winograd, G. (2002). Goal consensus and collaboration. In J. C. Norcross (Ed.), *Psychotherapy relationships that work* (pp. 109–125). New York: Oxford University Press.

Tschuschke, V., & Dies, R. R. (1994). Intensive analysis of therapeutic factors and outcome in long-term inpatient groups. *International Journal of Group Psychotherapy, 44,* 185–208.

Wampold, B. E. (2001). *The great psychotherapy debate: Models, methods, and findings.* Mahwah, NJ: Erlbaum.

Weinberger, J. (1995). Common factors aren't so common: The common factors dilemma. *Clinical Psychology: Science and Practice, 2,* 45–69.

Worthington, E. L., & Sandage, S. J. (2002). Religion and spirituality. In J. C. Norcross (Ed.), *Psychotherapy relationships that work* (pp. 383–399). New York: Oxford University Press.

Zuroff, D. C., & Blatt, S. J. (2006). The therapeutic relationship in the brief treatment of depression: Contributions to clinical improvement and enhanced adaptive capacities. *Journal of Consulting and Clinical Psychology, 74,* 130–140.

# 5

# PUTTING MODELS AND TECHNIQUES IN CONTEXT

TIMOTHY ANDERSON, KIRK M. LUNNEN, AND BENJAMIN M. OGLES

> Mental health care exerts an influence on the basis of its claim to scientific status, but that claim is false. What it actually does is induct people into understanding life in certain ways that are artifacts of the cultures of healing.
>
> —Robert Fancher

At first glance, this chapter may seem out of place. Why would a book with a focus on the common factors—the "Heart and Soul" of psychotherapy—include a chapter on factors as specific as models and techniques? Any confusion is entirely understandable. For many years, *common* (e.g., the therapeutic relationship) and *specific* (e.g., therapeutic models and techniques) have been the primary and traditional categories used for understanding psychotherapy research. In recent decades, the distinction has also been the major organizing scheme used by practitioners and researchers, many of whom feel compelled to represent their work either as primarily based on technique (e.g., empirically supported treatments; Chambless & Hollon, 1998; Task Force on Promotion and Dissemination of Psychological Procedures, 1995) or based on common relationship factors (e.g., empirically supported relationships; Norcross, 2002). However, the common versus specific divide emphasizes a fundamental misunderstanding, namely, that the treatment model and the common factors are separate and distinct. In point of fact, the therapeutic factors identified and discussed in this volume are intricately interwoven with the theoretical orientation of the therapist and the treatment provided (Wampold, 2007).

# DEFINING MODELS

Historically, there have been varied and often contradictory definitions for models. Some view them as specific to predicting change in therapy, whereas others consider them highly abstract formulations with applicability to all human behavior (Matarazzo & Garner, 1992; Poznanski & McLennan, 1995). The first therapy models were simply extensions of psychological theories. Early models of treatment were not merely a collection of techniques to be used with people in therapy but reflected an overarching worldview. Most were rational, quasiphilosophical formulations about individual development and personality that contained implicit assumptions and values about life, mental health, and mental illness.

In this chapter, a *model* is defined as a collection of beliefs or a unifying theory about what is needed to bring about change with a particular client in a particular treatment context. Models generally operate based on a set of core principles (Castonguay & Beutler, 2006; Goldfried, 1980) that lead to or include specific therapeutic *techniques*, defined here as actions that are local extensions of the beliefs or theory. Orlinsky, Grawe, and Parks (1994) summarized that "the particular techniques or methods employed by therapists can be thought of as tactical interventions made to implement heuristic goals. These [techniques and goals] vary according to the treatment model being followed" (p. 306). Models and techniques are, therefore, related but not identical, but one assumes that therapists implement techniques that originate from some sort of model. In other words, however implicit, all therapists operate according to certain beliefs or assumptions about what facilitates positive outcomes. Often, these models are aligned with a theoretical orientation.

In contrast to the contemporary focus on specificity, the earliest theories and techniques were thought to be universally applicable. Much of the early history of psychoanalysis involved Freud's efforts to establish that all mental disorders had libidinal causes; his theories were sufficiently expansive that they could explain cultural practices, history, and art (Makari, 2008). Skinner's theory of radical behaviorism not only served as the impetus for behavioral treatment but also as the inspiration for a utopian vision of a society based on the widespread application of behavioral principles (Skinner, 1948). Rogers's (1961) client-centered theory, on the other hand, served as a vision of society based on individual freedom and self-determination as well as underpinning a method of psychotherapy. Accordingly, these initial psychotherapy approaches were used widely to treat all distress, regardless of the disorder, cultural context, and client history. Of course, there was mutual antipathy between various approaches and even within approaches, as the proponents of a particular brand of psychotherapy believed fervently that theirs was the only legitimate approach and all others were misguided (Miller, Duncan, & Hubble, 1997)!

Although the proponents of various approaches fought bitter battles, a few scientists and theoreticians who approached psychotherapy as a contextual phenomenon suggested that the commonalities among the various psychotherapies were more important than the differences (Frank & Frank, 1991; Rosenzweig, 1936). Over the years, a number of common factors models have been proposed. The typical strategy has been to present a list of categorized components believed to account for the benefits of psychotherapy (cf. Garfield, 1995; Grencavage & Norcross, 1990; Hubble, Duncan, & Miller, 1999b; Imel & Wampold, 2008; Lambert, 1992; Lambert & Ogles, 2004).

It is unfortunate that the various categorization schemes, although providing a compelling argument that the common factors were the essence of therapeutic success, served to reinforce the mistaken impression that psychotherapy was primarily a technical endeavor. In place of a grand organizing theory applied to everyone seeking treatment or a specific treatment applied to a specific disorder, effective therapy was now a matter of mixing in the appropriate amounts of client strengths and resources, therapeutic relationship, hope and expectancy, and therapeutic techniques. However, as the authors of chapter 1 of this volume point out, such a conceptualization ignores that the common factors are embedded in the context of the delivery of specific treatments.

In this chapter, emphasis is placed on how the various therapeutic factors are organized around treatment. Without a treatment, the factors, like techniques, are simply ingredients; with a treatment, they form a coherent and viable package of what is known as psychotherapy. To explain the relationship between treatment models and other therapeutic factors, we now turn to a metaframework that has been termed the *contextual model*.

## THE CONTEXTUAL MODEL

The contextual model of psychotherapy (Frank & Frank, 1991; Wampold, 2001) is a superordinate or metamodel of psychotherapy. The contextual view holds that psychotherapy orientations (and other forms of healing) are equivalent in their effectiveness because of factors shared by all, in particular: (a) a healing setting; (b) a rationale, myth, or conceptual framework that provides an explanation for the client's presenting complaint and a method for resolving them; (c) an emotionally charged, confiding relationship with a helping person; and (d) a ritual or procedure that requires involvement of both the healer and client to bring about the "cure" or resolution.

In contrast to the traditional theoretical models described above, which propose that change is due either to specific technical operations or various common factors, the contextual model proposes that therapeutic change occurs because there is a single theory or rationale that is acceptable or believable to both the healer and client. The specifics of the theory and techniques are for all points and purposes irrelevant. Rather, the key is that there must be (a) a set of techniques or rituals that are consistent with shared cultural beliefs, (b) a theory that is understood and accepted by the client, and (c) a treatment that is implemented in a way that promotes a positive outcome.

As just one example, consider the treatment of depression and anxiety. Many different psychotherapeutic approaches exist. In cognitive therapy, for example, specific interventions such as identifying and altering automatic thoughts and core belief structures are believed to be responsible for change. At the same time, however, numerous other approaches based on entirely different and sometimes contradictory rationales (e.g., interpersonal therapy, process experiential therapy, short-term dynamic therapy) have been tested and proven effective (Wampold, 2007). Finally, many of the specific actions of different therapies can be explained through the mechanisms championed by rival therapies. A prominent example is the technique of psychoanalytic interpretation that when explained by Wachtel (1997) is nearly identical to behavioral exposure techniques. It is clear that the truth of any model and associated strategies is not critical to success. Rather, each merely offers an opportunity for engagement of the client and therapist in a process that promises to be helpful.

Figure 5.1 uses Orlinsky and Howard's (1986) generic model of psychotherapy to illustrate the relationship between the contextual model and traditional psychotherapy models, principles, and techniques. The rectangular shapes represent the four components of the contextual model. Treatment models and techniques are contained within the circular shapes. The more abstract aspects of psychotherapy models—including the healing setting or culture, the myth or rationale, and psychotherapy orientations—are found at the top of the diagram. Principles and processes are in the center, illustrating links between theory and technique as well as interconnections among theories that share principles. Rituals, or the procedures and techniques associated with specific models, are located at the bottom of the figure.

In the material that follows, each component of the contextual model is explored and connected to the delivery of specific treatments. As we see it, the various components of the model can be discussed separately but are held together by common principles that link these factors into a cohesive treatment (Wampold, 2007) that works best under specific cultural circumstances, problems, and shared beliefs. A metaphor for this dynamic connection among the various components of common factors is the three-legged stool. As used by Miller, Duncan, and Hubble (2005), the treatment methods and the emotional bond serve as two of the three supporting ingredients of a helping relationship; the third leg is agreement between client and therapist on the goals, meaning, or purpose of the therapy. Holding the legs in place is the seat or

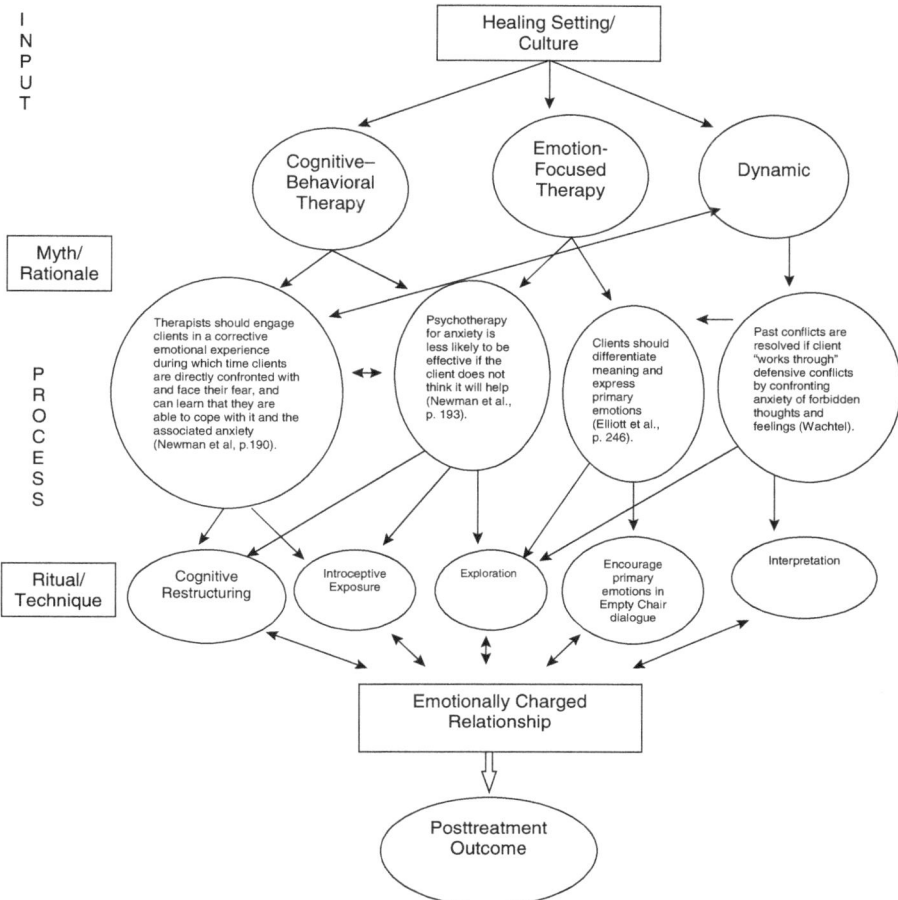

*Figure 5.1.* Examples of models and techniques in context from the contextual and generic models of psychotherapy. Rectangular boxes are the four factors from Frank and Frank's (1991) contextual model. Circular shapes represent specific examples of various models and techniques (i.e., myths and rituals), which are on a continuum of high (orientations) to low (specific techniques) levels of abstraction. Treatment principles (intermediate circular shapes) link orientations and techniques. Newman et al. = Newman, Stiles, Janeck, and Woody (2006); Elliott et al. = Elliott, Watson, Goldman, and Greenberg (2004); Wachtel = Wachtel (1997).

degree to which the three legs fit with the culture, worldview, circumstances, and preferences of the client (i.e., the client's theory of change; see Duncan & Miller, 2000).

The model described in Figure 5.1 is similar in that common factors are interdependent. When there are shifts within these treatment components (i.e., culture, myth or rationale, ritual or technique, relationship) or the connecting principles, the entire treatment must be brought into balance for the treatment to remain sustainable. In Miller et al.'s (2005) stool analogy, adjustments in the legs or seat of the stool have the potential to make "the stool uncomfortable or toppl[e] it completely" (p. 87). For the sake of parsimony, we review the components of this comprehensive model separately.

## Healing Setting or Culture

The first element of the contextual model refers to everything from the architecture of a clinic to the number and nature of the forms used to initiate services. Whether conducted in a shaman's hut or a Western hospital, the setting in which a treatment occurs imbues the process with power and prestige while simultaneously reminding the participants of the predominant cultural beliefs regarding effective care. That said, seeing the cultural influences in one's core beliefs is not easy, making it difficult (if not impossible) to clearly perceive the role of this critical factor in the operation of psychotherapy models.

To be persuasive, any intervention must first be meaningfully linked with shared communal beliefs (Wampold, 2007). As Frank and Frank (1998) noted, "The power of any therapeutic rationale to persuade is influenced by the culture from which it derives. In devout cultures, religious rationales may have the greatest therapeutic power. In our secular society, such power derives from science" (p. 590). In short, models must possess a rationale that strikes at the heart of what it means to be a person within a particular place and time.

The implications for treatment are clear. Clinicians not only need to be aware of the many meaningful cultural myths available but also should be open to altering techniques, style, and approach to achieve a better fit with the client. As Fischer, Jome, and Atkinson (1998) argued, therapists should use

> cultural (and individual) knowledge to be flexible—that is, to consider the role of culture (broadly construed)—in negotiating the structure of the relationship, the way that they and their clients communicate about that relationship and about the clients' experience (the worldview), the course of action and experience they anticipate (expectations for change), and the steps they and their clients take to help clients reach their goals (intervention). (p. 603)

## Myth or Rationale

Following setting and culture in the contextual model is myth or rationale. In the practice of psychotherapy, this aspect is most easy linked to theoretical orientation or therapeutic school. As can be seen in Figure 5.1, therapeutic theories or rationales serve an important function, acting as the "central station" between (a) the culture in which psychotherapy is embedded and (b) the principles of treatment and associated therapeutic techniques. The close relationship between these parts makes clear, as Wampold, Imel, Bhati, and Johnson-Jennings (2007) noted, that

> to be effective [the therapeutic rationale] must lie within the expected cultural frame in which the healing practice is most often conducted, should be proximal to the client's currently held explanation or expectation, and should not create dissonance with the attitudes and values of the client that would cause the client to reject the explanation outright. (p. 125)

The idea that client perceptions are critical to successful psychotherapy, Duncan and Miller (2000) pointed out, "has a rich, although somewhat ignored theoretical heritage" (p. 174; see also Duncan & Moynihan, 1994; Duncan, Solovey, & Rusk, 1992; Hubble, Miller, & Duncan, 1999a). As early as 1955, for example, psychiatrist Paul Hoch (1955) observed that "there are some patients who would like to submit to a psychotherapeutic procedure whose theoretical foundations are in agreement with their own ideas about psychic functioning" (p. 322). Others have hypothesized that problems in treatment were often the result of the "two parties . . . applying models that are out of phase with one another" (Brickman et al., 1982, p. 375).

Once again, the implications for psychotherapy are clear: The rationale for treatment should be selected and carefully tailored to the culture, worldview, circumstances, and preferences of the client (Hubble et al., 1999a). "Ideally," Frank and Frank (1991) argued, "therapists should select for each patient the therapy that accords, or can be brought to accord, with the patient's personal characteristics and view of the problem" (p. xv). Consistent with the history of the profession, the currency of particular explanations wax and wane as culture evolves and changes. To be sure, the notion that the "truth" of a particular treatment rationale is unimportant may be unsettling to some (Grawe, 2004). And yet, Duncan and Miller (2000) pointed out that key to finding what works for the individual client is found in this very indeterminacy.

## Ritual or Technique

The third component of the contextual model needs little introduction. Ritual or technique is the means by which a given cultural myth or therapeutic rationale is enacted. Where myth or rationale explains why, ritual or technique shows how. In the field of psychotherapy, practice and research have long been dominated by therapeutic technique. At the same time, it may be said, paraphrasing Winston Churchill, that never has a subject that contributes so little to outcome received so much professional attention and approbation.

As reviewed elsewhere in this volume, no differences in effectiveness have been found among treatment approaches intended to be therapeutic. The same body of evidence has also failed to find any connection between the techniques of a specific model and outcome (Ahn & Wampold, 2001). When combined with research showing that structurally equivalent sham treatments (e.g., placebo; technically inert comparison conditions designed to closely resemble real treatments) reliably produce effects as large as bona fide therapies (Baskin, Tierney, Minami, & Wampold, 2003), the conclusion is inescapable. As long as a treatment makes sense to, is accepted by, and fosters the active engagement of the client, the particular treatment approach used is unimportant. In other words, therapeutic techniques are placebo delivery devices (Kirsch, 2005). This is discussed further later in this chapter. At this point, suffice it to say that techniques work, in large part, if not completely, through the activation and operation of placebo, hope, and expectancy.

The saga of present-centered therapy is illustrative. As Wampold (2007) effectively described, the approach currently known as *present-centered therapy* (PCT) began its journey to empirically supported status as a lowly control group technique. Researchers testing the efficacy of cognitive–behavioral treatments (CBT) for posttraumatic stress disorder (PTSD) needed a comparison condition that contained curative factors shared by all treatment approaches (e.g., warm empathic relationship) while excluding those believed unique to CBT (e.g., exposure). This control treatment, described as *supportive counseling*, contained no treatment rationale and no therapeutic actions. Moreover, to rule out any possibility of exposure, even covert in nature, clients were not allowed to talk about the traumatic events that had precipitated treatment!

Needless to say, PCT was found to be less effective than CBT. However, when a manual containing a rationale and condition-specific treatment actions was added later to facilitate standardization in training and delivery, few differences in efficacy were found between PCT and CBT in the treatment of PTSD (McDonagh et al., 2005). In fact, significantly fewer clients dropped out of PCT than CBT. Thus, when PCT was made to resemble a bona fide treatment, it was not only as effective as but also more acceptable than CBT. Although recent findings were more favorable to CBT over PCT (Schnurr et al., 2007), the malleability of PCT illustrates our point. Specifically, the effect of a treatment likely depends on the extent to which the treatment matches shared social constructions about what it means to be remoralized within the culture in which it is practiced.

While discussing the qualities of effective rituals and techniques, we should also mention the impact of researcher or therapist allegiance on treatment outcome. Briefly, *allegiance* is the degree to which a practitioner delivering or a researcher investigating a treatment believes a particular therapy to be efficacious (Wampold, 1997). Considerable evidence now exists that belief in or commitment to a particular method of treatment has a significant influence on treatment outcome (Dush, Hirt, & Shroeder, 1983; Hoag & Burlingame, 1997; Luborsky et al., 1999, 2002; Paley & Shapiro, 2002; Robinson, Berman, & Neimeyer, 1990; D. A. Shapiro & Shapiro, 1982; Smith, Glass, & Miller, 1980). Indeed, allegiance effects appear to be greater than the effects produced by comparisons of treatments—as much as 3 times greater when the most liberal estimates are used (Wampold, 2001). As Frank and Frank (1991) observed, "A therapist who is convinced by personal experience of the validity of a particular method may be powerfully effective in persuading patients they too will benefit" (p. 161).

In sum, techniques are a necessary component of effective care. Fortunately, the evidence indicates that therapists need not spend any time searching for the right treatment for a particular disorder. Instead, the "best" methods are those (a) intended or believed to be therapeutic; (b) delivered with a cogent rationale; and, above all, (c) acceptable to the client.

## Emotionally Charged, Confiding Relationship

An emotionally charged, confiding relationship is the fourth and final component of the contextual model. Although little debate exists regarding the overall importance of the therapeutic relationship, there is considerable difference of opinion regarding its potency and place. Advocates of particular treatment approaches emphasize the specific ingredients of their chosen method, arguing that the relationship is necessary but not sufficient to bring about change. Barlow (2004), for example—although acknowledging the "strengths of traditional psychotherapy, including the importance of therapeutic alliance, the induction of positive expectancy of change, and remoralization"—argued that effective psychological treatments must contain "specific psychological procedures targeted at the psychopathology at hand" (p. 873). Others have disagreed sharply, downplaying the role of techniques and citing the primacy of the relationship in successful therapy. Thus, Jordan (2002) contended, treatment "is not based on a sophisticated set of techniques, but depends largely on an attitude of mutual respect and inquiry . . . brought to a therapy relationship" (p. 237). In each instance, the therapeutic relationship and treatment techniques are treated as separate, independent factors contributing to the outcome of psychotherapy.

The contextual model, by contrast, emphasizes the coordinated and synchronized interaction of technique and relationship factors (see Figure 5.1). In short, the two are inextricably linked, are mutually dependent, and must be delivered in a coordinated fashion with each other (Butler & Strupp, 1986; Duncan & Moynihan, 1994; Gelso & Hayes, 1998; Hatcher & Barends, 2006). Conceptualized in this way, there can be no alliance without a treatment.

Equally true, any technique is only as effective as its delivery through the context of the client–therapist relationship. Frank and Frank (1991) put it this way, "The success of all methods . . . depends on the patients' conviction that the therapist cares about them *and* [italics added] is competent to help" (p. 154).

## PLACEBOS: CULTURAL SYMBOLS THAT
## CREATE POWERFUL EXPECTATIONS

We have made allusions throughout this chapter to the role that hope and expectancy play in successful psychotherapy, a subject taken up in more detail here. We argue that many of the benefits of treatment occur via the installation of hope and changed expectations. We also argue that the primary means for inspiring hope; changing expectations; and facilitating belief in the therapist, treatment, and relationship is the therapeutic myth or rationale provided to or developed in conjunction with the client.

A brief review of placebos in medicine reveals the power of expectations. Modern medicine was established as a scientific endeavor, in part, by demonstrating that the administration of a substance or the application of a procedure had benefits over and above an inert substance or method; that is, the treatment was superior to a placebo (A. K. Shapiro & Shapiro, 1997a; Wampold, Minami, Tierney, Baskin, & Bhati, 2005). As a consequence, placebo effects were deemed unimportant. Occurring as they did in the psyche rather than in the soma, placebos were not considered real phenomena worthy of serious study (A. K. Shapiro & Shapiro, 1997b; Wampold, Imel, & Minami, 2007). As the name implies, the randomized, double-blind, placebo-controlled design was designed and widely adopted to eliminate the influence of positive expectations or other psychological mediators of outcome (e.g., a caring relationship with the practitioner)—the very ingredients research indicates are critical to successful psychotherapy.

Recent investigations establishing physiological as well as subjective psychological effects of placebos have led to renewed interest in the phenomenon. Data indicate, for example, that placebo analgesics increase natural opioids in the brain (Price, Finniss, & Benedetti, 2008). Physiological responses to placebos have been detected in other medical disorders as well. For example, people with Parkinson's disease who receive a placebo with the suggestion that motor performance will improve indeed show a marked improvement. A number of studies have demonstrated that the low levels of dopamine, which is hypothesized to be related to the motor deficits, increases in those exhibiting a placebo response (Price et al., 2008). Studies are underway to explicate placebo mechanisms in hypertension, gastrointestinal diseases, and asthma (Benedetti, Czajkowski, Kitt, Stefanek, & Sternberg, 2002).

Many models have been proposed for understanding placebo effects (Guess, Kleinman, Kusek, & Engel, 2002; Harrington, 2008; Price et al., 2008), some of which are particularly informative when psychotherapy models and associated techniques are considered among many shared therapeutic factors. Some of the models suggest that the placebo response is embedded in culture (Brody, 1997; Morris, 1997). According to these models, a treatment has symbolic value. Pills, syringes, stethoscopes, and white coats are the symbols of modern medicine and as such they can be powerful placebos without much adornment (for a discussion of placebo effects and psychiatric drugs, see chap. 7, this volume). Psychotherapy, accepted by many, may have healing power simply because of its cultural status as a healing practice. Two research results support this contention. Frank noticed several decades ago that psychotherapy clients improve greatly from the time they make an appointment to the time they present for the first session (Frank & Frank, 1991), underscoring the notion that even the expectation of psychotherapy is in and of itself potent. Furthermore, the form of psychotherapy, without any particular active ingredients, is moderately effective. "Placebo" psychotherapies in which there is no rationale or therapeutic actions produces effects about half as large as a treatment intended to be therapeutic (Wampold, 2001).

In many ways, cultural symbols create expectations, leading some to argue that placebos act through expectations (Kirsch, 1997, 2005; Price et al., 2008). Expectations can be created by the context in which the treatment is administered. As an example, consider a series of ingenious experiments by Benedetti and colleagues. In the studies, the researchers administered an analgesic in open and hidden formats (Benedetti et al., 2003; Price et al., 2003). It is not surprising that when people were aware a drug was being administered, it was experienced as more effective. Accumulating evidence corroborates that the degree to which expectations are induced, the larger the effects that follow (Montgomery & Kirsch, 1997; Nitschke et al., 2006; Price et al., 2008).

Typically, expectations are created in a verbal context; in practice, the clinicians' explanations to the client are powerful. Thomas (1987) demonstrated that simple verbal explanations can result in the reduction of certain symptoms. In the study, people suffering from problems such as pain, cough, or tiredness were assigned either to a placebo treatment or a no treatment condition (e.g., some inert treatment or no treatment at all) and a positive versus negative consultation context (e.g., "You will soon be well" or "I am not sure this treatment will help"). Results indicated no differences in outcome between the placebo treatment and no treatment but a significant difference between the positive and negative explanations.

A comprehensive review of available psychotherapy research has found that therapist explanations influence clients' experience of and benefit from psychotherapy (Greenberg, Constantino, & Bruce, 2006). The same body of evidence shows that clients' pretreatment expectations regarding both the process and outcome of psychotherapy interact in significant ways with engagement, retention, and outcome (Arnkoff, Glass, & Shapiro, 2002; Constantino & DeGeorge, 2008; Greenberg et al., 2006). In their succinct and clinically oriented summary of both areas of research, Constantino and DeGeorge (2008) observed that although expectancy "has been traditionally undervalued across all psychotherapy orientations," the strength of the data makes clear that therapists should "heed the expectancy literature and, if they have not already, incorporate expectancy-based strategies into their clinical repertoires." That not only includes, the authors go on to say, "explicitly assess[ing] patients' expectations at the treatment's launch . . . [but also] . . . work to change their patients' expectations . . . and/or, if appropriate, alter the nature of treatment to better meet patients' expectations" (pp. 2–3).

## IMPLICATIONS FOR RESEARCH AND PRACTICE

In this chapter, we have provided support for a contextual model of psychotherapy, not just as an appealing alternative to any theoretical orientation but more broadly as a superordinate explanation for the effectiveness of therapy that incorporates the importance of theoretical orientations (myths) and their related principles and techniques (rituals). Discussion was purposefully limited to models and techniques. Other chapters in the book provide additional evidence for the importance of other therapeutic factors along with expanding philosophical and theoretical musings about the central ingredients for psychotherapy. With the conceptual framework squarely in place, one might reasonably ask what the implications of this model are for research and practice.

### Implications for Research

Understanding the importance of explanation and therapeutic action as a central therapeutic factor has implications for the study of psychotherapy. Clinical trials in psychotherapy often use a type of control condition that involves an interaction with an empathic healer but contains no treatment, at least not a treatment that a clinician would deem legitimate. The therapists in these comparison conditions might be allowed to respond empathically but prevented from offering explanation for the client's distress or suggesting actions to overcome that distress; these conditions lack the myth and ritual components of the contextual model. These control conditions—often called *alternative treatment*, *supportive counseling*, and *common factor controls*—therefore lack one of the most important ingredients of successful psychotherapy, regardless of school or theoretical orientation (Wampold, 2001; Wampold, Imel, Bhati, & Johnson-Jennings, 2007). Moreover, in such conditions, the therapeutic relationship is itself artificially constrained, lacking essential qualities such as agreement on the tasks and goals of therapy. Is it any surprise really that treatments intended to be therapeutic are more effective than such controls (Baskin et al., 2003; Wampold, 2001)? With shocking frequency, the superiority of a treatment over such a control condition is (inappropriately) cited as evidence for the importance of the specific ingredients of the investigated approach (e.g., Stevens, Hynan, & Allen, 2000).

A more productive research program could be fashioned by using what is known about the delivery of effective treatments. Much variability in outcomes, for example, is attributable to the therapist who provides a treatment (Wampold, 2006). As discussed in this chapter, it may well be that these super therapists select treatments that are compatible with clients' attitudes, values, and cultural context (Miller, Hubble, & Duncan, 2007). There is in fact a modest, although somewhat ambiguous, literature on client preferences for treatment that appears to indicate that providing the preferred treatment results in increased engagement and stronger alliances (Arnkoff et al., 2002; Elkin et al., 1999; Iacoviello et al., 2007; Leykin et al., 2007; Lyddon, 1989). This is a perspective that is compatible with the idea of client-directed services (Bohart & Tallman, 1999; Duncan et al., 1992; Duncan, Miller, & Sparks, 2004). Clearly, further research is needed in this area.

As the expectancy research cited earlier indicates, therapist explanations influence clients' experience of and benefit from psychotherapy. Clients may have some preconceived notions about psychotherapy, but the effective therapist creates positive expectations for an alternative approach. An old literature on therapy induction (i.e., a pretreatment session to explain how psychotherapy works) seems to indicate that it improved outcomes (Frank & Frank, 1991). There is also some research to indicate that clients prefer treatments delivered by credible therapists; that is, preference follows credibility (Goates-Jones & Hill, 2008). Therapist credibility is the extent to which the therapist can don the mantel of socially shared expectations for a healer who provides the client solutions to problems that fit within a broadly accepted cultural change narrative. Again, an examination of how effective therapists both accommodate and influence client expectations in the delivery of treatment is critically needed.

Clients drop out of treatment for many reasons, but one good candidate reason is that they find the treatment rationale and actions unacceptable. In clinical trials, therapists have less latitude to modify treatments, and this suggests that if clients do not find the treatment agreeable, they drop out of treatment. In general, dropout rates in clinical trials are quite high (Wampold,

2007; Westen, Novotny, & Thompson-Brenner, 2004). For example, in a trial of CBT for PTSD, an empirically supported treatment, the dropout rate was approximately 40% (McDonagh et al., 2005). Research could be productively focused on whether effective therapists are flexible in their approach so that when resistance to the treatment is expressed, the therapist alters the treatment or uses a different treatment altogether.

### Implications for Practice

One might think the contextual model would lead to downplaying the necessity of training in techniques. However, training in the specific techniques (or rituals) and a given orientation (or myth) is important for the cultural belief systems of both the healer and client. As indicated throughout the chapter, models and techniques are important and necessary ingredients of successful therapies. That said, having an understanding of the importance of the myth and ritual within any given social context may enhance effective practice. Contrary to the claims of critics of common factor models, therapists need to be able to deliver many different kinds of treatments. To ensure a good fit with the individual consumer of psychological services, therapists need to carefully monitor client acceptance of and agreement with the treatment and agreement about the tasks and goals of therapy (i.e., the alliance). Resistance to the treatment provided is viewed as a function of the type of treatment delivered or the manner in which it is delivered rather than the result of a "resistant" client; that is, it is the therapist's responsibility to address resistance to treatment, and it is not the fault of the client.

Lambert and colleagues (Lambert, Hansen, & Finch, 2001; Lambert, Harmon, Slade, Whipple, & Hawkins, 2005) have shown that therapists often are poor judges of therapy process and outcome. To aid in monitoring therapy process and outcome, researchers have designed a number of measures and systems to help therapists be aware of these important aspects of psychotherapy (Duncan et al., 2004; Hannan et al., 2005; Lambert et al., 2001; Miller et al., 2005; for a full discussion, see chap. 8, this volume). Feedback systems of this sort may assist therapists in becoming more flexible in their styles and encourage earlier referrals when there is a mismatch. Although the most effective therapists may naturally monitor process and outcome, it is clear that providing such information to therapists generally increases the quality of services (Anker, Duncan, & Sparks, 2009; Lambert et al., 2001; Miller et al., 2005).

Additional tools may be needed to assist practitioners to integrate facets of the healing setting. Working within the cultural context of the healing setting requires therapists to be empathically attuned to the client's cultural experiences, beliefs, and values. Both the client's and the therapist's cultural identities are likely to be a significant influence on how the healing myth is negotiated and ritualized. Failing to be aware of cultural differences may enhance the likelihood of stereotype beliefs and inappropriate therapist behaviors. As Sue and Lam (2002) noted, conforming to "politically correct" behaviors with diverse groups alone suggests that the "intrinsic appropriateness of the behavior" (p. 416) may be lost. Therapists who primarily are driven by appearing socially desirable, without internalized cultural beliefs, may unknowingly inject needless tension in the therapeutic relationship and thus damage the persuasiveness of the myth and ritual.

In conclusion, one should keep in mind the following points:

- The complex interplay of a therapeutic orientation (myth), including its specific techniques (ritual), within the context of a healing setting and relationship provide the needed ingredients for successful psychotherapy.
- Whether specific ingredients are highly idiosyncratic or aligned with one of the dominant therapeutic orientations does not matter. The cogency of the rationale for the treatment and its acceptance by the client are the critical aspects of a successful treatment.
- Effective therapists and therapy provide a culturally acceptable rationale for change that leads to altered expectations and enhanced well-being.
- As future research and practice continue to evolve, the contextual model will provide a coherent metatheory for ongoing exploration.
- In the final analysis, the beauty of a treatment, or the efficacy established in a clinical trial, is not important; the important issue is whether for a particular client, the treatment as delivered by the therapist is successful. This success can only be established by monitoring the outcomes for this particular client.

## QUESTIONS FROM THE EDITORS

1. *You make clear in this chapter that specific factors associated with treatments are not responsible for treatment outcome. If the therapist knows that his or her treatment is a myth, then how can the therapist generate belief (e.g., allegiance) sufficient to create a credible treatment? That is, if he or she knows that the explanation is not true, how does he or she convince the client that it is true?*

Awareness that contemporary healing practices are infused with the culture's mythology does not necessarily diminish one's ability to participate in and use them in treatment. Therapists who gain an appreciation for the myths of treatment are perhaps similar to the film critic who becomes savvy to the many devices that filmmakers use to entice the typical moviegoer into the narrative. Certainly, one can become jaded and cynical as a result of this knowledge, but many film critics seem to believe that their participation in film is enhanced by their knowledge and expertise. However, just because a therapist might have an awareness of treatment as myth does not reduce the therapist into a detached and cynical critic who is playing a charade. As noted throughout, effective therapy requires emotional investment and commitment to some shared cultural values. That is, the therapist who cannot summon a passionate commitment to his or her core beliefs will ultimately fail to engage the patient in an emotionally charged relationship. The therapist's own emotion and commitment serve to weave treatment myth, treatment principles, and ritual into a powerful and persuasive communication that, in turn, enhances the therapeutic relationship (see Figure 5.1). Knowledge that these values are culturally dependent need not be a forbidden fruit that bans the therapist from participation in his or her own culture, nor from conducting good psychotherapy!

For many therapists, adherence to their practices seems to be based on both literal and historical sense. Therapists may believe just as stridently that only the client's narrative construction is true in its own right. With regard to the latter, narrative truth is no less real than the physical and historical reality, such as in the prior discussion of placebo effects. Part of the delight in thinking contextually about psychotherapy can be the discovery of how our healing rituals are linked to myth, which no doubt can be a lifelong journey and occupational benefit. Knowledge of how psychological treatments are grounded in myth and how those myths translate into real-world change should actually serve to enhance the beliefs of the proponents of various psychotherapies.

2. *If therapy works in the way you describe, how can or should the field distinguish between therapists, religious ministers, and native healers? Put another way, is the professional psychotherapist (regardless of degree, training, or licensure) a mere player in a historical context—in our particular case, an epiphenomenon of Western, Enlightenment-based cultures?*

We believe that psychotherapy is indeed an epiphenomenon of Western, Enlightenment-based cultures. Tracing the evolution of the need for and current role of psychotherapy and psychotherapists would require significantly more space than is allotted here, however. Suffice it to say, we can imagine a time in the future when, as in the past, clinicians delivering psychotherapy as presently practiced would not be necessary. The "secular priesthood" (London, 1986) has a place in our time because the culture creates a place for it. And as soon as the culture does not have a place for it, it will be replaced.

It is also clear that religious ministers and native healers are connected with therapists whether the "professionals" like it or not. Even if one ignores the obvious connection between psychotherapy and religious healing through the myth, ritual, setting, and relationship of the contextual model, it is obvious to astute observers that religious ministers and native healers capitalize on many of the techniques and beliefs that are effectively used by therapists (or is it the other way around?). Perhaps the difference lies in the fact that therapists, for the most part, form a society-sanctioned profession with associated rules of operation, laws to govern practice, and guidelines for handling problems. In addition, psychotherapists typically adhere to the scientific model of evidence, whereas religious ministers and native healers may have a different standard and source of evidence demonstrating effective practice.

3. *As a follow-up, are all treatments provided by psychotherapists legitimate? Are some therapies simply too "crazy" to be used by psychotherapists? If so, how does one discriminate between legitimate and illegitimate psychotherapies?*

According to the model described in this chapter, a therapy would be defined as too alien only when it fails to include a belief that is meaningfully linked to larger cultural beliefs. Specifically, the belief has to not only be meaningful but also, as stated in the body of the chapter, acceptable and helpful to the client. Obviously, treatments that do not engage the client, however well intentioned, will only serve to diminish hope.

Discriminating therapies that are legitimate from those that are not is a more difficult task. New therapies must be allowed to flourish if psychotherapy is allowed to keep pace with social evolutionary changes within society. A natural evolutionary course will take place in which inert treatments, those that fail to make meaningful connections to core contextual beliefs held by the client patient and his or her community, will naturally drop out of use. Similarly, therapies that are not effective will likely fall out of use naturally because the rationale behind the treatment is not believable to clients. Consider the bounty of remedies that are no longer used in therapy: primal scream, nude marathon and encounter group therapies, Orgone therapy, transactional analysis, prolonged bathing, nasal surgery, and even tooth extractions for treatment of psychosis (Scull, 2005). Such treatments were used in the United States in the 20th century but are now viewed as quaint, out of date, simplistic, and even torturous.

Given the large number of therapies that have been introduced in the past 20 to 30 years, legitimate concerns have been raised about ethical practice. It seems that these judgments could be made through a consensus from committees of distinguished therapists and researchers. We believe that such monitoring would be best if cautious and limited to excluding therapies that are suspect, ethically questionable, or not likely to be effective. Monitoring does not guarantee discontinuation of treatments that harm. For instance, the example of repeated, drastic surgery and tooth removal (Scull, 2005) was based on a stated rationale of benevolence (i.e., certain limbs, organs, etc., must be removed because of pockets of infection believed to be causing insanity). Although some professionals publicly voiced concerns, those who could have halted this practice believed the theory of focal infection. The prominence of those who voiced support for radical surgeries illustrates the power of the rationale behind any treatment and the inherent problems with oversight and monitoring myths. Even so, such examples give us reason to hope that future oversight will be more reflective of the context in which these myths arise.

It seems reasonable (from the current place and time) that therapies whose myth does not appear believable could be required to be submitted for empirical study and support. Asking that a handful of therapies be submitted to a clinical trial to demonstrate empirical support (i.e., equivalent effectiveness with other therapies) seems to us a more parsimonious solution to the problem of illegitimate treatments. Such a solution would seem both practically and scientifically more reasonable than asking that all treatments undergo clinical trials to demonstrate that they are just as effective as almost all other forms of therapy (see the overview of this research in this chapter). This solution would free practitioners to engage in treatment development. It would also free scientists to study legitimately framed research issues (e.g., search for active ingredients common to all therapies). As a field, psychotherapy will be in much better position to distinguish legitimate from illegitimate treatments once our research advances enough to determine how common factors are used as active ingredients in circumstances and contexts.

## REFERENCES

Ahn, H. & Wampold, B. E. (2001). Where oh where are the specific ingredients? A meta-analysis of component studies in counseling and psychotherapy. *Journal of Counseling Psychology, 48*, 251–257.

Anker, M., Duncan, B., & Sparks, J. (2009). Using client feedback to improve couples therapy outcomes: A randomized clinical trial in a naturalistic setting. *Journal of Consulting and Clinical Psychology, 77*, 693–705.

Arnkoff, D. B., Glass, C. R., & Shapiro, S. J. (2002). Expectations and preferences. In J. C. Norcross (Ed.), *Psychotherapy relationships that work: Therapists contributions and responsiveness to patients* (pp. 325–346). New York: Oxford University Press.

Barlow, D. H. (2004). Psychological treatments. *American Psychologist, 59*, 869–878.

Baskin, T. W., Tierney, S. C., Minami, T., & Wampold, B. E. (2003). Establishing specificity in psychotherapy: A meta-analysis of structural equivalence of placebo controls. *Journal of Consulting and Clinical Psychology, 71*, 973–979.

Benedetti, F., Czajkowski, S. M., Kitt, C. A., Stefanek, M., & Sternberg, E. M. (2002). Recommendations for research to further elucidate the nature of the placebo. In H. A. Guess, A. Kleinman, J. W. Kusek, & L. W. Engel (Eds.), *The science of the placebo: Toward an interdisciplinary research agenda* (pp. 286–292). London: BMJ Books.

Benedetti, F., Maggi, G., Lopiano, L., Lanotte, M., Rainero, I., Vighetti, S., et al. (2003). Open versus hidden medical treatments: The patient's knowledge about therapy affects the therapy outcome. *Prevention & Treatment, 6,* Article 1. Available at http://content2.apa.org/journals/pre/6/1/1

Bohart, A. C., & Tallman, K. (1999). *How clients make therapy work: The process of active self-healing.* Washington, DC: American Psychological Association.

Brickman, P., Rabinowitz, V., Karuza, J., Coates, D., Cohn, E., & Kidder, L. (1982). Models of helping and coping. *American Psychologist, 37,* 368–384.

Brody, N. (1997). The doctor as therapeutic agent: A placebo effect research agenda. In A. Harrington (Ed.), *The placebo effect: An interdisciplinary exploration* (pp. 77–92). Cambridge, MA: Harvard University Press.

Butler, S. F., & Strupp, H. H. (1986). "Specific" and "nonspecific" factors in psychotherapy: A problematic paradigm for psychotherapy research. *Psychotherapy, 23,* 30–40.

Castonguay, L. G., & Beutler, L. E. (2006). *Principles of therapeutic change that work.* Oxford, England: Oxford University Press.

Chambless, D. L., & Hollon, S. D. (1998). Defining empirically supported therapies. *Journal of Consulting and Clinical Psychology, 66,* 7–18.

Constantino, M. J., & DeGeorge, J. (2008). Believing is seeing: Clinical implications of research on patient expectations. *Psychotherapy Bulletin, 43,* 1–6.

Duncan, B. L., & Miller, S. D. (2000). The client's theory of change. *Journal of Psychotherapy Integration, 10,* 169–187.

Duncan, B. L., Miller, S. D., & Sparks, J. A. (2004). *The heroic client: A revolutionary way to improve effectiveness through client-directed, outcome-informed therapy* (Rev. ed.). San Francisco: Jossey-Bass.

Duncan, B. L., & Moynihan, D. (1994). Applying outcome research: Intentional utilization of the client's frame of reference. *Psychotherapy, 31,* 294–301.

Duncan, B. L., Solovey, A., & Rusk, G. (1992). *Changing the rules: A client-directed approach.* New York: Guilford Press.

Dush, D. M., Hirt, D. M., & Schroeder, H. E. (1983). Self-statement modification with adults: A meta-analysis. *Psychological Bulletin, 94,* 408–422.

Elkin, I., Yamaguchi, J. L., Arnkoff, D. B., Glass, C. R., Sotsky, S. M., & Krupnick, J. L. (1999). Patient–treatment fit and early engagement in therapy. *Psychotherapy Research, 9,* 437–451.

Elliott, R., Watson, J. C., Goldman, R. N., & Greenberg, L. S. (2004). *Learning emotion-focused therapy: The process–experiential approach to change.* Washington, DC: American Psychological Association.

Fischer, A. R., Jome, L. M., & Atkinson, D. R. (1998). Back to the future of multicultural psychotherapy with a common factors approach. *The Counseling Psychologist, 26,* 602–606.

Frank, J. D., & Frank, J. B. (1991). *Persuasion and healing: A comparative study of psychotherapy*. Baltimore: The Johns Hopkins University Press.

Frank, J. D., & Frank, J. B. (1998). Comments on "Reconceptualizing multicultural counseling: Universal healing conditions." *The Counseling Psychologist, 26,* 589–591.

Garfield, S. L. (1995). *Psychotherapy: An eclectic–integrative approach*. New York: Wiley.

Gelso, C. J., & Hayes, J. A. (1998). *The psychotherapy relationship: Theory, research, and practice*. New York: Wiley.

Goldfried, M. R.. (1980). Toward the delineation of therapeutic change principles. *American Psychologist, 35,* 991–999.

Grawe, K. (2004). *Psychological therapy*. Cambridge, MA: Hogrefe & Huber.

Greenberg, R. P., Constantino, M. J., & Bruce, N. (2006). Are patient expectations still relevant for psychotherapy process and outcome? *Clinical Psychology Review, 26,* 657–678.

Grencavage, L. M., & Norcross, J. C. (1990). Where are the commonalities among the therapeutic common factors? *Professional Psychology: Research and Practice, 21,* 372–378.

Guess, H. A., Kleinman, A., Kusek, J. W., & Engel, L. W. (2002). *The science of placebo: Toward an interdisciplinary research agenda*. London: BMJ Books.

Hannan, C., Lambert, M. J., Harmon, C., Nielsen, S. L., Smart, D. W., Shimokawa, K., et al. (2005). A lab test and algorithms for identifying clients at risk for treatment failure. *Journal of Clinical Psychology: In Session, 61,* 1–9.

Harrington, A. (2008). *The cure within: A history of mind–body medicine*. New York: Norton.

Hatcher, R. L., & Barends, A. W. (2006). How a return to theory could help alliance research. *Psychotherapy: Theory, Research, & Practice, 43,* 292–299.

Hoag, M. J., & Burlingame, G. M. (1997). Evaluating the effectiveness of child and adolescent group treatment: A meta-analytic review. *Journal of Clinical Child Psychology, 26,* 234–246.

Hoch, P. (1955). Aims and limitations of psychotherapy. *American Journal of Psychiatry, 112,* 321–327.

Hubble, M. A., Duncan, B. L., & Miller, S. D. (1999a). Directing attention to what works. In M. A. Hubble, B. L. Duncan, & S. D. Miller (Eds.), *The heart and soul of change: What works in therapy* (pp. 407–448). Washington, DC: American Psychological Association.

Hubble, M. A., Duncan, B. L., & Miller, S. D. (Eds.). (1999b). *The heart and soul of change: What works in therapy*. Washington, DC: American Psychological Association.

Iacoviello, B. M., McCarthy, K. S., Barrett, M., S., Rynn, M., Gallop, R., & Barber, J. P. (2007). Treatment preferences affect the therapeutic alliance: Implications for randomized controlled trials. *Journal of Consulting and Clinical Psychology, 75,* 194–198.

Imel, Z. E., & Wampold, B. E. (2008). The common factors of psychotherapy. In S. D. Brown & R. W. Lent (Eds.), *Handbook of counseling psychology* (4th ed., pp. 249–266). New York: Wiley.

Jordan, J. V. (2002). *Comprehensive handbook of psychotherapy: Interpersonal/humanistic/existential* (Vol. 3). Hoboken, NJ: Wiley.

Kirsch, I. (1997). Specifying nonspecifics: Psychological mechanisms of placebo effects. In A. Harrington (Ed.), *The placebo effect: An interdisciplinary exploration* (pp. 166–186). Cambridge, MA: Harvard University Press.

Kirsch, I. (2005). Placebo psychotherapy: Synonym or oxymoron? *Journal of Clinical Psychology, 61,* 791–803.

Lambert, M. J. (1992). Implications for outcome research for psychotherapy integration. In J. C. Norcross & S. L. Garfield (Eds.), *Handbook of psychotherapy integration* (pp. 94–129). New York: Wiley.

Lambert, M. J., Hansen, N. B., & Finch, A. E. (2001). Patient-focused research: Using patient outcome data to enhance treatment effects. *Journal of Consulting and Clinical Psychology, 69,* 159–172.

Lambert, M. J., Harmon, C., Slade, K., Whipple, J. L., & Hawkins, E. J. (2005). Providing feedback to psychotherapists on their patients' progress: Clinical results and practice suggestions. *Journal of Clinical Psychology, 61,* 165–174.

Lambert, M. J. & Ogles, B. M. (2004). The efficacy and effectiveness of psychotherapy. In M. J. Lambert (Ed.), *Bergin and Garfield's handbook of psychotherapy and behavior change* (5th ed., pp. 139–193). New York: Wiley.

Leykin, Y., DeRubeis, R. J., Gallop, R., Amsterdam, J. D., Shelton, R. C., & Hollon, S. D. (2007). The relation of patients' treatment preferences to outcome in a randomized clinical trial. *Behavior Therapy, 38,* 209–217.

London, P. (1986). *The modes and morals of psychotherapy.* Washington, DC: Hemisphere Publishing.

Luborsky, L., Diguer, L., Seligman, D. A., Rosenthal, R., Krause, E. D., Johnson, S., et al. (1999). The researcher's own therapy allegiances: A "wild card" in comparisons of treatment efficacy. *Clinical Psychology: Science and Practice, 6,* 95–106.

Luborsky, L., Rosenthal, R., Diguer, L., Andrusyna, T. P., Berman, J. S., Levitt, J. T., et al. (2002). The dodo bird verdict is alive and well—mostly. *Clinical Psychology: Science and Practice, 9,* 2–12.

Lyddon, W. J. (1989). Personal epistemology and preference for counseling. *Journal of Counseling Psychology, 36,* 423–429.

Makari, G. (2008). *Revolution in mind: The creation of psychoanalysis.* New York: HarperCollins.

Matarazzo, R. G., & Garner, A. M. (1992). Research on training of psychotherapy. In D. K. Freedheim (Ed.), *History of psychotherapy* (pp. 850–877). Washington, DC: American Psychological Association.

McDonagh, A., Friedman, M., McHugo, G., Ford, J., Sengupta, A., Mueser, K., et al. (2005). Randomized trial of cognitive–behavioral therapy for chronic posttraumatic stress disorder in adult female survivors of childhood sexual abuse. *Journal of Consulting and Clinical Psychology, 73,* 515–524.

Miller, S. D., Duncan, B. L., & Hubble, M. A. (1997). *Escape from Babel: Toward a unifying language for psychotherapy practice.* New York: Norton.

Miller, S. D., Duncan, B. L., & Hubble, M. A. (2005). Outcome-informed clinical work. In J. C. Norcross & M. R. Goldfried (Eds.), *Handbook of psychotherapy integration* (2nd ed., (pp. 84–102). New York: Oxford University Press.

Miller, S., Hubble, M., & Duncan, B. (2007). Supershrinks. *Psychotherapy Networker, 31,* 27–35, 56.

Montgomery, G. H., & Kirsch, I. (1997). Classical conditioning and the placebo effect. *Pain, 72,* 107–113.

Morris, D. B. (1997). Placebo, pain, and belief: A biocultural model. In A. Harrington (Ed.), *The placebo effect: An interdisciplinary exploration* (pp. 187–207). Cambridge, MA: Harvard University Press.

Newman, M. G., Stiles. W. B., Janeck, A., & Woody, S. R. (2006). Integration of therapeutic factors in anxiety disorders. In L. G. Castonguay & L. E. Beutler (Eds.), *Principles of therapeutic change that work* (pp. 187–200). Oxford, England: Oxford University Press.

Nitschke, J. B., Dixon, G. E., Sarinopoulos, I., Short, S. J., Cohen, J. D., Smith, E. E., et al. (2006). Altering expectancy dampens neural response to aversive taste in primary taste cortex. *Nature Neuroscience, 9,* 435–442.

Norcross, J. C. (2002). *Psychotherapy relationships that work: Therapist contributions and responsiveness to patients.* Oxford, England: Oxford University Press.

Orlinsky, D. E., Grawe, K., & Parks, B. K. (1994). Process and outcome in psychotherapy—Noch einmal. In S. L. Garfield & A. E. Bergin (Eds.), *Handbook of psychotherapy and behavior change* (4th ed., pp. 270–376). New York: Wiley.

Orlinsky, D. E., & Howard, K. I. (1986). Process and outcome in psychotherapy. In S. L. Garfield & A. E. Bergin (Eds.), *Handbook of psychotherapy and behavior change* (3rd ed., pp. 311–381). New York: Wiley.

Paley, G., & Shapiro, D.A. (2002). Lessons from psychotherapy research for psychological interventions for people with schizophrenia. *Psychology and Psychotherapy: Theory, Research, and Practice, 75,* 5–17.

Price, D. P., Finniss, D. G., & Benedetti, F. (2008). A comprehensive review of the placebo effect: Recent advances and current thought. *Annual Review of Psychology, 59,* 565–590.

Poznanski, J. J., & McLennan, J. (1995). Conceptualizing and measuring counselors' theoretical orientation. *Journal of Counseling Psychology, 42,* 411–422.

Robinson, L. A., Berman, J. S., & Neimeyer, R. A. (1990). Psychotherapy for the treatment of depression: A comprehensive review of controlled outcome research. *Psychological Bulletin, 53,* 294–302.

Rogers, C. (1961). *On becoming a person.* New York: Norton.

Rosenzweig, S. (1936). Some implicit common factors in diverse methods of psychotherapy. *American Journal of Orthopsychiatry, 6,* 412–415.

Schnurr, P. P., Friedman, M. J., Engel, C. C., Foa, E. B., Shea, M. T., Chow, B. K., et al. (2007) Cognitive behavioral therapy for posttraumatic stress disorder in women: A randomized controlled trial. *JAMA, 297,* 820–830.

Scull, A. (2005). *Madhouse: A tragic tale of megalomania and modern medicine.* New Haven, CT: Yale University Press.

Shapiro, A. K., & Shapiro, E. S. (1997a). The placebo: Is it much ado about nothing? In A. Harrington (Ed.), *The placebo effect: An interdisciplinary exploration* (pp. 12–36). Cambridge, MA: Harvard University Press.

Shapiro, A. K., & Shapiro, E. S. (1997b). *The powerful placebo: From ancient priest to modern medicine.* Baltimore: The Johns Hopkins University Press.

Shapiro, D. A. & Shapiro, D. (1982). Meta-analysis of comparative therapy outcome studies: A replication and refinement. *Psychological Bulletin, 92,* 581–604.

Skinner, B. F. (1948). *Walden two.* New York: Macmillan.

Smith, M. L., Glass, G. V., & Miller, T. I. (1980). *The benefits of psychotherapy.* Baltimore: The Johns Hopkins University Press.

Stevens, S. E., Hynan, M. T., & Allen, M. (2000). A meta-analysis of common factor and specific treatment effects across domains of the phase model of psychotherapy. *Clinical Psychology: Science and Practice, 7,* 273–290.

Sue, S., & Lam, A. G. (2002). Cultural and demographic diversity. In J. C. Norcross (Ed.), *Psychotherapy relationships that work: Therapist contributions and responsiveness to patients* (pp. 401–422). Oxford, England: Oxford University Press.

Task Force on Promotion and Dissemination of Psychological Procedures. (1995). Training in and dissemination of empirically-validated psychological treatment: Report and recommendations. *The Clinical Psychologist, 48,* 2–23.

Thomas, K. B. (1987). General practice consultations: Is there any point in being positive? *British Medical Journal, 294,* 1200–1202.

Wachtel, P. L. (1997). *Psychoanalysis, behavior therapy, and the relational world.* Washington DC: American Psychological Association.

Wampold, B. E. (1997). Methodological problems in identifying efficacious psychotherapies. *Psychotherapy Research, 7,* 21–43.

Wampold, B. E. (2001). *The great psychotherapy debate: Models, methods, and findings.* Mahwah, NJ: Erlbaum.

Wampold, B. E. (2006). The psychotherapist. In J. C. Norcross, L. E. Beutler, & R. F. Levant (Eds.), *Evidence-based practices in mental health: Debate and dialogues on the fundamental questions* (pp. 200–208). Washington, DC: American Psychological Association.

Wampold, B. E. (2007). Psychotherapy: The humanistic (and effective) treatment. *American Psychologist, 62,* 857–873.

Wampold, B. E., Imel, Z. E., Bhati, K. S., & Johnson-Jennings, M. D. (2007). Insight as a common factor. In L. G. Castonguay & C. E. Hill (Eds.), *Insight in psychotherapy* (pp. 119–139). Washington, DC: American Psychological Association.

Wampold, B. E., Imel, Z. E., & Minami, T. (2007). The story of placebo effects in medicine: Evidence in context. *Journal of Clinical Psychology, 63,* 379–390.

Wampold, B. E., Minami, T., Tierney, S. C., Baskin, T. W., & Bhati, K. S. (2005). The placebo is powerful: Estimating placebo effects in medicine and psychotherapy from clinical trials. *Journal of Clinical Psychology, 61,* 835–854.

Westen, D., Novotny, C. M., & Thompson-Brenner, H. (2004). The empirical status of empirically supported psychotherapies: Assumptions, findings, and reporting in controlled clinical trials. *Psychological Bulletin, 130,* 631–663.

# 6

# EVIDENCE-BASED PRACTICE: EVIDENCE OR ORTHODOXY?

JULIA H. LITTELL

Believe those who are seeking the truth; doubt those who find it.

—André Gide

The hope that clinical practice will be informed by the results of empirical research is not new, but this ideal has been difficult to attain. Reformers have tried to use scientific knowledge to improve the human condition since the late 19th century. Early reformers embraced "a rather sweeping trust in science to guide the hand of the practitioner" (Zimbalist, 1977, p. 32), but their use of science was rhetorical. Scientific therapeutics have come and gone, yet the desire to build empirical foundations for the helping professions remains. A new breed of scientist–practitioner emerged in psychology and social work in the 1960s and 1970s. A product of academics, the scientist–practitioners' designs were not sustained in practice, thwarted by lack of agency support (Reid, 1994).

Much has been written about tensions that divide clinical work and research. Clinicians and social scientists have distinct imperatives and sensibilities. Therapy requires action and faith in the process, whereas science demands observation and skepticism. Most scientific knowledge is tentative and nomothetic, not directly applicable to individual cases. Experts have stepped into this breach by packaging empirical evidence for use in practice. Sometimes this is little more than a ruse to promote favorite theories and therapies. Yet, wrapped in scientific rhetoric, some authoritative pronouncements have become orthodoxy.

Now evidence-based practice (EBP) is in vogue in the helping professions. Are its scientific claims genuine? Can its methods be seamlessly integrated into practice? Or is EBP just a new orthodoxy?

Two fundamentally different approaches to EBP and their influence on the marketing and regulation of clinical practice are described in this chapter. Because both approaches rely on summaries of empirical evidence, methods of research synthesis are examined, using case examples to illustrate the promise and problems of these methods. This leads to a discussion about the current state of the science, the premature closure of inquiry about what works, and the requirements for firm empirical foundations. Recommendations are offered to enhance critical evaluation of research so that EBP is not interpreted in a way that unfairly restricts treatments.

## WHAT IS EVIDENCE-BASED PRACTICE?

EBP evolved from evidence-based medicine (EBM). EBM was developed at McMaster University in the 1980s in response to concerns that knowledge derived from medical research was not routinely used in clinical practice. Sackett and colleagues defined EBM as the integration of the best research evidence with clinical expertise, including patient values, to make informed decisions about individual cases (Sackett, Rosenberg, Gray, Haynes, & Richardson, 1996). EBM is a process driven by clinicians who pose specific questions that have practical value for a patient, seek available research evidence to address their questions, act, and assess the results.

Interest in EBM grew in the 1990s, spawning many workshops for physicians on how to find, critically appraise, and incorporate empirical evidence in clinical decisions. EBM also propelled efforts to synthesize research results and make rigorous evidence summaries readily available to patients and physicians. Now the international Cochrane Collaboration, the U.K. Centre for Review and Dissemination, the U.S. Evidence-Based Practice Centers (funded by the U.S. Agency for Healthcare Research and Quality [AHRQ]), and others produce and disseminate systematic reviews and meta-analyses of clinical trials on the effectiveness of interventions in health care.

The process of EBM was adopted in models of EBP for human services (Gibbs, 2003) and public policy (Davies, 2004). The 2005 American Psychological Association (APA) Presidential Task Force on Evidence-Based Practice (2006) adopted the following definition: "Evidence-based practice in psychology . . . is the integration of the best available research with clinical expertise in the context of patient characteristics, culture, and preferences" (p. 273).

Like EBM, EBP rests on the assumption that many sources and types of evidence are material for clinicians and other decision makers. As Gibbs (2003) and Davies (2004) have noted, evidence is needed about a variety of topics, including the following: the client's condition, values, and preferences; the knowledge and skills the practitioner possesses or can find in colleagues; available resources, opportunities, and contextual constraints; the efficacy and effectiveness of interventions; and larger policy and programmatic goals. What counts as credible evidence depends on the question. To find out which treatments are preferred in a particular community, we might survey community members. If we want to know why people prefer one treatment over another, qualitative analysis of interviews would be useful. When we need to know about an individual's preferences, anecdotal information from (or about) that individual may suffice.

Much of the discussion of EBP has focused on what is known about the efficacy and effectiveness of interventions. These topics are not inherently more important than others, but intervention effects do matter. This chapter focuses on evidence of intervention effects for the following reasons. As noted previously, the EBP literature has been concerned with efficacy and effectiveness. Second, knowledge of intervention effects is difficult to obtain; it requires causal inferences that are among the hardest to confirm scientifically. Third, there is much room for improvement in how people analyze, synthesize, and disseminate evidence about intervention effects.

## EVIDENCE-BASED TREATMENTS

Criteria for evaluating the efficacy and effectiveness of therapeutic interventions have been developed by many professional and government organizations. Diverse criteria have been applied to bodies of empirical evidence to determine what works for various conditions. Results have been used to create lists of effective or model programs, called evidence-based treatments (EBTs), empirically supported treatments (ESTs), or empirically validated treatments (EVTs). Here the term *evidence-based treatments* is used to distinguish programs that meet certain evidentiary criteria from EBP as a model of practice.

Examples of the EBT approach include the prestigious Blueprints for Violence Prevention series (Mihalic, Fagan, Irwin, Ballard, & Elliott, 2004); the National Registry of Evidence-Based Programs and Practices (Substance Abuse and Mental Health Services Administration [SAMSHA], 2007); the Society for Prevention Research standards for efficacy, effectiveness, and broad dissemination (Flay et al., 2005); and the APA Society of Clinical Psychology (Division 12; Chambless et al., 1998). According to Chambless et al.'s (1998) criteria, "probably efficacious" programs are those with at least two "good between group experiments" or three single-subject experiments showing evidence of positive effects (compared with a pill, placebo, or other treatment) or effects that are equivalent to those of an already established treatment. If the experiments were conducted by at least two different investigators or if there are nine single-subject experiments, the program is regarded as "well-established" (Chambless et al., 1998, p. 4). The debate over such standards of evidence has been overshadowed by efforts to implement EBTs "however they are defined" (New Freedom Commission on Mental Health, 2005, p. 3).

Chambless and Ollendick (2001) described the "drive to identify and disseminate ESTs" (p. 686). Although the authors claim that it stems from EBM, the EBT movement seized on the notion that clinicians need summaries of evidence provided by expert reviews. This is not compatible with Sackett's (2000) skeptical view of reliance on experts, which is discussed later. In contrast to EBP models, the EBT approach has been largely top-down. That is, emphasis is on widespread implementation of EBTs, largely through state and national initiatives.

### The "Know–Do" Gap

In 2001, a U.S. Surgeon General report suggested "a terrifying gap between what we know and how we act" exists in the treatment and prevention of youth violence (U.S. Department of Health and Human Services [DHHS], 2001, p. 15). This sentiment has been echoed through the work of the U.S. National Institutes of Health (NIH) and in many publications and official pronouncements. The failure to provide EBTs on a wider scale has been the subject of recent inquiry. Limited use of EBTs is seen as a result of faulty graduate education, resistance among clinicians and community agencies, or ineffective dissemination practices.

Some training in EBTs is required in graduate programs in clinical psychology (APA, 1996), but proponents argue there is a need for greater emphasis on EBTs. Presumably, graduate training should reflect "the scientific basis of the discipline" (Woody, Weisz, & McLean, 2005, p. 11). Woody and colleagues described barriers to training in EBTs.

Some of this opposition was based on the idea that lists of ESTs reflect a political or theoretical bias more than they reflect treatments that work. Others opposed what they see as an erosion of their autonomy as professionals because of pressure to limit their interventions to ESTs. In this view, the manualized approach is seen as too rigid and as objectifying rather than humanizing clients. Some training directors also expressed a lack of trust in researchers, pointing to stories of misleading reporting of clinical trials from the drug industry in support of this view (Woody et al., 2005, p. 11).

Nevertheless, current theory and research focus not on limitations of EBTs but on clinician and agency characteristics associated with resistance to their adoption. Clinicians' attitudes toward EBTs, executive leadership styles, organizational climate, and organizational readiness for change have been the focus of some of this work (Aarons, 2006; Simpson & Flynn, 2007). Dissemination theories from other fields have been tapped to develop strategies to successfully transfer EBTs to practice settings (Stirman, Crits-Christoph, & DeRubeis, 2004).

## If We Fund It, They Will Come

The President's New Freedom Commission on Mental Health (2005) identified a need for organizational and financial incentives to implement EBTs. Consistent with their emphasis on the translation and transfer of empirical knowledge to practice, NIH and the DHHS funded state implementation of EBTs, research on the transportability of EBTs, and studies of organizational factors associated with readiness to adopt EBTs. The Centers for Disease Control and Prevention is funding *translational research,* which it defines as the process by which a "proven scientific discovery" is successfully institutionalized (Centers for Disease Control and Prevention, 2007). This includes dissemination, implementation, and diffusion of EBTs.

By 2002, 49 state mental health agencies had implemented one or more EBTs (Ganju, 2003). In 2003, the state of Oregon mandated use of EBTs in their mental health and addiction service systems. In 2004, Iowa legislation required 70% of block grant funds to go to community mental health centers, and all of these funds were to be used to support EBTs. The State of Washington assigns letter grades to services on the basis of a hierarchy of evidence that reflects the extent to which the service has some "proven benefit" to clients (Washington State Administrative Code; also see Washington Department of Social and Health Services, 2005). These grades affect coverage decisions.

Given funding and regulatory mandates for the inclusion of EBTs, they are now inextricably woven into the fabric of mental health and substance abuse practice. But are such mandates empirically justified? It is argued here that the prominent approaches used to accumulate evidence of intervention effects of EBTs are unscientific and inadequate.

## THE ACHILLES HEEL OF EVIDENCE-BASED PRACTICE AND EVIDENCE-BASED TREATMENTS

Arguments have been made for and against EBP and EBTs (e.g., Gambrill, 2006; Gibbs & Gambrill, 2002; Hubble, Duncan, & Miller, 1999; Wampold, 2001; Westen, Novotny, & Thompson-Brenner, 2004). EBP reflects the understanding that scientific evidence is tentative, whereas EBTs depict confidence in available evidence. EBP appeals to those who value clinicians' autonomy and individualized treatment decisions. EBTs appeal to those who believe that more structure and consistency is needed in mental health services.

EBP and EBTs both share an Achilles heel: reliance on unscientific syntheses of evidence about what works. Today, when clinicians look for evidence of effectiveness and when policy makers select services from a list of EBTs, the information they find is likely to be incomplete and potentially misleading. It is ironic that the results that clinicians and policymakers are urged to use have been compiled in a manner that reflects a lack of awareness of the empirical evidence about the process and methods of research synthesis.

The proliferation of unscientific research syntheses poses a much more serious problem for ESTs because they depend on evidence of efficacy and effectiveness. EBP includes a broader array of evidence, but practitioners can be misinformed by unscientific syntheses.

## METHODS OF RESEARCH SYNTHESIS

The synthesis of results across studies is important for many reasons. A single study provides only one of many possible answers that could be gleaned from a population. As one does not take one person's view on politics as a reliable indicator of public opinion, one cannot rely on any single study to provide definitive information about treatment effects. Outcome studies vary in their methodology and credibility and sometimes produce conflicting evidence. A careful synthesis of results across studies places the findings of each in context and provides an opportunity to investigate reasons for variations in outcomes across samples, treatments, measures, and settings.

### Traditional, Narrative Reviews

Typically, research synthesis begins with a question about available evidence on a certain question or topic. The reviewer seeks pertinent published studies using an electronic keyword search in one or more bibliographic databases, such as PsycINFO. The reviewer might consult other sources (e.g., Dissertation Abstracts International). He or she reads the material at hand and then writes a narrative summary of the studies and their results. The reviewer draws conclusions about similarities and differences among the studies, central patterns, and the overall weight of the evidence. Some of the most influential reviews of EBTs have used traditional, narrative methods (e.g., Brestan & Eyberg, 1998; Burns, Hoagwood, & Mrazek, 1999; Chambless & Ollendick, 2001; Hoagwood, Burns, Kiser, Ringeisen, & Schoenwald, 2001; Kazdin & Weisz, 1998).

Traditional reviews have well-known limitations. They are based on unspecified samples that are not representative of all of the credible studies conducted on a topic. For example, many reviewers rely on convenience samples of published studies. These samples are often biased toward positive results. Narrative reviews rarely explain how studies were selected. Thus, readers may be unable to tell whether studies were selected because they supported a favored position or for some other reason.

Second, reviewers rarely explain how they sifted through evidence and drew conclusions about overall trends. This is not an easy task. The synthesis of results of multiple studies involves several complex operations that are not performed easily with college algebra. Studies show that reviewers' conclusions can be influenced by trivial properties of research reports (Bushman & Wells, 2001). To address this issue, some reviewers use a process called *vote counting*. In this procedure, studies are sorted into two or three categories according to their results and the reviewer tallies the number of studies with significant positive results, negative results, and null findings (sometimes the negative and null categories are combined). Several problems exist with this approach. Vote counting relies on tests of statistical significance in the original studies. Those significance tests are heavily influenced by sample size, so clinically significant results are missed in small studies and trivial results appear statistically significant in large studies. A vote count is a tally of results that are not inherently meaningful. Carlton and Strawderman (1996) showed that vote counting can lead to the wrong conclusions.

Unless the methods of selecting and synthesizing research results are explicit, readers cannot tell whether the review is a comprehensive and fair appraisal of the evidence. "Ideally, practitioners should be able to rely on reviewers to isolate the best evidence for them and to distill it for its essence to guide practice decision-making. Unfortunately, conventional reviews have fallen far short of such expectations" (Gibbs, 2003, p. 153).

## Bias in Research Synthesis

Research synthesis can be affected by biases from three sources: those that arise in the original studies, in the reporting and dissemination of results, and in the review process itself. Owing to design and implementation problems, outcome studies can systematically overestimate or underestimate effects, thereby making conclusions vulnerable to threats to validity (Shadish, Cook, & Campbell, 2002). Related to experimenter expectancies, allegiance effects may appear when interventions are studied by their advocates (Luborsky et al., 1999; see chap. 11 and 12, this volume, for allegiance bias examples).

Investigators are more likely to report results that are statistically significant and positive (Dickersin, 2005). Negative and null results are apt to be underreported (i.e., presented with missing information) when they are reported at all (A. W. Chan, Hróbjartsson, Haar, Gøtzsche, & Altman, 2004). Studies with significant positive results are more likely to be accepted for publication than studies with null or negative results (Dickersin, 2005; Scherer, Langenberg, & von Elm, 2007). Although investigators are the primary source of publication bias (Dickersin, 2005), peer reviewers may be biased against manuscripts that counter their expectations or theoretical perspectives (Mahoney, 1977). After acceptance for publication, the studies with significant, positive results are published more rapidly (Hopewell, Clarke, Stewart, & Tierney, 2001) and cited more often (Egger & Smith, 1998). The selective reporting, publication, dissemination, and citation of positive results make them more visible and available than other, equally valid findings. These biases are likely to affect research synthesis unless reviewers take precautions to avoid them (Rothstein, Sutton, & Bornstein, 2005).

The review process is most vulnerable to bias when reviewers sample studies selectively, rely only on published studies, fail to consider variations in study qualities that may affect their validity, and selectively report results. The same biases that affect primary research may be present in a research synthesis. Moreover, the same principles used to minimize bias in primary research apply to the synthesis of research findings. Research synthesis is, after all, a form of research, akin to a survey or observational study of previous research.

## Systematic Reviews

The term *systematic review* refers to "a process involving measures to control biases in research synthesis" (Chalmers, Hedges, & Cooper, 2002, p. 16). Systematic reviews follow basic steps in the research process, using explicit and replicable procedures to minimize bias at each step (Higgins & Green, 2008; Littell, Corcoran, & Pillai, 2008).

### Transparent Intentions and Methods

A protocol for the review is developed in advance, specifying central objectives and methods. Steps and decisions are carefully documented so readers can follow and evaluate reviewers' methods (Moher et al., 1999). Conflicts of interest and sponsorship arrangements are disclosed because these issues can affect reviewers' decisions and conclusions (e.g., Jørgensen, Hilden, & Gøtzsche, 2006).

### Explicit Inclusion and Exclusion Criteria

Reviewers specify, in advance, the study designs, populations, interventions, comparisons, and outcome measures that will be included and excluded.

Reasons for exclusion are documented for each excluded study. This limits reviewers' freedom to select studies on the basis of their results or on some other basis. Systematic reviews have clear boundaries so they can be replicated or extended by others.

## Search Strategies

Reviewers use a systematic approach and a variety of sources to try to locate all potentially material studies. In collaboration with information retrieval specialists, they identify electronic databases and develop appropriate keyword strings to use in each database. Hand searching of the contents of journals is often needed to find eligible studies that are not properly indexed (Hopewell, Clarke, Lefebvre, & Scherer, 2006). Reviewers must make vigorous efforts to locate the *gray literature* (i.e., unpublished and hard-to-find studies) to avoid the file drawer problem (Hopewell, McDonald, Clarke, & Egger, 2006; Rothstein et al., 2005). This involves personal contacts with experts, along with scanning conference abstracts and reference lists. The search process and its results are carefully documented.

## Interrater Agreement on All Key Decisions

Two or more raters review all citations and abstracts. Decisions on full-text retrieval, study inclusion and exclusion, and study coding are made by at least two independent raters. These raters compare notes, resolve differences, and document reasons for their decisions.

## Systematic Extraction of Data From Original Studies

Raters extract data from study reports onto paper or electronic coding forms. These data are then available for use in the analysis and synthesis of results. The data forms provide a bridge between the primary research studies and the research synthesis, and a historical record of reviewers' decisions (Higgins & Green, 2008).

## Analysis of Study Qualities

Aspects of methodology that relate to the validity of a study's conclusions are assessed individually. Reviewers are encouraged to use separate assessments of different study qualities, instead of an overall study quality score. Campbell's threats-to-validity approach is a useful framework in this regard, as is the assessment of potential sources and types of bias in the primary studies (Higgins & Green, 2008). These assessments may be useful in analysis and interpretation of data on treatment effects.

## Analysis of Study Results

Study findings are represented as effect sizes whenever possible. The term *effect size* refers to a group of statistics that express the strength and direction of an effect or relationship between variables. Most effect sizes are standardized to facilitate synthesis of results across studies. Examples include the standardized mean difference (the difference between two group means divided by their pooled standard deviation), odds ratio, risk ratio, and correlation coefficient. Raters document the data and formulas used for effect size calculations.

## Synthesis of Results

Transparent methods are used to combine results across studies. Quantitative methods lend themselves to this purpose. Meta-analysis is a set of statistical techniques used to estimate combined effect sizes, account for variations in the precision of effect size estimates drawn from different samples, explore potential moderators of effects, and examine potential effects of publication bias (Lipsey & Wilson, 2001; Littell et al., 2008). It is noteworthy that some meta-analyses are not embedded in systematic reviews. For example, a meta-analysis of a convenience sample of published studies is not a systematic review. Systematic reviews do not always include meta-analysis.

## Reporting of Results

Moher et al. (1999) developed the Quality of Reporting of Meta-analyses (QUOROM) statement to improve reports on systematic reviews and meta-analyses. The QUOROM statement includes a checklist of items that should be reported and a flow diagram for authors to use to describe how studies were identified, screened, and selected.

## Updating

To remain current and germane for policy and practice, systematic reviews need to be updated regularly. Systematic approaches to reviewing research are not new, nor did they originate in the biomedical sciences (Chalmers et al., 2002; Petticrew & Roberts, 2006). Two international, interdisciplinary collaborations of scholars, policy makers, clinicians, and consumers have emerged to bridge the science and practice of research synthesis. The Cochrane Collaboration produces systematic reviews of studies on effects of interventions in health care (see http://www.cochrane.org). The Campbell Collaboration synthesizes results of interventions in social care (education, social welfare, mental health, and crime and justice; http://www.campbellcollaboration.org). These groups produce guidelines for research synthesis that are based on methodological research where that research is available.

# CURRENT PRACTICE

The practice of research synthesis—as represented by the proliferation of published narrative reviews and lists of EBTs—is not well connected to the science of research synthesis. That is, most research reviews are not informed by the growing body of research on the advantages and disadvantages of different approaches to the identification, analysis, and synthesis of empirical evidence (Littell, 2005). As Chalmers et al. (2002) observed, "science is supposed to be cumulative, but scientists only rarely cumulate evidence scientifically" (p. 12). They noted that academics are usually unaware of the fundamental methodological and practical issues in research synthesis.

Systematic reviews and meta-analyses are becoming more common, but traditional reviews prevail in the social sciences. Many publications that are called systematic reviews or meta-analyses bear little resemblance to standards set by the Cochrane and Campbell Collaborations and the QUOROM statement. Studies of the quality of systematic reviews and meta-analyses exist in the medical literature (e.g., Jadad et al., 2000; Shea, Moher, Graham, Pham, & Tugwell, 2002), but scant attention has been paid to the methods used in reviews in psychology and other social and behavioral sciences.

## A CASE STUDY: THE QUALITY OF PUBLISHED REVIEWS OF AN EVIDENCE-BASED TREATMENT

What criteria and methods have reviewers used to locate, analyze, and synthesize evidence for EBTs? How systematic are these reviews? To find out, I conducted a case study of published reviews of effects of a model program, Multisystemic Therapy (MST). This case was prompted by discrepancies between results of a Cochrane and Campbell systematic review (Littell, Popa, & Forsythe, 2005) and conclusions of prior reviews (Littell, 2005).

MST is a short-term, home- and community-based program that addresses complex psychosocial problems. It also provides alternatives to out-of-home placement for youth with social, emotional, and behavioral problems (Henggeler, Schoenwald, Borduin, Rowland, & Cunningham, 1998; Henggeler, Schoenwald, Rowland, & Cunningham, 2002). It is one of the model programs identified by SAMSHA (2007) and by the Blueprints for Violence Prevention (Henggeler, Mihalic, Rone, Thomas, & Timmons-Mitchell, 1998). MST has been cited as an effective treatment by the National Institute on Drug Abuse (1999, 2003), National Institute of Mental Health (2001), and the Surgeon General's office (U.S. DHHS, 1999, 2001). Licensed MST programs exist in more than 30 states in the United States and in Canada,

Australia, New Zealand, England, Ireland, Norway, Sweden, Denmark, and the Netherlands.

## A Systematic Review

The Cochrane and Campbell review included eight randomized controlled trials (RCTs) of licensed MST programs for youth with social, emotional, and behavioral problems (Littell et al., 2005). Reviewers found problems in some RCTs that had not been previously identified, including discrepancies across published reports, ambiguous or substandard research procedures, and systematic omission of participants who did not complete treatment (inability to support intent-to-treat analysis). Results were synthesized across all studies on 21 distinct outcome measures. These included the following: incarceration, other restrictive out-of-home placements, arrest or conviction, self-reported delinquency, peer relationships, behavior problems, substance use, youth psychiatric symptoms, parent psychiatric symptoms, and family functioning. Forest plots showed results from each study that provided data on an outcome measure (examples are shown in Figures 6.1 and 6.2). Overall (mean) effects were estimated using random effect models.

Results were inconsistent across studies on every outcome measure. No significant differences between MST and treatment as usual were obtained in the largest and most rigorous study: a multi-site trial conducted by independent investigators with full intent-to-treat analysis (Leschied & Cunningham, 2002). The results of this study are public but not published. A few significant effects of MST were found in weaker studies; none of the overall effects were statistically significant.

These results suggest that MST is not consistently better or worse than other services. This does not mean that MST is ineffective. Low statistical power (too few studies) is a plausible explanation for the null results. In any case, these conclusions are contrary to those of many published reviews that claim that the effectiveness of MST is well-established.

## Published Reviews

Elsewhere, I analyzed the methods and conclusions of 37 reviews published after 1996. These reviews cited one or more MST studies, providing some analysis or synthesis of results on effects of MST (Littell, 2008). Most (22) of the 37 reviews relied solely on narrative synthesis of convenience samples of studies. One provided a narrative synthesis on the basis of a systematic search for published studies (Brestan & Eyberg, 1998). Five described studies and their results in tables and text. Three reviews provided study-level effect sizes, five included quantitative synthesis (meta-analysis), and one included

Review: Multisystemic Therapy for social, emotional, and behavioral problems in youth aged 10-17
Comparison: 01 Out-of-home placement
Outcome: 01 Incarceration

| Study or sub-category | Treatment n/N | Control n/N | OR (random) 95% CI | Weight % | OR (random) 95% CI |
|---|---|---|---|---|---|
| 01 Leschied 2002 | 70/211 | 63/198 | | 28.61 | 1.06 [0.70, 1.61] |
| 04 Henggeler 1997 | 31/82 | 37/73 | | 26.00 | 0.59 [0.31, 1.12] |
| 05 Henggeler 1999a | 19/58 | 16/60 | | 24.00 | 1.34 [0.61, 2.96] |
| 06 Henggeler 1992 | 9/43 | 28/41 | | 21.39 | 0.12 [0.05, 0.33] |
| Total (95% CI) | 394 | 372 | | 100.00 | 0.61 [0.27, 1.39] |

Total events: 129 (Treatment), 144 (Control)
Test for heterogeneity: Chi² = 18.18, df = 3 (P = 0.0004), I² = 83.5%
Test for overall effect: Z = 1.18 (P = 0.24)

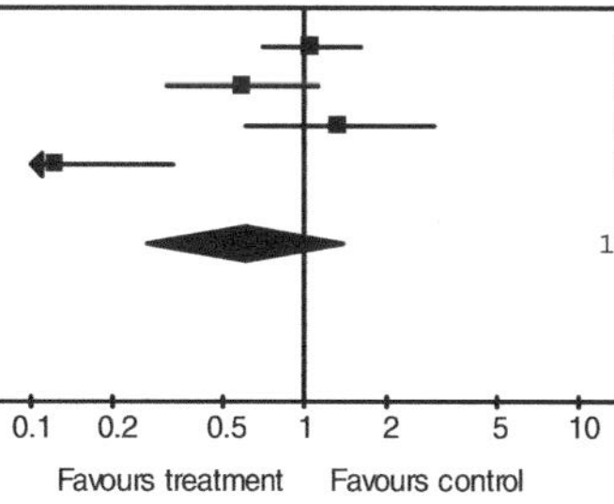

0.1 0.2 0.5 1 2 5 10

Favours treatment    Favours control

*Figure 6.1.* Effects of multisystemic therapy (MST) on the odds of incarceration. Adapted from "Multisystemic Therapy for Social, Emotional, and Behavioral Problems in Youth Aged 10–17," by J. H. Littell, M. Popa, & B. Forsythe, 2005, *Cochrane Database of Systematic Reviews*, Issue 4, Art. No. CD004797, doi: 10.1002/14651858.cd004797.pub4. Copyright 2005 by Cochrane Collaboration. Used with permission.

Review:  Multisystemic Therapy for social, emotional, and behavioral problems in youth aged 10-17
Comparison:  09 Family functioning
Outcome:  02 FACES Adaptability

| Study or sub-category | N | Treatment Mean (SD) | N | Control Mean (SD) | SMD (random) 95% CI | Weight % | SMD (random) 95% CI |
|---|---|---|---|---|---|---|---|
| 03 Henggeler 1999b | 57 | 22.40 (6.85) | 56 | 23.10 (6.20) | | 21.35 | -0.11 [-0.48, 0.26] |
| 04 Henggeler 1997 | 75 | 29.00 (5.02) | 65 | 29.75 (4.21) | | 23.32 | -0.16 [-0.49, 0.17] |
| 06 Henggeler 1992 | 33 | -0.32 (1.79) | 23 | -0.67 (1.27) | | 14.29 | 0.22 [-0.32, 0.75] |
| 07 Borduin 1995 | 70 | 0.13 (0.86) | 56 | -0.16 (0.71) | | 22.13 | 0.36 [0.01, 0.72] |
| 08 Ogden 2004 | 61 | 25.96 (3.95) | 35 | 27.43 (4.80) | | 18.91 | -0.34 [-0.76, 0.08] |
| Total (95% CI) | 296 | | 235 | | | 100.00 | -0.01 [-0.27, 0.24] |

Test for heterogeneity: Chi² = 8.36, df = 4 (P = 0.08), I² = 52.1%
Test for overall effect: Z = 0.10 (P = 0.92)

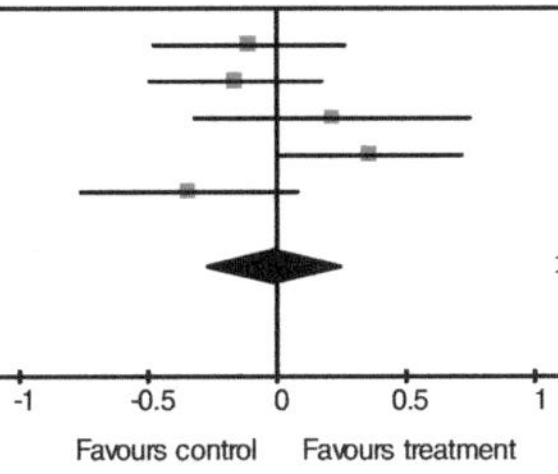

-1 -0.5 0 0.5 1
Favours control Favours treatment

*Figure 6.2.* Effects of Multisystemic Therapy (MST) on the Family Adaptability and Cohesion Evaluation Scales family adaptability scores Adapted from "Multisystemic Therapy for Social, Emotional, and Behavioral Problems in Youth Aged 10–17," by J. H. Littell, M. Popa, & B. Forsythe, 2005, *Cochrane Database of Systematic Reviews*, Issue 4, Art. No. CD004797, doi: 10.1002/14651858.cd004797.pub4. Copyright 2005 by Cochrane Collaboration. Used with permission.

both meta-analysis and cost–benefit analysis (Aos, Phipps, Barnoski, & Lieb, 2001).

Only eight reviews used explicit inclusion or exclusion criteria. Nine used systematic keyword searches of electronic databases. Most distinguished randomized and nonrandomized studies, but variations in study quality within these categories rarely were considered.

Several reviews summarized evidence in tables of key findings or selected outcomes. In some, evidence was organized by outcome domains, and tables showed which studies provided evidence of favorable effects on outcomes for MST (e.g., Corcoran, 2003). Others organized the evidence by study, highlighting positive results from each (e.g., Burns, Schoenwald, Burchard, Faw, & Santos, 2000; Henggeler et al., 2002). Notably, null results and negative effects were not mentioned in these summaries. A similar approach was used in some narrative syntheses (e.g., Henggeler & Sheidow, 2003; Letourneau, Cunningham, & Henggeler, 2002). Several reviews reported the number of studies that showed statistically significant differences favoring the MST group on one or more outcome measures (e.g., Burns et al., 1999; Miller, Johnson, Sandberg, Stringer-Seibold, & Gfeller-Strouts, 2000; U.S. DHHS, 1999). The practice of highlighting positive or favorable outcomes is an example of *confirmation bias*, the tendency to emphasize results that confirm a hypothesis and ignore evidence to the contrary (see Nickerson, 1988).

Considerable variation was seen in the methods used and studies included in the reviews, with more consistency in their conclusions. Several reviews classified MST as a "probably efficacious" treatment according to Chambless et al.'s (1998) criteria mentioned earlier (Brestan & Eyberg, 1998; Burns, 2003; Burns et al., 1999, 2000; Chorpita et al., 2002). Nine reviews provided a caveat about the evidence (e.g., results were not well-established, appeared related to fidelity, and had not been replicated by independent teams). Only three mentioned negative or null effects in their conclusions (Farrington & Welsh, 2003; Swenson & Henggeler, 2003; Woolfenden, Williams, & Peat, 2003). Most (25) reviews offered unqualified support for MST.

Because all reviews included studies that had mixed results, it is uncertain whether or how these results were factored into reviewers' conclusions. How did reviewers determine whether positive results outweighed negative or null findings, especially when they did not use quantitative methods to pool results across studies? The next section takes a closer look at these issues.

## Research Reports and Reviews: Lost in Translation?

There is one published RCT of the effects of MST in a sample of families of abused or neglected children (Brunk, Henggeler, & Whelan, 1987). This study was not included in the Cochrane and Campbell review (Littell et al.,

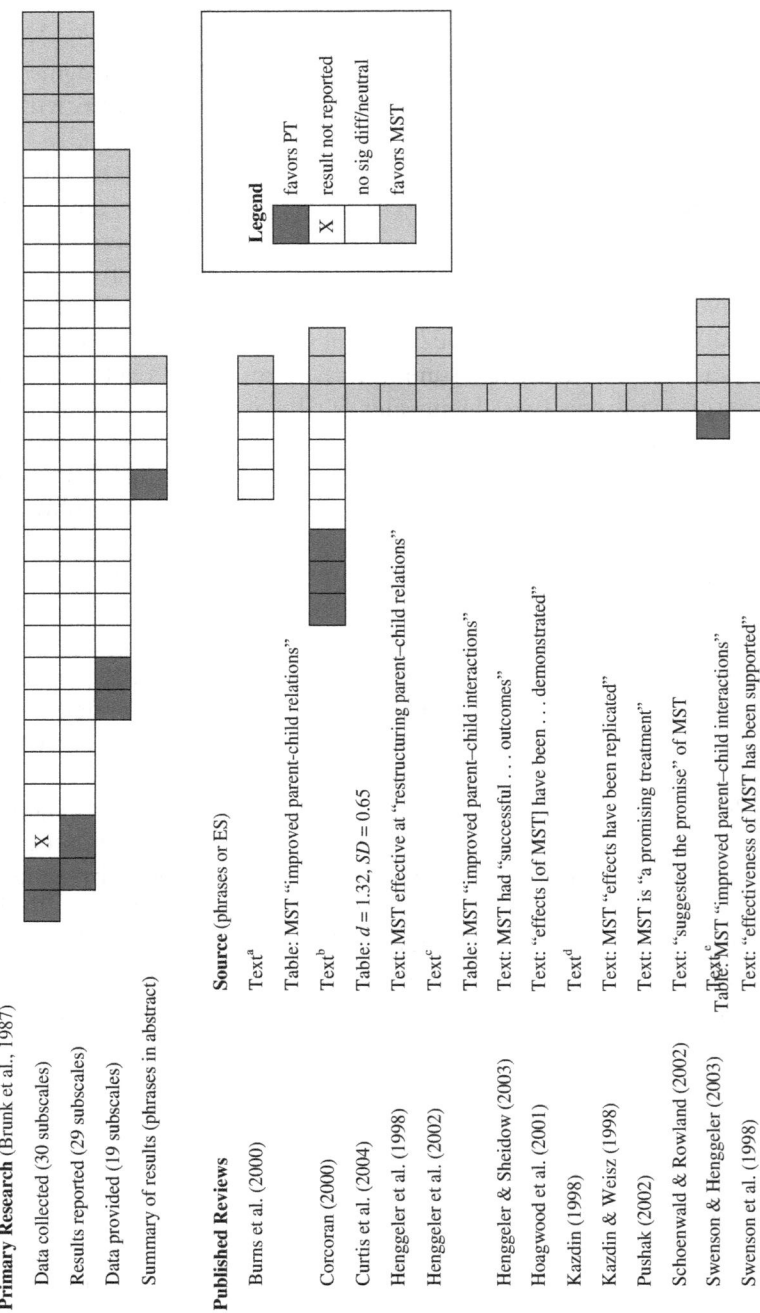

**Primary Research** (Brunk et al., 1987)

Data collected (30 subscales)

Results reported (29 subscales)

Data provided (19 subscales)

Summary of results (phrases in abstract)

**Published Reviews**          **Source** (phrases or ES)

Burns et al. (2000)            Text[a]

                               Table: MST "improved parent–child relations"

Corcoran (2000)                Text[b]

Curtis et al. (2004)           Table: $d = 1.32$, $SD = 0.65$

Henggeler et al. (1998)        Text: MST effective at "restructuring parent–child relations"

Henggeler et al. (2002)        Text[c]

                               Table: MST "improved parent–child interactions"

Henggeler & Sheidow (2003)     Text: MST had "successful . . . outcomes"

Hoagwood et al. (2001)         Text: "effects [of MST] have been . . . demonstrated"

Kazdin (1998)                  Text[d]

Kazdin & Weisz (1998)          Text: MST "effects have been replicated"

Pushak (2002)                  Text: MST is "a promising treatment"

Schoenwald & Rowland (2002)    Text: "suggested the promise" of MST

Swenson & Henggeler (2003)     Table[c]: MST "improved parent–child interactions"

Swenson et al. (1998)          Text: "effectiveness of MST has been supported"

*Figure 6.3.* Results and reviews of Brunk, Henggeler, and Whelan (1987). ES = effect size; PT = parent training; no sig diff = no significant difference. [a]"Parents in both groups reported decreases in psychiatric symptomatology and *(Continues)*

2005) because the main effects of MST could not be calculated from available data. Brunk et al.'s (1987) study was cited by published reviews as evidence for the effectiveness of MST in cases of child maltreatment. To understand how reviewers arrived at this conclusion, I conducted a content analysis of Brunk et al.'s study and published reviews that cited this study (Littell, 2008). Results are illustrated in Figure 6.3.

In Brunk et al.'s (1987) study, 43 families were randomly assigned to MST or parent training (PT) groups. Immediate posttreatment outcome data were reported for 33 (77%) of these families. Mean scores were presented for subgroups of abuse cases and neglect cases. Brunk and colleagues reported that they collected data on 30 measures or subscales (client self-reports on 16 items, therapist reports on 3 measures, and 11 observational measures of parent–child interactions). Results were reported on 29 of the 30 measures; subgroup means were provided for 19. As shown in the top portion of Figure 6.3, the pattern of results was mixed. Two comparisons (one self-report and one observational measure) favored PT, five observational measures favored MST, and the rest showed no significant differences between groups overall. The investigators described results in the abstract of the article as follows:

> Families who received either treatment showed decreased parental psychiatric symptomology, reduced overall stress, and a reduction in the severity of identified problems. Analyses of sequential observational mea-

---

*(Continued)*

reduced overall stress. . . . both groups demonstrated decreases in the severity of the identified problems. . . . [MST] improved [parent–child] interactions, implying a decreased risk for maltreatment of children in the MST condition" (p. 293). [b]"Both approaches acted to reduce psychiatric symptoms in parents and parental stress, as well as to alleviate individual and family problems. . . . [MST] was more effective in improving parent-child interactions, helping physically abusive parents manage child behavior, and assisting neglectful parents in responding more appropriately to their child's needs. Surprisingly, [PT] was more advantageous for improving parents' social lives. The hypothesis is the group setting for parent training reduced isolation and improved parents' support system." (p. 568). [c]"MST has consistently produced improvements in family functioning across outcome studies with juvenile offenders and maltreating families. Several of these studies used observational methods to demonstrate increased positive family interactions and decreased negative interactions" (p. 209). [d]"[MST] outcome studies have extended to . . . parents who engage in physical abuse or neglect. . . . Thus, the model of providing treatment may have broad applicability across problem domains among seriously disturbed children" (p. 79). [e]"MST was more effective than [PT] for improving parent-child interactions associated with maltreatment. Abusive parents showed greater progress in controlling their child's behavior, maltreated children exhibited less passive noncompliance, and neglecting parents became more responsive to their child's behavior. [PT] was superior to MST [in] decreasing social problems (i.e., social support network)" (pp. 75–76).

sures revealed that multisystemic therapy was more effective than parent training at restructuring parent–child relations. Parent training was more effective than multisystemic therapy at reducing identified social problems. The differential influences of the two treatments were probably associated with differences in their respective treatment contexts and epistemologies. (Brunk et al., 1987, p. 171)

The coding of this passage is shown in Figure 6.3. There are five distinct phrases describing outcomes: One favors PT, three phrases (in the first sentence) indicate similarities between groups, and one phrase favors MST. This is a balanced abstract.

Now consider how the results of this small RCT are characterized in later, published reviews. The bottom portion of Figure 6.3 shows coding of phrases used to describe results of Brunk et al.'s (1987) study in the tables and text of 13 published reviews. Of the 37 reviews analyzed above, these are the only reviews that provided specific comments on the results of Brunk et al.'s study. Most reviewers emphasized statistically significant differences that favored the MST group. In fact, 11 of 13 reviews used a single number or phrase (in the text or tables) to characterize results of this study. All 11 indicate that MST had favorable outcomes.

Figure 6.3 shows three trends as research results are reported and reviewed. The first pattern is data reduction; the number of comparisons is reduced from 30 to a smaller, more manageable number. Second, there is an apparent reduction in uncertainty, as many of the null results were underreported in the original study and ignored in most reviews. Finally, reviewers highlighted positive results that confirm expected effects of MST; this is a clear example of confirmation bias.

## Selective Citation and Repetition

In addition to the 37 reviews described above, I found 19 that relied primarily (or solely) on other reviews (Littell, 2008). These include often-cited reviews by Lehman, Goldman, Dixon, and Churchill (2004), Mihalic et al. (2004), the Office of the Surgeon General (U.S. DHHS, 2001) and the NIH State-of-the-Science Conference Statement on Preventing Violence (National Institutes of Health [NIH], 2004). Frequent repetition of the same conclusions may be mistaken for replication.

The NIH statement cited the Blueprints group as their source of information on effective treatments and concluded that MST "evaluations demonstrated reductions in long-term rates of rearrest, violent crime arrest, and out-of-home placements" and "positive results were maintained for nearly 4 years after treatment ended" (NIH, 2004, p. 12). The statement did not mention negative or null results, nor did it indicate that only one study had a multiyear follow-up. Moreover, the NIH statement did not rely on the systematic review that was commissioned especially for its purposes. Produced by independent authors (under a contract with the U.S. AHRQ), that review did not assess effects of specific interventions because the number of studies was too small to detect differences between programs (L. S. Chan et al., 2004).

Critical appraisal of the research base for EBTs is scant, but MST and Brunk et al.'s (1987) study are not unique. Gorman and others have criticized research on school-based drug abuse and violence prevention programs that appear on many lists of EBTs. Additionally, Gorman identified problems similar to those found in MST trials, including substandard research practices that compromised the internal validity of RCTs (Gorman, 2002, 2003a, 2003b, 2005a). Gandhi, Murphy-Graham, Petrosino, Chrismer, and Weiss (2006) found a low threshold for evidence of effectiveness.

## Evidence, Experts, and Orthodoxy

Questions about the scientific bases of EBTs have been met with appeals to consensus and authority, resistance to criticism, outright hostility, and ad hominem responses (Gorman, 2003a, 2003b, 2005c; Littell, 2006). Gorman (2005b) argued that some proponents of EBTs are "abandoning the critical underpinnings of science in favor of verification and affirmation . . . [which] leads to intellectual stagnation and dogma." These conditions are antithetical to serious empirical inquiry, practice-based research, and EBP.

Researchers must distinguish empirical evidence from expert opinion. That is difficult to do when experts claim their opinions are based on sound scientific evidence and when their conclusions are often repeated and endorsed by others. Sackett (2000) said that too many experts impede the healthy advancement of science. It is interesting that he stopped writing about EBM after he discovered the term *Sackettisation* had been coined to connote "the artificial linkage of a publication to the evidence based medicine movement in order to improve sales" (Sackett, 2000, p. 1283). Equally important, researchers must critically appraise evidentiary claims and be wary of experts, junk science, and pseudoscience. Pseudoscience sells. It appeals to the desire for quick fixes and certainty, whereas science leaves probability and doubt (Tavris, 2003).

It is inevitable that the dialectic between EBP and EBTs involves power and influence. Each approach enhances the power, influence, and wealth of some individuals and groups, reducing that of others. EBP "directly challenges the authority of expert opinion" and is "a threat to the power of consultants" (Lipman, 2000, p. 557). The drive to implement EBTs provides new funding opportunities for promoters of EBTs (e.g., in the form of research grants to study knowledge transfer, transportability, and implementation). The linkage of federal, state, and private insurance (managed care) resources to the provision of EBTs restricts practice. This is the creation of orthodoxy.

## DISCUSSION AND CONCLUSIONS

There are two fundamentally different approaches to EBP. One emphasizes processes clinicians can use to integrate empirical evidence with clinical expertise and client preferences to make informed judgments in individual cases (EBP). The other seeks to identify treatments that are effective for specific conditions and ensure the widespread availability of these treatments (EBTs).

The EBP and EBT movements share a common weakness: reliance on unscientific syntheses of evidence about treatment effects. These syntheses are vulnerable to biases that may pose a threat to the validity of EBTs. EBP may be less affected because it considers other sources of evidence. Published reviews and lists of EBTs are based on outdated methods of research synthesis. The previous section demonstrated that evidence available to advocates of EBP and EBTs is tainted by publication, dissemination, and confirmation biases. The extent of these problems is not known, but there is cause for concern about the state of the science.

Greenwood (2006) called for a new culture of accountability that rewards the production and replication of valid evidence, instead of novelty and promotional efforts. The emphasis on novelty (statistically significant results that confirm new hypotheses) distorts the scientific literature. In fact, Ioannidis (2005a) showed that 32% of the most widely cited medical studies in high impact journals did not hold up in later studies (44% were replicated, and another 24% remained unchallenged). He then showed that it is likely that most published research findings are false (Ioannidis, 2005b). Chalmers et al. (2002) predicted that soon the public will begin to ask why it has taken academia so long to begin to practice scientific self-discipline. Why do researchers not routinely make raw data public and available for systematic reviews?

Concerns about the problems that plague the development and dissemination of scientific knowledge—selective reporting, publication bias, lack of critical appraisal, and lack of transparency—have led to several strategies for improving the state of the science. These include the following: standards for reporting results of clinical trials (Moher, Schultz, Altman, & the CONSORT Group, 2001), systematic reviews and meta-analyses (Moher et al., 1999), and other types of studies; development and application of methods to detect data fabrication (Al-Marzouki, Evans, Marshall, & Roberts, 2005); requirements for prospective registration of clinical trials before data collection as a condition of publication in scientific journals (De Angelis et al., 2004); and development of a global platform for prospective registers of treatment research (World Health Organization, 2006).

Recent emphasis on EBP may have increased the demand for scientific evidence of intervention effects, but it has done little to increase the supply. Policymakers could fund more rigorous research and syntheses, instead of scores of unscientific reviews of a handful of available studies. Attempts to achieve some consensus on "what works" based on "what we already know" led to adoption of a very low threshold for EBTs (Gandhi et al., 2006; Jensen, Weersing, Hoagwood, & Goldman, 2005). The standard of accepting two studies with positive results on virtually any outcome measure is too low. More than two studies are needed to establish credible evidence of effects (Gandhi et al., 2006). Indeed, effect sizes for mental health treatments decrease with the accumulation of studies over time (Trikalinos et al., 2004). Too little attention has been paid to possible adverse effects of mental health treatments (Papanikolaou, Churchill, Wahlbeck, & Ioannidis, 2004), and there has been far too little critical appraisal of the evidence for EBTs.

This erosion of standards of evidence may be a natural outcome when groups feel pressure to make definitive statements on the basis of insufficient evidence. Such statements may be made to demonstrate expertise and authority and to gain or maintain control over resources. Campbell (1988) noted that when policymakers asked them what to do, social scientists would respond with far greater assurances than the data warrant. Promoters of EBTs have fallen into the overadvocacy trap Campbell identified. This has hidden costs.

If orthodox assurances about EBTs do not hold up—and there is reason to think they will not—a backlash against EBP and EBTs may occur. This could have lasting negative impacts on practice and policy, but it is understandable. Why should practitioners and policy makers trust purveyors of biased evidence? How does our track record compare with that of pharmaceutical companies?

Other opportunity costs of the EBT movement relate to premature closure of inquiry, including the belief that EBTs, once identified, "are not likely to lose their status, that is, be removed from the list" (Kazdin, 2004, p. 552). Insufficient attention has been paid to interventions that are not yet tested, and there is a failure to attend to the influence of common factors in studies of EBTs (Hubble et al., 1999; Jensen et al., 2005; Wampold, 2001).[1]

In conclusion, wide-scale adoption of EBTs is scientifically premature (Garske & Anderson, 2003) and may waste valuable resources. EBP cannot become a reality until social scientists and policymakers adopt safeguards that

[1]It is not clear whether publication bias and confirmation bias are serious threats to the validity of syntheses of research on the common factors of therapy, but there is reason for concern here. Meta-analyses of studies of therapeutic relationship variables have relied on published journal articles.

ensure complete reporting and open, critical appraisal of scientific evidence. This is consistent with our ethical obligations to clients and the public right to know about all the results of all studies that involve human participants (De Angelis et al., 2004).

## IMPLICATIONS

EBP models can provide useful guidance about how to ask and answer clinically relevant questions, how to identify and critically appraise relevant research and research reviews, and how to incorporate empirical evidence along with other considerations (such as client values) to make good practice decisions. Gibbs (2003) and others (e.g., Straus, Richardson, Glaziou, & Haynes, 2005) have provided detailed suggestions in this regard. Some general principles for clinicians are as follows.

- Evidence from multiple studies is always preferred to results of a single study. Systematic reviews of research are preferable to traditional narrative reviews. Thus, clinicians should look for systematic reviews, mindful of the fact that these reviews vary in quality.
- The Cochrane and Campbell Collaborations are good sources of high-quality systematic reviews. Clinicians can and should assess potential sources of bias in any review. The characteristics of systematic reviews described in this chapter can be used as a yardstick that clinicians can use to judge how well specific reviews measure up. The QUOROM statement (Moher et al., 1999) provides guidance about what to look for in reports on systematic reviews, as does a recent report by Shea et al. (2007).
- When relevant reviews are not available, out of date, or potentially biased, clinicians can identify individual studies and assess the credibility of those studies, using one of many tools developed for this purpose (e.g., Gibbs, 2003). It would be ideal if clinicians were able to rely on others to produce valid research syntheses.
- Above all, clinicians should remember that critical thinking is crucial to understanding and using evidence. Authorities, expert opinion, and lists of ESTs provide insufficient evidence for sound clinical practice. Further, clinicians must determine how credible evidence relates to the particular needs, values, preferences, circumstances, and ultimately, the responses of their clients.

Clinicians and researchers also need to have an effect on policy so that EBP is not interpreted in a way that unfairly restricts treatments.

- Policymakers and others can be educated about the nature of EBP. EBP is a process aimed at informing the choices that clinicians make. It should inform and enhance practice, "increasing, not dictating, choice" (Dickersin, Straus, & Bero, 2007, p. s10). EBP supports choices among alternative treatments that have similar effects. It supports the choice of a less effective alternative, when an effective treatment is not acceptable to a client.
- Policymakers and others can be educated about the nature of evidence and methods of research synthesis. Empirical evidence is tentative, and it evolves over time as new information is added to the knowledge base. At present, there is insufficient evidence about the effectiveness of most psychological and psychosocial treatments (including some so-called empirically supported treatments). Policymakers need to understand that most lists of effective treatments are not based on rigorous systematic reviews; thus, they are not necessarily based on sound evidence. It makes little sense to base policy decisions on lists of preferred treatments because this limits consumer choice.
- Lists of selected or preferred treatments should not restrict the use of other potentially effective treatments. Policies that restrict treatments that have been shown to be harmful or ineffective, however, are of benefit. Lists of harmful or wasteful treatments could be compiled to discourage their use.

## QUESTIONS FROM THE EDITORS

*1. Given the concerns about the dissemination of incorrect conclusions, is it time for greater oversight of publications? That is, is the peer review system as currently practiced flawed?*

Publication and dissemination biases have been recognized for decades (for reviews, see Dickersin, 2005; Torgerson, 2006). Flaws in the peer review system are also well documented. I think a peer review system is necessary, but the current system has not been sufficient to prevent widespread bias against findings that are not statistically significant and those that contradict prevailing beliefs. Journal editors should pay much more attention to this problem and devise ways to ensure that null and negative results are reviewed fairly.

The problem extends well beyond publication practices, however. Incorrect information is disseminated by government agencies, professional organizations, experts, and others through many formal and informal channels. I see two solutions to this problem. First, consumer education can enhance critical appraisal skills so that policymakers, practitioners, and clients can judge evidence on its merits. Second, radical changes are needed in the norms and practices of science. These include the routine registration of studies in prospective registers so that the public has access to information about data collection and increased scrutiny of micro (raw) data. In my view, raw data should be available to other investigators for reanalysis, particularly when these data have been gathered with public funds.

2. *Proponents of EBTs often argue that treatment fidelity improves outcomes. Did your analysis of MST address the fidelity–outcome claim?*

Yes, but perceived fidelity is confounded with the relationship between program developers and evaluators. That is, programs evaluated by their developers are reported (by the developers) to have higher fidelity than those evaluated by independent investigators. In the absence of valid, independently verifiable data on fidelity, it is not possible to determine whether differences in outcomes may be due to fidelity or allegiance bias (for further discussion, see Littell, 2006, 2008).

## REFERENCES

Aarons, G. A. (2006). Transformational and transactional leadership: Association with attitudes toward evidence-based practice. *Psychiatric Services, 57,* 1162–1169.

Al-Marzouki, S., Evans, S., Marshall, T., & Roberts, I. (2005). Are these data real? Statistical methods for the detection of data fabrication in clinical trials. *British Medical Journal, 331,* 267–270.

American Psychological Association. (1996). *Guidelines and principles for accreditation of programs in professional psychology.* Washington, DC: Author.

American Psychological Association Presidential Task Force on Evidence-Based Practice. (2006). Evidence-based practice in psychology. *American Psychologist, 61,* 271–285.

Aos S., Phipps, P., Barnoski, R., & Lieb, R. (2001). *The comparative costs and benefits of programs to reduce crime* (Version 4.0, Document Number 01-05-1201). Olympia: Washington State Institute for Public Policy.

Brestan, E. V., & Eyberg, S. M. (1998). Effective psychosocial treatments of conduct-disordered children and adolescents: 29 years, 82 studies, and 5,272 kids. *Journal of Clinical Child Psychology, 27,* 180–189.

Brunk, M., Henggeler, S. W., & Whelan, J. P. (1987). A comparison of multisystemic therapy and parent training in the brief treatment of child abuse and neglect. *Journal of Consulting and Clinical Psychology, 55,* 171–178.

Burns, B. J. (2003). Children and evidence-based practice. *Psychiatric Clinics of North America, 26,* 955–870.

Burns, B. J., Hoagwood, K., & Mrazek, P. J. (1999). Effective treatment for mental disorders in children and adolescents. *Clinical Child and Family Psychology Review, 2*, 199–244.

Burns, B. J., Schoenwald, S. K., Burchard, J. D., Faw, L., & Santos, A. B. (2000). Comprehensive community-based interventions for youth with severe emotional disorders: Multisystemic Therapy and the wraparound process. *Journal of Child and Family Studies, 9*, 283–314.

Bushman, B. J., & Wells, G. L. (2001). Narrative impressions of literature: The availability bias and the corrective properties of meta-analytic approaches. *Personal and Social Psychology Bulletin, 27*, 1123–1130.

Campbell, D. T. (1988). The experimenting society. In E. S. Overman (Ed.), *Methodology and epistemology for social science: Selected papers* (pp. 290–314). Chicago: University of Chicago Press.

Carlton, P. L., & Strawderman, W. E. (1996). Evaluating cumulated research: I. The inadequacy of traditional methods. *Biological Psychiatry, 39*, 65–72.

Centers for Disease Control and Prevention. (2007). *Request for proposals: Improving public health practice through translation research* (Funding Opportunity Announcement RFA-CD-07-005). Retrieved July 6, 2009, from http://grants.nih.gov/grants/guide/rfa-files/RFA-CD-07-005.html

Chalmers, I., Hedges, L. V., & Cooper, H. (2002). A brief history of research synthesis. *Evaluation & the Health Professions, 25*, 12–37.

Chambless, D. L., Baker, M. J., Baucom, D. H., Beutler, L. E., Calhoun, K. S., Crits-Christoph P., et al. (1998). Update on empirically validated therapies: II. *The Clinical Psychologist, 51*, 3–16.

Chambless, D. L., & Ollendick, T. H. (2001). Empirically supported psychological interventions: Controversies and evidence. *Annual Review of Psychology, 52*, 685–716.

Chan, A. W., Hróbjartsson, A., Haar, M. T., Gøtzsche, P. C., & Altman, D. G. (2004). Empirical evidence for selective reporting of outcomes in randomized trials: Comparison of protocols to published articles. *JAMA, 291*, 2457–2465.

Chan, L. S., Kipke, M. D., Schneir, A., Iverson, E., Warf, C., Limbos, M. A., et al. (2004). *Preventing violence and related health-risking social behaviors in adolescents* (AHRQ Publication No. 04-E032-2). Rockville, MD: Agency for Healthcare Research and Quality.

Chorpita, B. F., Yim, L. M., Donkervoet, J. C., Arensdorf, A., Amundsen, M. J., McGee, C., et al. (2002). Toward large-scale implementation of empirically supported treatments for children: A review and observations by the Hawaii empirical basis to services task force. *Clinical Psychology: Science and Practice, 9*, 165–190.

Corcoran, J. (2000). Family interventions with child physical abuse and neglect: A critical review. *Children and Youth Services Review, 22*, 563–591.

Corcoran, J. (2003). *Clinical applications of evidence-based family interventions*. New York: Oxford University Press.

Curtis, N. M., Ronan, K. R., & Borduin, C. M. (2004). Multisystemic treatment: A meta-analysis of outcome studies. *Journal of Family Psychology, 18*, 411–419.

Davies, P. (2004, February). *Evidence-based government . . . Is it possible?* Paper presented at the 4th Annual Campbell Collaboration Colloquium, Washington, DC.

De Angelis, C., Drazen, J. M., Frizelle, F. A., Haug, C., Hoey, J., Horton, R., et al. (2004). Clinical trial registration: A statement from the International Committee of Medical Journal Editors. *New England Journal of Medicine, 351*, 1250–1251.

Dickersin, K. (2005). Publication bias: Recognizing the problem, understanding its origins and scope, and preventing harm. In H. R. Rothstein, A. J. Sutton, & M. Borenstein (Eds.), *Publication bias in meta-analysis: Prevention, assessment, and adjustments* (pp. 11–33). Chichester, England: Wiley.

Dickersin, K., Straus, S. E., & Bero, L. (2007). Evidence based medicine: Increasing, not dictating, choice. *British Medical Journal, 334*, s10.

Egger, M., & Smith, G. D. (1998). Bias in location and selection of studies. *British Medical Journal, 316*, 61–66.

Farrington, D. P., & Welsh, B. C. (2003). Family-based prevention of offending: A meta-analysis. *Australian and New Zealand Journal of Criminology, 36*, 127–151.

Flay, B. R., Biglan, A., Boruch, R. F., Castro, F. G., Gottfredson, D., Kellam, S., et al. (2005). Standards of evidence: Criteria for efficacy, effectiveness and dissemination. *Prevention Science, 6*, 151–175.

Gambrill, E. (2006). Evidence-based practice and policy: Choices ahead. *Research on Social Work Practice, 16*, 338–357.

Gandhi, A. G., Murphy-Graham, E., Petrosino, A., Chrismer, S. S., & Weiss, C. H. (2006). The devil is in the details: Examining the evidence for "proven" school-based drug abuse prevention programs. *Evaluation Review, 31*, 43–74.

Ganju, V. (2003). Implementation of evidence-based practices in state mental health systems: Implications for research and effectiveness studies. *Schizophrenia Bulletin, 29*, 125–131.

Garske, J. P., & Anderson, T. (2003). Toward a science of psychotherapy research: Present status and evaluation. In S. O. Lilienfeld, S. J. Lynn, & J. M. Lohr (Eds.), *Science and pseudoscience in clinical psychology* (pp. 145–175). New York: Guilford Press.

Gibbs, L. E. (2003). *Evidence-based practice for the helping professions: A practical guide with integrated multimedia.* Pacific Grove, CA: Brooks/Cole-Thompson Learning.

Gibbs, L., & Gambrill, E. (2002). Evidence-based practice: Counterarguments to objections. *Research on Social Work Practice, 12*, 452–476.

Gorman, D. M. (2002). The "science" of drug and alcohol prevention: The case of the randomized trial of the Life Skills Training program. *International Journal of Drug Policy, 13*, 21–26.

Gorman, D. M. (2003a, February/March). Prevention programs and scientific nonsense. *Policy Review*, 65–75.

Gorman, D. M. (2003b). The best of practices, the worst of practices: The making of science-based primary prevention programs. *Psychiatric Services, 54*, 1087–1089.

Gorman, D. M. (2005a). Does measurement dependence explain the effects of the Life Skills Training program on smoking outcomes? *Preventive Medicine, 40*, 479–487.

Gorman, D. M. (2005b). Drug and violence prevention: Rediscovering the critical rational dimension of evaluation research. *Journal of Experimental Criminology, 1*, 39–62.

Gorman, D. M. (2005c). The centrality of critical rational reasoning in science: A response and further comments on the Life Skills Training program, the Seattle Social Development Project, and prevention studies. *Journal of Experimental Criminology, 1*, 263–275.

Greenwood, P. W. (2006). *Changing lives: Delinquency prevention as crime-control policy*. Chicago: The University of Chicago Press.

Henggeler, S. W., Mihalic, S. F., Rone, L., Thomas, C., & Timmons-Mitchell, J. (1998). *Blueprints for Violence Prevention: Book Six. Multisystemic therapy*. Boulder, CO: Center for the Study and Prevention of Violence.

Henggeler, S. W., Schoenwald, S. K., Borduin, C. M., Rowland, M. D., & Cunningham, P. B. (1998). *Multisystemic treatment of antisocial behavior in children and adolescents*. New York: Guilford Press.

Henggeler, S. W., Schoenwald, S. K., Rowland, M. D., & Cunningham, P. B. (2002). *Serious emotional disturbances in children and adolescents: Multisystemic therapy*. New York: Guilford Press.

Henggeler, S. W., & Sheidow, A. J. (2003). Conduct disorder and delinquency. *Journal of Marital and Family Therapy, 29*, 505–522.

Higgins J. P. T., & Green, S. (Eds.). (2008). Cochrane handbook for systematic reviews of interventions (Version 5). Retrieved July 6, 2009, from http://www.cochrane-handbook.org/

Hoagwood, K., Burns, B. J., Kiser, L., Ringeisen, H., & Schoenwald, S. K. (2001). Evidence-based practice in child and adolescent mental health services. *Psychiatric Services, 52*, 1179–1189.

Hopewell, S., Clarke, M., Lefebvre, C., & Scherer, R. (2006). Handsearching versus electronic searching to identify reports of randomized trials. *Cochrane Database of Systematic Reviews*, Issue 4, Art. No. 000001. doi: 10.1002/14651858.mr000001.pub2

Hopewell, S., Clarke, M., Stewart, L., & Tierney, J. (2001). Time to publication for results of clinical trials. *Cochrane Database of Methodology Reviews*, Issue 3, Art. No. MR000011. doi: 000010.001002/14651858.mr14000011

Hopewell, S., McDonald, S., Clarke, M., & Egger, M. (2006). Grey literature in meta-analyses of randomized trials of health care interventions. *Cochrane Data-*

base of *Systematic Reviews*, Issue 2, Art No. MR000010. doi: 10.102/14651858. mr000010.pub3

Hubble, M. A., Duncan, B. L., & Miller, S. D. (1999). *The heart and soul of change: What works in therapy.* Washington, DC: American Psychological Association.

Ioannidis, J. P. (2005a). Contradicted and initially stronger effects in highly cited clinical research. *JAMA, 294,* 218–228.

Ioannidis, J. P. (2005b). Why most published research findings are false. *PLoS Medicine, 2*(8), e124.

Jadad, A. R., Moher, M., Browman, G. P., Booker, L., Sigouin, C., Fuentes, M., et al. (2000). Systematic reviews and meta-analyses on treatment of asthma: Critical evaluation. *British Medical Journal, 320,* 537–540.

Jensen, P. S., Weersing, R., Hoagwood, K. E., & Goldman, E. (2005). What is the evidence for evidence-based treatments? A hard look at our soft underbelly. *Mental Health Services Research, 7,* 53–74.

Jørgensen, A. W., Hilden, J., & Gøtzsche, P. G. (2006). Cochrane reviews compared with industry supported meta-analyses and other meta-analyses of the same drugs: Systematic review. *British Medical Journal, 333,* 782–785.

Kazdin, A. E. (1998). Psychosocial treatments for conduct disorder in children. In P. E. Nathan & J. M. Gorman (Eds.), *A guide to treatments that work* (pp. 65–89). New York: Oxford University Press.

Kazdin, A. E. (2004). Psychotherapy for children and adolescents. In M. J. Lambert (Ed.), *Bergin and Garfield's handbook of psychotherapy and behavior change* (5th ed., pp. 543–589). New York: Wiley.

Kazdin, A. E., & Weisz, J. R. (1998). Identifying and developing empirically supported child and adolescent treatments. *Journal of Consulting and Clinical Psychology, 66,* 19–36.

Lehman, A. F., Goldman, H. H., Dixon, L. B., & Churchill, R. (2004). *Evidence-based mental health treatments and services: Examples to inform public policy.* New York: Milbank Memorial Fund.

Leschied, A. W., & Cunningham, A. (2002). Seeking effective interventions for young offenders: Interim results of a four-year randomized study of multisystemic therapy in Ontario, Canada. London, Ontario, Canada: Centre for Children and Families in the Justice System.

Letourneau, E. J., Cunningham, P. B., & Henggeler, S. W. (2002). Multisystemic treatment of antisocial behavior in adolescents. In S. G. Hofmann, & M. C. Tompson (Ed.), *Treating chronic and severe mental disorders: A handbook of empirically supported interventions* (pp. 364–381). New York: Guilford Press.

Lipman, T. (2000). Power and influence in clinical effectiveness and evidence-based medicine. *Family Practice, 17,* 557–563.

Lipsey, M. W., & Wilson, D. B. (2001). *Practical meta-analysis.* Thousand Oaks, CA: Sage.

Littell, J. H. (2005). Lessons from a systematic review of effects of Multisystemic Therapy. *Children and Youth Services Review, 47*, 445–463.

Littell, J. H. (2006). The case for multisystemic therapy: Evidence or orthodoxy? *Children and Youth Services, 28*, 458–472.

Littell, J. H. (2008). Evidence-based or biased? The quality of published reviews of evidence-based practices. *Children and Youth Services Review, 30*, 1299–1317.

Littell, J. H., Corcoran, J., & Pillai, V. (2008). *Systematic reviews and meta-analysis.* New York: Oxford University Press.

Littell, J. H., Popa, M., & Forsythe, B. (2005). Multisystemic therapy for social, emotional, and behavioral problems in youth aged 10–17. *Cochrane Database of Systematic Reviews*, Issue 4. Art. No. CD004797. doi: 10.1002/14651858. cd004797.pub4

Luborsky, L., Diguer, L., Seligman, D. A., Rosenthal, R., Krause, E. D., Johnson, S., et al. (1999). The researcher's own therapy allegiances: A "wild card" in comparisons of treatment efficacy. *Clinical Psychology: Science and Practice, 6*, 95–106.

Mahoney, M. J. (1977). Publication prejudices: An experimental study of confirmatory bias in the peer review system. *Cognitive Therapy and Research, 1*, 161–175.

Mihalic, S., Fagan, A., Irwin, K., Ballard, D., & Elliott, D. (2004). *Blueprints for Violence Prevention* (No. NCJ 204274). Washington, DC: U.S. Department of Justice Office of Juvenile Justice and Delinquency Prevention.

Miller, R. B., Johnson, L. N., Sandberg, J. G., Stringer-Seibold, T. A., & Gfeller-Strouts, L. (2000). An addendum to the 1997 outcome research chart. *American Journal of Family Therapy, 28*, 347–354.

Moher, D., Cook, D. J., Eastwood, S., Olkin, I., Rennie, D., Stroup, D. F., et al. (1999). Improving the quality of reports of meta-analyses of randomised controlled trials: The QUOROM statement. *The Lancet, 354*, 1896–1900.

Moher, D., Schultz, K. F., Altman, D. G., & the CONSORT Group (2001). The CONSORT statement: Revised recommendations for improving the quality of reports of parallel-group randomized trials. *The Lancet, 357*, 1191–1194.

National Institute of Mental Health. (2001). *Youth in a difficult world* (NIH Publication No. 01-4587). Bethesda, MD: National Institutes of Health.

National Institute on Drug Abuse. (1999). *Principles of drug addiction treatment: A research-based guide* (NIH Publication 99-4180). Bethesda, MD: Author.

National Institute on Drug Abuse. (2003). Effective drug abuse treatment approaches: Multisystemic therapy. Retrieved March 1, 2004, from http://www.nida.nih.gov/BRDP/Effective/Henggeler.html

National Institutes of Health. (2004). NIH state-of-the-science conference statement on preventing violence and related health-risking social behaviors in adolescents. *NIH Consensus and State-of-the-Science Statements 2004, 21*(2), 1–34.

New Freedom Commission on Mental Health. (2005). *Subcommittee on evidence-based practices: Background paper* (DHHS Pub. No. SMA-05-4007). Rockville, MD:

Author. Retrieved July 6, 2009, from http://www.mentalhealthcommission.gov/reports/EBP_Final_040605.pdf

Nickerson, R. S. (1998). Confirmation bias: A ubiquitous phenomenon in many guises. *Review of General Psychology, 2*, 175–220.

Papanikolaou, P. N., Churchill, R., Wahlbeck, K., & Ioannidis, J. P. A. (2004). Safety reporting in randomized trials of mental health interventions. *American Journal of Psychiatry, 161*, 1692–1697.

Petticrew, M., & Roberts, H. (2006). *Systematic reviews in the social sciences: A practical guide*. Oxford, England: Blackwell.

Pushak, R. E. (2002). The dearth of empirically supported mental health services for children: Multisystemic Therapy as a promising alternative. *Scientific Review of Mental Health Practice, 1*(2). Available at http://www.srmhp.org/0102/multisystemic-therapy.html

Reid, W. J. (1994). The empirical practice movement. *Social Service Review, 68*, 165–184.

Rothstein, H. R., Sutton, A. J., & Bornstein, M. (Eds.). (2005). *Publication bias in meta-analysis: Prevention, assessment, and adjustments*. Chichester, England: Wiley.

Sackett, D. L. (2000). The sins of expertness and a proposal for redemption. *British Medical Journal, 320*, 1283.

Sackett, D. L., Rosenberg, W. M. C., Gray, J. A. M., Haynes, R. B., & Richardson, W. S. (1996). Evidence based medicine: What it is and what it isn't. *British Medical Journal, 312*, 71–72.

Scherer, R. W., Langenberg, P., & von Elm, E. (2007). Full publication of results initially presented in abstracts. *Cochrane Database of Systematic Reviews*, Issue 2, Art. No. MR000005. doi: 10.1002/14651858.mr000005.pub3

Schoenwald, S. K., & Rowland, M. S. (2002). Multisystemic therapy. In B. J. Burns & K. Hoagwood (Eds.), *Community treatment for youth: Evidence-based interventions for severe emotional and behavioral disorders* (pp. 91–116). New York: Oxford University Press.

Shadish, W. R., Cook, T. D., & Campbell, D. T. (2002). *Experimental and quasi-experimental designs for generalized causal inference*. Boston: Houghton Mifflin.

Shea, B. J., Grimshaw, J. M., Wells, G. A., Boers, M., Andersson, N., Hamel, C., et al. (2007). Development of AMSTAR: A measurement tool to assess the methodological quality of systematic reviews. *BMC Medical Research Methodology, 7*, 10. Retrieved July 6, 2009, from http://www.biomedcentral.com/1471-2288/7/10 ; doi: 10.1186/1471-2288-7-10

Shea, B., Moher, D., Graham, I., Pham, B., & Tugwell, P. (2002). Comparison of the quality of Cochrane reviews and systematic reviews published in paper-based journals. *Evaluation & The Health Professions, 25*, 116–129.

Simpson, D. D., & Flynn, P. M. (2007). Moving innovations into treatment: A stage-based approach to program change. *Journal of Substance Abuse Treatment, 33*, 111–120.

Stirman, S. W., Crits-Christoph, P., & DeRubeis, R. J. (2004). Achieving successful dissemination of empirically supported psychotherapies: A synthesis of dissemination theory. *Clinical Psychology: Science and Practice, 11*, 343–359.

Straus, S. E., Richardson, W. S., Glasziou, P., & Haynes, R. B. (2005). *Evidence-based medicine: How to practice and teach EBM* (3rd ed.). Edinburgh, Scotland: Churchill Livingston.

Substance Abuse and Mental Health Services Administration. (2007). *National registry of evidence-based programs and practices*. Retrieved August 1, 2007, from http://www.nrepp.samhsa.gov/

Swenson, C. C., & Henggeler, S. W. (2003). Multisystemic therapy (MST) for maltreated children and their families. In B. E. Saunders, L. Berliner, & R. F. Hanson (Eds.), *Child physical and sexual abuse: Guidelines for treatment (Final report: January 15, 2003)* (pp. 75–77). Charleston, SC: National Crime Victims Research and Treatment Center.

Swenson, C. C., Henggeler, S. W., Schoenwald, S. K., Kaufman, K. L., & Randall, J. (1998). Changing the social ecologies of adolescent sexual offenders: Implications of the success of multisystemic therapy in treating serious anti-social behavior in adolescents. *Child Maltreatment, 3*, 330–338.

Tavris, C. (2003). Forward: The widening scientist–practitioner gap: A view from the bridge. In S. O. Lilienfeld, S. J. Lynn, & J. M. Lohr (Eds.), *Science and pseudoscience in clinical psychology* (pp. ix–xviii). New York: Guilford Press.

Torgerson, C. J. (2006). Publication bias: The Achilles' heel of systematic reviews? *British Journal of Educational Studies, 54*, 89–102.

Trikalinos, T. A., Churchill, R., Ferri, M., Leucht, S., Tuunainen, A., Wahlbeck, K., et al. (2004). Effect sizes in cumulative meta-analyses of mental health randomized trials evolved over time. *Journal of Clinical Epidemiology, 57*, 1124–1130.

U.S. Department of Health and Human Services. (1999). *Mental health: A report of the Surgeon General*. Rockville, MD: Author.

U.S. Department of Health and Human Services. (2001). *Youth violence: A report of the Surgeon General*. Washington, DC: Author.

Wampold, B. E. (2001). *The great psychotherapy debate: Models, methods, and findings*. Mahwah, NJ: Erlbaum.

Washington Department of Social and Health Services. (2005). Permanent rules, WSR 05-23-031, Section (6)(b). Retrieved July 6, 2009 from http://apps.leg.wa.giv/documents/laws/wsr/2005/23/05-23-031.htm

Washington State Administrative Code 388-501-0165, Section (6)(b), 2005. Retrieved July 6, 2009, from http://apps.leg.wa.gov/WAC/default.aspx?cite=3898-501-0165

Westen, D., Novotny, C. M., & Thompson-Brenner, H. (2004). The empirical status of empirically supported psychotherapies: Assumptions, findings, and reporting in controlled clinical trials. *Psychological Bulletin, 130*, 631–663.

Woody, S. R., Weisz, J., & McLean, C. (2005). Empirically supported treatments: 10 years later. *The Clinical Psychologist, 58*, 5–11.

Woolfenden, S., Williams, K., & Peat, J. (2003). Family and parenting interventions in children and adolescents with conduct disorder and delinquency aged 10–17. *Cochrane Database of Systematic Reviews*, Issue 2, Art. No. CD003015. doi: 10.1002/14651858.cd003015

World Health Organization. (2006). *International Clinical Trials Registry Platform (ICTRP)*. Retrieved July 6, 2009, from http://www.who.int/ictrp/en/

Zimbalist, S. E. (1977). *Historic themes and landmarks in social welfare research*. New York: Harper & Row.

# 7

# PSYCHIATRIC DRUGS AND COMMON FACTORS: AN EVALUATION OF RISKS AND BENEFITS FOR CLINICAL PRACTICE

JACQUELINE A. SPARKS, BARRY L. DUNCAN, DAVID COHEN, AND DAVID O. ANTONUCCIO

Having heard all of this, you may choose to look the other way . . . but you can never say again that you did not know.
—William Wilberforce,
*Address to the English Parliament Regarding the Slave Trade*

According to the Agency for Healthcare Research and Quality, the number of people using psychiatric drugs in the United States increased from 21 million in 1997 to 32.6 million in 2004, and spending climbed from $7.9 billion to $20 billion during the same period (Stagnitti, 2007). A 2004 review of prescription data for 300,000 children concluded that for the first time, spending for medications for childhood behavior problems eclipsed expenditure for any other drug category, including antibiotics (Medco Health Solutions, Inc., 2004). In 2008, antipsychotics ranked number one in total prescription sales in the U.S. market (IMS Health, n.d.), with antidepressants third in the numbers of prescriptions written in that same year. Although psychotropic drug use has risen, community behavioral intervention has remained flat or declined (Case, Olfson, Marcus, & Siegel, 2007). More and more, treatment means medication.

But are the skyrocketing rates of prescription justified by clinical trial evidence? This chapter addresses this fundamental question via a risk–benefit analysis of the major drug classes for all age groups and provides a template for clinicians to both evaluate the drug literature and facilitate medication decisions with their clients. This chapter also places medication treatment, like other interventions, within a common factors context, asserting that like psychotherapy, pantheoretical elements are unacknowledged linchpins behind improvement. As a basis for this position, we first review the evidence for efficacy and safety of major drug classes for all age groups. Next, we illustrate a critical flaws analysis for evaluating conclusions made in the trial literature and popular press. We conclude by discussing the implications of a critical common factors perspective of psychiatric medication in everyday practice.

## ANTIDEPRESSANTS

Antidepressants accounted for the greatest single expenditure for any form of mental health care and 66.7% of all psychotropic drugs in a sample of 5.5 million private health insurance enrollees (Larson, Miller, & Fleming, 2007). The National Institute of Mental Health (NIMH) has asserted that although a variety of antidepressants and psychotherapies are useful treatments for depression, "people with moderate to severe depression most often benefit from antidepressants. Most do best with combined treatment" (NIMH, 2008). The NIMH also stated that "antidepressants may cause mild and, usually, temporary side effects. . . . Typically these are annoying, but not serious." In short, according to the government agency tasked with researching and disseminating state-of-the-art treatment information, antidepressants are the treatment of choice for all but mild depressions and are both effective and safe.

Empirical evidence paints a different picture. The only large-scale population-based study of antidepressants found that for users of antidepressants, compared with nonusers, the duration of depression episodes was longer and the number of episodes was higher for users (Patten, 2004). The author of this study suggested that although this finding may represent a methodological artifact (e.g., users may have been more severely depressed), the common assumption of antidepressant efficacy is inconsistent with emerging observational and meta-analytic data. Kirsch and Sapirstein (1998), in a meta-analytic review of 19 studies involving 2,318 people, showed that 75% of the response to antidepressants was duplicated by placebo. They speculated that the remaining 25% of the positive antidepressant effect may be attributable to the unblinding power of side effects. Adding to the critique, Kirsch, Moore, Scoboria, and Nicholls (2002) analyzed the efficacy data submitted to the U.S. Food and Drug Administration (FDA) for the six most widely prescribed antidepressants approved between 1987 and 1999. Approximately 82% of the response to medication was duplicated by placebo control groups; 57% of the studies failed to show a drug versus placebo difference. When a difference was found, the drug–placebo difference was only, on average, 1.8 points on the clinician-rated Hamilton Depression Rating Scale. FDA memoranda intimated that the clinical significance of such a small difference was questionable (Laughren, 1998).

In a review of antidepressant trials involving 12,564 persons (Turner, Matthews, Eftihia Linardatos, Tell, & Rosenthal, 2008), 94% of published trials had favorable results, whereas the percentage of positive results for published and unpublished trials together dropped to 51%. The authors warned that publication bias of this magnitude dramatically distorts reported effect sizes and has serious implications for researchers, health care professionals, and clients. Kirsch et al. (2008) provided further evidence that the belief in antidepressant efficacy is scientifically unfounded. Meta-analytically examining all trials submitted to the FDA for the licensing of four popular SSRIs, the authors found no clinically significant differences between placebo and the drugs, with the exception of the most distressed in the severely depressed group. Even this negligible difference was found to be due not to the drug but to a decreased response to placebo.

"Treatment resistant depression" prompted the Sequenced Treatment Alternatives to Relieve Depression (STAR*D; Rush et al., 2004), a 6-year, $35 million NIMH-funded study with nearly 2,900 participants (complete data available for analysis) at Level 1 examining the impact of sequenced augmentation or drug switching strategies on depression when a traditional regimen of a single SSRI failed. STAR*D was an unblinded, non-placebo-controlled trial designed to simulate conditions faced in daily practice. The sample, however, did not represent a general clinical population because it excluded those with a history of intolerance or nonresponse to any SSRI and included only those who preferred a medication intervention. As a result of the lack of a placebo and double blind, the authors acknowledged that "nonspecific treatment effects [e.g., the expectation of improvement] undoubtedly accounted for some unknown proportion of the acute response or remission rates" (Trivedi, Rush, et al., 2006, p. 37).

Even though the design favored a drug response, the results were disappointing. In the STAR*D, the average remission rate based on the primary outcome measure was 28% and 25% on the first two levels, and 14% and 13% on the last two—particularly unimpressive considering the typical 30% placebo response in antidepressant trials (Thase & Jindal, 2004). At Level 1, 28% experienced moderate to intolerable side effects (Trivedi, Rush, et al., 2006). At Level 2 (participants augmented or switched), 51% experienced side effects ranging from moderate to intolerable (Rush, Trivedi, Wisniewski, Stewart, et al., 2006; Trivedi, Fava, et al., 2006). For all levels, 24% exited because of drug intolerability (Rush, Trivedi, Wisniewski, Nierenberg, et al., 2006). Data from the 12-month follow-up of those who either remitted or responded indicated a relapse rate of 58% (Rush, Trivedi, Wisniewski, Nierenberg, et al., 2006).[1]

---

[1]Various other psychotropic medications, aimed at reducing SSRI-induced agitation or sexual dysfunctions, were concomitantly prescribed to an unknown proportion of the participants.

The conventional assumption that both psychotherapy and pharma-cotherapy combined produce better outcomes for depression also has gar-nered scant empirical support. Early reviews demonstrated no advantage for combining approaches (e.g., Antonuccio, Danton, & DeNelsky, 1995), but Thase et al. (1997) found that combining the two offered some added ben-efit for the minority suffering with severe, recurrent depressions. Support for a combined regimen for more chronic depressions is also found in Keller et al.'s (2000) trial. The combined group improved more than the medica-tion or psychotherapy groups at 12 weeks. Results were weakened by the lack of a placebo control group and the use of only a single clinician-rated outcome measure.[2] In a recent meta-analysis, combined medication–psychotherapy was better than psychotherapy alone in acute phases of depres-sion but not at follow-up (Cuijpers, van Straten, Warmerdam, & Andersson, 2009). The authors noted that the findings should be considered with cau-tion given the impossibility of placebo blinding, the suboptimal quality of many of the studies, and the relatively small number of studies included in the analysis. The authors further questioned the clinical significance of the results, given that no differences were found between conditions at follow-up.

The negligible advantage of SSRIs over placebo underlines the impor-tance of detecting their adverse effects. Common side effects, including agita-tion, sleep disruption, gastrointestinal complications, and sexual problems reach upwards of 40% of SSRI takers (Antonuccio, Danton, DeNelsky, Green-berg, & Gordon, 1999). SSRI-induced mania (Preda, MacLean, Mazure, & Bowers, 2001) and suicidality (Healy, 2003) have been concerns since the early 1990s. The FDA reviewed 295 antidepressant trials of more than 77,000 adults to examine the risk of suicidality (U.S. Food and Drug Administration, 2007a) and found that the relationship between antidepressants and reported suicidal-ity is strongly related to age. The risk associated with drug treatment relative to placebo was elevated for those under age 25 but reduced for those 65 or older. As a result, the FDA proposed that manufacturers update the existing black box warning (which currently warns about the higher risk for youths taking anti-depressants) to include the increased risks of suicidal thinking and behavior in young adults during initial treatment.

---

[2]The authors of this study (Keller et al., 2000), published in the *New England Journal of Medicine*, were so heavily tied to the pharmaceutical industry that the editors stated the following in a note within the article: "Our policy requires authors of Original Articles to disclose all financial ties with companies that make the products under study or competing products. In this case, the large number of authors and their varied and extensive financial associations with relevant companies make a detailed listing here impractical" (Keller et al., 2000, p. 1462). Additionally, the study's investigative drug (nefazodone) has since been recalled because of unacceptable liver toxicities.

# ANTIPSYCHOTICS

Antipsychotic use has expanded beyond hospital wards and after-care clinics to include the young and old, in all walks of life, many diagnosed with bipolar disorder, irritability, disruptive behaviors, and other nonpsychotic problems (Aparasu, Bhatara, & Gupta, 2005; Moreno et al., 2007). Prescription rates for second-generation antipsychotics (SGAs) tripled in the 5-year time frame from 1998 to 2002 (Aparasu et al., 2005). According to Aparasu et al. (2005), the shift from first to second generation agents is not "unambiguously supported by extant safety and efficacy data [but] is endorsed by guidelines based on expert-consensus and limited data" (p. 147).

Antipsychotic medication is viewed not as a choice but as a requirement (Thase & Jindal, 2004): Those diagnosed with severe psychiatric disorders purportedly need continuous medication to manage a presumed lifelong struggle with mental illness. However, studies have discredited the medication necessity myth, indicating improved outcomes (e.g., lower rates of relapse, better overall global functioning) for persons either never on drugs or weaned from them than for those continually medicated (e.g., Bola & Mosher, 2003; de Girolamo, 1996; Harding, Zubin, & Strauss, 1987; Harrow & Jobe, 2007).

Even with evidence that recovery need not entail drugs, diagnoses such as schizophrenia and bipolar disorder are generally considered "untreated" unless the person is compliant with an antipsychotic regimen. SGAs are often credited as presenting fewer side effects than first generation antipsychotics (FGAs), thereby improving both compliance and treatment longevity. Indeed, medication compliance, inextricably tied to client experiences of side effects, is widely considered the benchmark of successful treatment. The degree to which this factor defines outcome is reflected in the largest study of these medications to date, the NIMH-funded Clinical Antipsychotic Trials of Intervention (CATIE; Lieberman et al., 2005). In CATIE, the primary outcome measure was not clinical improvement or remission—it was simply discontinuation of treatment for any reason. CATIE enrolled 1,400 participants at 57 U.S. sites and used a triple blind: Clinicians, raters, and participants did not know which drug participants were taking. However, CATIE had no placebo group, allowed clinicians to make flexible dosing decisions, and permitted multiple additional drugs (excluding antipsychotics). The goal of CATIE was to evaluate how well SGAs (olanzapine [Zyprexa], quetiapine [Seroquel], risperidone [Risperdal]) compared with one another and an FGA (perphenazine [Etrafon]) in real-world conditions.

Results from the CATIE trials confirmed what many clients report anecdotally: Antipsychotics do not improve general life domains and carry a significant side effect burden. Overall, a disconcerting 74% of CATIE participants discontinued before 18 months, largely because of inefficacy and intolerable side effects (Lieberman et al., 2005). Lieberman et al. (2005) noted that these rates are consistent with those observed in previous anti-psychotic drug trials. Psychosocial functioning improved only modestly for the one third of CATIE participants who reached the primary Quality of Life Scale end point at 12 months (Swartz et al., 2007). Rates of moderate to severe adverse events revealed through systematic inquiry ranged from 42% to 69% (Zyprexa was the worst; Stroup et al., 2007). Hospitalization rates ranged from 11% to 20% over the study period, and a weight gain of more than 7% occurred in 14% to 36% of participants (Zyprexa was the worst). The lead author of the CATIE studies admitted that

> the claims of superiority for [SGAs] were greatly exaggerated. This may have been encouraged by an overly expectant community of clinicians and patients eager to believe in the power of new medications. At the same time, the aggressive marketing of these drugs may have contributed to this enhanced perception of their effectiveness in the absence of empir-ical information (Lieberman, 2006, p. 1070).

The Systematic Treatment Enhancement Program for Bipolar Disorder (STEP-BD), another major investigation funded by the NIMH, examined the effectiveness of SGAs and anticonvulsants for persons diagnosed with bipolar disorder (Sachs et al., 2003). In one of two outcome reports, only 30% experi-enced no recurrences of symptoms (Perlis et al., 2006); the second (Nierenberg et al., 2006) found even lower rates of recovery (just under 15%). Furthermore, results of the Work and Social Adjustment Scale evaluated during a period of remission revealed "considerable functional impairment" (Fagiolini et al., 2005, p. 284). Similar to CATIE findings, remission from clinically defined symptoms, even for the few who achieved this, did not mean adequate social functioning. Of note, in both STEP-BD outcome publications, no details were provided regarding treatment-induced adverse effects.

## CHILDREN AND ANTIDEPRESSANTS

STAR*D, CATIE, and STEP-BD substantially weaken the position that antidepressants, antipsychotics, and anticonvulsants are effective for adults. Several large trials, often cited as evidence justifying child psychotropic prescription, follow suit. Consider, for example, two randomized, placebo-controlled trials of fluoxetine (Prozac; Emslie et al., 1997, 2002). The Emslie trials gained FDA approval for Prozac for young people aged 8 to 17 years diag-nosed with depression (FDA, 2003). Given the failure of tricyclic antidepres-sants to show efficacy for this age group (Fisher & Greenberg, 1997), Prozac's approval was widely considered a breakthrough for the treatment of youth depression. However, both Emslie studies failed to find a statistical difference between Prozac and placebo on primary outcome measures.[3] Additionally, in both trials, manic reactions and suicidality were notably higher in the drug group compared with the placebo group (for an analysis of the Emslie trials, see Sparks & Duncan, 2008).

The NIMH-funded Treatment for Adolescents With Depression Study (TADS; TADS Team, 2004) again evaluated Prozac for the youth age group. TADS compared the efficacy of four treatment conditions: Prozac alone, cognitive–behavioral therapy (CBT) alone, CBT plus Prozac, and placebo. Despite media claims, (e.g., the *New York Times* front page headline, "Antidepressants Seen as Effective for Adolescents"; Harris, 2004), the good news seems less so on examination. The FDA did not count TADS as a positive study for SSRIs because of the negative findings on its primary outcome measure. Other end-point comparisons in TADS favored the combined medication and CBT arm. However, treatment was unblind, and only the combined group received all intervention components (drug, psychotherapy, psychoeducation and family therapy, and supportive pharmacotherapy monitoring), creating a significant disparity in favor of the combination arm. Adding to the bad news, the TADS recorded six suicide attempts by Prozac takers compared with one by non-Prozac takers, with more than double the incidence of harmful behavior in the Prozac conditions compared with placebo groups (despite the exclusion of youths deemed at high risk for suicidal behavior). Nevertheless, the authors recommended that "medical management of MDD [major depressive disorder] with fluoxetine, including careful monitoring for adverse events, should be made widely available, not discouraged" (TADS Team, 2004, p. 819), a challengeable conclusion given its inconsistency with the study's own harm data.

The long-term TADS efficacy and safety trial contains similar problems. In this 36-week study, partial and nonresponders to placebo, and responders and partial responders to Prozac, CBT, and combination treatments in the 12-week trial were openly treated (TADS Team, 2007). As in Phase 1, Prozac and combination groups received additional encouragement and contact (medication management). Despite this, all treatment conditions converged by 30 weeks and remained so by Week 36, with significantly more suicidal ideation in the Prozac-alone group. The percentage of suicidal events for those on Prozac, whether in combined or alone groups, was nearly 12%, double the 6% in the CBT group. Despite the convergence of efficacy and continued risks, TADS is often cited as evidence that combining psychotherapy and medication produce superior results (e.g., NIMH, n.d.).

---

[3]Jureidini et al. (2004) reported that the first Emslie trial changed its primary outcome measure between the trial's beginning and publication, using secondary measures to show superiority.

Jureidini et al. (2004) questioned the clinical significance of results that show no gains on primary or client- or parent-rated measures and highlight other design weaknesses, including relying on the last observation carried forward, emphasizing secondary end points, and transforming continuous into categorical outcomes, thereby inflating small differences. Moreover, *publication bias*—studies finding in favor of the investigative drug are published whereas unfavorable studies are not—clouds the picture of SSRI efficacy for youth depression. An independent analysis by the FDA concluded that only 3 out of 15 published and unpublished trials of SSRIs showed them to be more effective than placebo on primary outcome measures (Laughren, 2004). None of the 15 found differences on client- or parent-rated measures.

The risks noted in published and unpublished data prompted the FDA to issue a black box warning on all antidepressants for youth for increased risk of suicidality and clinical worsening (FDA, 2004). Further support of the warning emerged from an analysis of placebo-controlled trials of nine antidepressants: a total of 24 trials involving more than 4,400 children and adolescents (Hammad, Laughren, & Racoosin, 2006). The investigation revealed an average risk of suicidality of 4% in drug-treated youth, twice the 2% placebo risk.[4]


## CHILDREN AND STIMULANTS

In the first 3 years of this decade, spending for attention-deficit/ hyperactivity disorder (ADHD) drugs, including amphetamine (Adderall), methylphenidate (Concerta, Ritalin), and atomoxetine (Strattera) increased 183% for children overall and 369% for children under 5 (Medco Health Solutions, Inc., 2004). Although the United States continues to lead the world, global use of ADHD drugs has increased by 274% (Scheffler, Hinshaw, Modrek, & Levine, 2007). The empirical literature, however, is equivocal regarding stimulant benefits. A review of 40 years of trials supporting stimulant prescription (primarily Ritalin) found overall effect sizes in the moderate range, with low to moderate ranges for academic productivity and in the zero range for academic achievement (Conners, 2002). The report of the American Psychological Association (APA) Working Group on Psychoactive Medications for Children and Adolescents (APA Working Group; 2006) noted the lack of data supporting long-term efficacy or safety. Further highlighted

---

[4]The Medicines and Healthcare Products Regulatory Authority in the United Kingdom has banned all antidepressants for those under 18 with the exception of Prozac, which can only be used for those over 8 years of age and only in conjunction with continued psychotherapy and when the psychosocial intervention by itself has failed.

was that stimulants, although reducing symptoms, show minimal efficacy in general life domains of the child, including social and academic success.

Stimulant advocates, however, point to the Multimodal Treatment Study of Children with ADHD (MTA; MTA Cooperative Group, 1999), the largest, most complexly designed trial of interventions for ADHD, as proof that stimulants are more effective than behavioral approaches. Much like the Emslie studies are used to justify antidepressants for youth, the MTA is the supportive infrastructure of stimulant prescription. Yet, just like the Emslie trials, the MTA is far from persuasive. Only 3 of 19 measures, all unblinded, found differences favoring Ritalin. Neither blinded classroom observers, the children themselves, nor their peers found medication better than behavioral interventions. Moreover, 14-month endpoint assessments compared those actively medicated and those who had ended therapy (4 to 6 months after the last, face-to-face therapeutic contact; Pelham, 1999). Given this unfair comparison, the fact that only 3 unblinded measures found an advantage for Ritalin is telling. At the same time, 64% of MTA children were reported to have adverse drug reactions, 11% rated as moderate and 3% as severe.

A 24-month follow-up showed that group differences were even smaller; the medication and combined groups lost much of their effect (up to 50%), whereas behavioral treatment and community groups retained theirs (MTA Cooperative Group, 2004). At 36 months, treatment groups did not differ significantly on any measure (Jensen et al., 2007). Medicated children averaged 2.0 centimeters and 2.7 kilograms less growth than non-medicated groups, without evidence of growth rebound at 3 years (Swanson et al., 2007).

To address concerns about the use of stimulants without FDA approval with children under the age of 6 years, the Preschool ADHD Treatment Study investigated the efficacy and safety of Ritalin for preschoolers aged 3 to 5.5 years (Greenhill et al., 2006). Only 21% of the children achieved MTA-defined criterion for remission. In addition, rates of adverse events, including irritability, repetitive behaviors, tics, and emotional outbursts were significantly higher in the Ritalin group. Annual growth rates for the children who remained on medication were 20.3% less than expected for height and 55.2% less for weight (Swanson et al., 2006).

In March of 2006, a safety advisory committee of the FDA urged stronger warnings on ADHD drugs, citing reports of serious cardiac risks, psychosis or mania, and suicidality. Despite this recommendation, the FDA elected to forgo a black box warning for most ADHD drugs,[5] choosing instead to highlight risks on the label and include information with each prescription.

---

[5]Aderall has a black box for cardiac risk and Strattera for suicidality.

# CHILDREN, ANTIPSYCHOTICS, AND OTHER PSYCHOTROPICS

Prescriptions for children do not stop with antidepressants or stimulants. Prescribers increasingly select from antipsychotics, anticonvulsants, hypertensives, and novel agents (Zito & Safer, 2005). A 2007 study compared the rates of diagnosis of bipolar disorder for ages 0 to 19 years for the years 1994–1995 and 2002–2003 (Moreno et al., 2007). Investigators found a 40-fold increase in this diagnosis. Of these, more than 90% were treated with psychoactive drugs, approximately one half an antipsychotic and one third an anticonvulsant. Most of the children were prescribed more than one medication, and only 4 out of 10 received psychotherapy. According to another study of a large national sample, diagnoses of ADHD or conduct disorder were frequently associated with antipsychotic prescription, suggesting the use of these drugs for control of aggression, irritability, and other unwanted behaviors (Cooper et al., 2006). Two diagnostic categories, ADHD and bipolar disorder, accounted for 50% of all antipsychotic use in this sample (ages 2–18 years), despite the fact that these disorders are a far cry from the psychotic symptoms that have traditionally justified prescription of these drugs.

The APA Working Group found that studies supporting the use of antipsychotics to treat children were plagued with methodological limitations, including small sample sizes, open trials, and lower tier evidence (e.g., retrospective chart reviews and case reports). Nevertheless, on the basis of a series of industry-sponsored studies, the FDA recently issued an approval for Risperdal for children diagnosed with autism and exhibiting irritability or aggression, even though these studies were limited in design and scope and indicated significant rates of somnolence, weight gain, and movement disorders (see the section Flaw #7: Constructing Evidence later in this chapter for an analysis of these studies).

Moreover, in August 2007, the FDA also approved Risperdal for the treatment of adolescents aged 13 to 17 years diagnosed with schizophrenia and for children and teens aged 10 to 17 years diagnosed with bipolar disorder (FDA, 2007b). The approval was based on four trials conducted by Janssen, maker of Risperdal: a 6-week double-blind placebo-controlled trial (for schizophrenia), a 3-week double-blind placebo-controlled trial (for bipolar I), an 8-week comparison of two Risperdal doses, and a 6-month open-label safety trial. We located information regarding these trials in a memorandum written by the FDA Deputy Director of the Division of Psychiatry Products (Mathis, 2007) and documents faxed by Janssen in response to a request for information. All the trials were unpublished poster presentations (Haas et al., 2007; Kushner et al., 2007; Pandina, DelBello, Kushner, et al., 2007; Pandina, Kushner, Singer, et al., 2007).

The decision to approve Risperdal is cause for concern. The number of serious adverse events for youths on Risperdal in the short-term trials was more than 6 times that of placebo, and in at least two instances, hospitalization was required. In the 3-week trial, there were six suicide attempts for Risperdal takers compared with one in the placebo group. Also in this study, the incidence of *extrapyramidal symptoms* (EPSs; uncontrolled body movements) was 23% and 12% for the high- and low-dose Risperdal, respectively, compared with 5% for placebo. Adverse events occurring with rates at least twice those of placebo in the two placebo-controlled trials included somnolence, anxiety, hypertonia, dizziness, and EPSs. In the 6-month open-label study, 32% dropped out (reason not given), one third of participants experienced EPSs, 27% experienced somnolence, and 15% had weight increase. A significant increase in body weight also occurred in the 6-week trial (16% Risperdal, 2% placebo) and in the 8-week comparison study (39% high dose, 16% low dose). In the study, 97% of youths had prolactin levels above normal in the high-dose group and 64% in the low-dose group.

The approval of Risperdal expands SGA prescription for a wide spectrum of child behaviors. For young people falling under the popular bipolar umbrella, a 3-week trial sufficed as evidence of efficacy. Of the 10- to 17-year-olds in this study, only 36% were enrolled because of manic episodes. The remaining 64% were described as experiencing a behavior disorder, and 50% had a diagnosis of ADHD. The use of this antipsychotic as a behavior management tool warrants examination of the boundary between treatment and control. The memorandum reassured the regulatory agency that Risperdal is "reasonably safe" (Mathis, 2007, p. 16). Yet evidence from safety assessments contradicts this conclusion. The conclusion that "there were no unexpected adverse events" (Mathis, 2007, p. 16) is ironic: The troubling side effect profile of this drug has been well publicized in the child and adult literature. The FDA's decision to approve Risperdal is a risky and potentially harmful action not supported by the data.[6]

Finally, consider the NIMH-funded trial Treatment of Early Onset Schizophrenia Spectrum Disorders (TEOSS; Sikich et al., 2008). Described as a landmark trial (McClellan et al., 2007), TEOSS sought to examine the efficacy, tolerability, and safety of two SGAs (Risperdal and Zyprexa) for youths diagnosed with early-onset schizophrenia spectrum disorder and to compare these with an FGA (molindone [Moban]). Fewer than 50% of subjects com-

---

[6]Abilify, an SGA, has recently been approved for adolescents aged 13 to 17 years diagnosed with schizophrenia and children aged 10 to 17 years diagnosed with bipolar I, despite commonly observed adverse reactions of extrapyramidal disorder, somnolence, and tremor and documented evidence of additional serious reactions in adult trials (see Flaw #4: Minimization of Risks section).

pleted 8 weeks of treatment, and response rates were low and not significantly different for all three groups (Sikich et al., 2008). Participants in the study were allowed concomitant use of antidepressants, anticonvulsants, and benzodiazepines, compromising even these disappointing findings. A 17-year-old boy committed suicide, and an unspecified number of participants were hospitalized because of suicidality or worsening psychosis. These events are particularly disturbing in light of the fact that youths considered at risk for suicide were excluded from the study. Weight gain was deemed serious enough to warrant suspension of the Zyprexa arm (McClellan et al., 2007). Editorializing in the *American Journal of Psychiatry*, Ross (2008) summarized five arms of active antipsychotic medications for youths in two major studies, including TEOSS: "The effect size of antipsychotic medications in child and adolescent patients is thus relatively low. Furthermore, only ≤50% of subjects responded, regardless of treatment" (p. 1370).

## A CRITICAL FLAWS ANALYSIS

The fact that a for-profit industry plays a role in fashioning what counts as evidence may no longer surprise many. The former editor of the *New England Journal of Medicine* called attention to the problem of "ubiquitous and manifold . . . financial associations" authors of drug trials had to the companies whose drugs were being studied (Angell, 2000, p. 1516). The result is a direct correlation between who funds the study and its outcome. For example, Heres et al. (2006) looked at published comparisons of five antipsychotic medications. In 9 out of 10 studies, the drug made by the company that sponsored the study was found to be superior.

Government agencies and academic advisory panels, presumably the watchdogs over industry-sponsored research, are not the firewalls many assume. In a Pulitzer Prize–winning report, Willman (2003) investigated the National Institutes of Health and found widespread ties to pharmaceutical money. Financial conflicts of interest among FDA advisory members are common (Lurie, Almeida, Stine, Stine, & Wolfe, 2006). Cosgrove, Krimsky, Vijayaraghavan, and Schneider (2006) noted "strong financial ties between the industry and those who are responsible for developing and modifying the diagnostic criteria for mental illness" (p. 154). Experts who formulate practice parameters often serve as consultants for drug companies (Choudhry, Stelfox, & Detsky, 2002).

Antonuccio, Danton, and McClanahan (2003) detailed the vast reach of the pharmaceutical industry from internet, print, and broadcast media; direct-to-consumer advertising; grass-roots consumer advocacy organizations; and professional guilds to medical schools, prescribing physicians, and research—even into the board rooms of the FDA. They concluded, "It is difficult to think of any arena involving information about medications that does not have significant industry financial or marketing influences" (p. 1030). Given the infiltration of industry influence, reliance on press reports, Web sites, and even the academic literature as a basis for sound decision making is unwise. Discerning good science from good marketing requires a willingness to engage primary source material and a critical flaws analysis.

### Flaw #1: Compromises to the Blind

Fisher and Greenberg (1997) asserted that the validity of studies in which a placebo is compared with an active medication depends on the "blindness" of participants who rate the outcomes. They note that inert sugar pills, or inactive placebos, do not produce the standard side effect profile of actual drugs—dry mouth, weight loss or gain, dizziness, headache, nausea, insomnia, and so on. Because study participants must be informed of the possibility and nature of side effects in giving consent, they are necessarily alert for these events, enabling them to correctly identify their study group. In addition, interviews that listen for or elicit side effect information easily reveal active versus inactive pill takers, effectively unblinding the study for clinical raters and skewing results. Moreover, many trial participants in placebo groups have previously been on drug regimens, even some just prior to entering the trial, and are therefore familiar with medication effects. In support of this theory, a meta-analysis of Prozac found a significant correlation between reports of side effects and outcome (Greenberg, Bornstein, Zborowski, Fisher, & Greenberg, 1994). A meta-analytic review of studies using active placebos (side effects mimic active drug) also supports this hypothesis, finding negligible differences between medication and placebo groups (Moncrieff, Wessely, & Hardy, 2004).

Maintenance versus withdrawal trials can also compromise double blinds. The emergence of somatic discontinuation syndrome on withdrawal of many classes of psychiatric drugs include both original and new symptoms, suggesting not relapse but a response associated with biological adaptation after a period of drug exposure (Moncrieff, 2006). Consider, for example, a recent study of long-term use of Risperdal for children and adolescents diagnosed with disruptive behavior disorders (Reyes, Buitelaar, Toren, Augustyns, & Eerdekens, 2006). All children (ages 5–17 years) who had responded to the drug in an open label, 12-week trial prior to the study's start were randomized to 6 months of double-blind treatment of either Risperdal or placebo. There was no down-titration of medication for those switched to placebo. At the end of the study, the groups were evaluated based on time to symptom recurrence. As might be expected, time to recurrence was significantly shorter for those who were abruptly withdrawn than for those who continued without change. In this trial and others like it, not only does the design ensure an outcome favorable to the drug, the blind between groups is likely compromised because of the predictable responses of those experiencing a precipitous withdrawal.

## Flaw #2: Reliance on Clinician Measures

Fisher and Greenberg (1997) demonstrated that clinicians and clients often differ substantially in their judgment of improvement in clinical trials. A meta-analysis of 22 antidepressant studies involving 2,230 persons found that both tricylics and SSRIs showed an approximate 20% advantage over placebo on clinician-rated measures, but none on client-rated measures (Greenberg, Bornstein, Fisher, & Greenberg, 1992). In the Emslie studies, the MTA, and the TADS, client-rated measures found no difference between the placebo and SSRIs and among the conditions in the MTA. The lack of endorsement of efficacy by clients in clinical trials begs the question: If clients don't notice improvements, how significant can those rated by others be?

In addition, clinician-rated scales are often categorical, allowing a subjective range of responses to participant interviews and potential bias because of compromised blind conditions. Moreover, continuous data are often converted into discrete categories (e.g., response and nonresponse), further magnifying differences (Kirsch et al., 2002). Finally, some clinician-rated measures tilt toward specific domains of discomfort that favor the investigative drug, potentially distorting findings. For example, the Hamilton Rating Depression Scale contains 6 points that favor medications with sedative properties, and many trials add sedatives or use drugs with sedative effects (Moncrieff, 2001).

## Flaw #3: Time of Measurement

Psychiatric drugs are often prescribed for long periods of time. This suggests that most clinical trials, which last for 6 to 8 weeks, are not measuring how well the drugs do in actual settings. Additionally, differences between medication and placebo groups often dissolve over time (Fisher & Greenberg, 1997). Without longer term follow-ups, conclusions about effectiveness in real life cannot be determined. Authors of many short-term clinical trials fail to discuss time-frame limitations or to modify accordingly claims made in conclusions. For example, Emslie et al. (1997), in an 8-week study, concluded that "fluoxetine in 20 mg/d is safe and effective in children and adolescents" (p. 1036), without mentioning time.

It could be argued that time limitations favor placebo, and given enough time, antidepressants, for example, will prove their superiority. However, data from the NIMH Treatment of Depression Collaborative Research Project (TDCRP) suggest otherwise. The 18-month follow-up data (Shea et al., 1992) found clients assigned to placebo (plus clinical management) had intent-to-treat outcomes comparable to that of the active drug condition (plus clinical management). Even with maintenance antidepressants, up to 33% of remitted clients experienced a return of depressive symptoms (Byrne & Rothschild, 1998). The significant rates of relapse in STAR*D (58%) underscore the inability of antidepressants to provide long-term relief for many. Similarly, the MTA and CATIE showed that differences with nondrug treatments tend to dissipate over time and that initial effects of drug treatment must be weighed in terms of long-term tolerability and impact beyond symptom remission. Moreover, a meta-analysis of placebo-controlled antidepressant trials found that the durability of placebo was substantial: Four out of five placebo responders remained well during continuation phases (Khan, Redding, & Brown, 2008). Time, therefore, is a principal consideration in assessing clinical trial findings, and claims of superiority for the investigative drug on the basis of results of 8-week (or shorter) trials must be interpreted within the context of what longer term studies have shown.

### Flaw #4: Minimization of Risks

Many psychiatric drug studies downplay or fail to assess adverse drug reactions. As a result, rates of side effects may be substantially underreported (Safer, 2002). Moreover, clinical trial publications typically do not give adverse events the same status as efficacy data. Instead of detailed tables, adverse events may be described in a narrative rather than tabulated formats (e.g., Emslie et al., 1997). Statistical significance for safety comparisons, unlike efficacy comparisons, may not be reported. Authors of trials often confidently assert in abstracts and discussion sections that the drug is safe when the data, in fact, show otherwise.

Consider a 26-week randomized, double-blind placebo-controlled trial designed to evaluate the safety and efficacy of the antipsychotic aripiprazole (Abilify) to prevent relapse of mood episodes for persons diagnosed with bipolar I disorder (Keck et al., 2006). No less than 88% of participants dropped out of the study. Reports of *akathisia* (pronounced inner restlessness), tremor, and pain in the extremities in the Abilify group were at least twice that of placebo. The authors mentioned that there were "more" adverse events related to EPSs for those on Abilify than placebo but failed to analyze this difference statistically. Significant weight gain was also seen for 13% of those taking Abilify versus none for those on placebo. In their conclusions, the authors blandly stated that during the trial, "aripiprazole exhibited no unusual or unexpected adverse events," and the tolerability profile was consistent with that found in other trials of the drug (Keck et al., 2006, p. 636). On the surface, this sounds reassuring. However, a consideration of the 88% dropout rate combined with a consistent pattern of increased incidence of akathisia, EPSs, and weight gain is anything but reassuring.

## Flaw #5: Conflicts of Interest

Richard Smith (2003), who resigned as editor-in-chief of the *British Medical Journal* because of rampant industry influence in academic research, explained that the number one aim of industry-sponsored trials is to find favorable results for the company drug. He noted a host of strategies that help accomplish this goal, including comparing the industry drug against another known to be inferior, comparing a low dose of a competitor's drug to prove efficacy and a high dose to prove less toxicity, using multiple end points and then picking the one that casts the drug in the best light, or conducting subgroup analyses and selecting for publication those that are favorable. According to Smith, the design, conduct, analysis, and publication of clinical trials are, essentially, marketing issues.

Knowing that a meaningful boundary between science and industry no longer exists is essential for evaluating any study's findings. Most academic journals now recommend transparency regarding funding sources and author affiliations. With these as caveats, readers can approach the study with a warranted skepticism and a more careful analysis of trial methods and conclusions. For example, financial disclosures at the end of the Keck et al. (2006) study of Abilify are telling. Lead investigators Keck and Calabrese were identified as consultants or members of the scientific advisory boards of Bristol-Myers Squibb, the makers of Abilify; the remaining six authors were identified as employees (three also are major stock shareholders) of Bristol-Mayers Squibb/Otsuka. For those studies conducted before disclosure recommendations, an online database published by a nonprofit health advocacy group documents researcher conflicts (see Integrity in Science, http://www.cspinet.org/integrity/).

## Flaw #6: Biased Samples, Unfair Comparisons

Random assignment to either a placebo or drug group attempts to ensure that both groups are relatively equal in important attributes and differ only in the presence or absence of the drug being tested. Randomization in drug trials, however, does not mean that the groups are representative samples of real-world populations or that the groups are equal. Most often, a larger percentage of persons in drug trials are likely to respond favorably to the investigative drug than a sample of the general population. For example, trials that use placebo washouts eliminate short-term placebo responders before the study begins. Thus, both study groups will be skewed toward placebo nonresponders. On the face of it, this arbitrary exclusion makes no sense, given that the purpose of the study is to determine whether a drug is superior to placebo. This systematic bias favoring the drug is compounded in studies that exclude those who have failed to respond to the investigative drug (or one in its class) but allow successful responders.

For example, in Reyes et al.'s (2006) study of long-term Risperdal use in children and adolescents, the original pool of participants contained only those determined to be positive responders. The authors noted this as a potential source of selection bias. Exclusionary criteria and placebo washouts, common elements of many clinical trials, increase the chances that the medication group will significantly differentiate from the control group on crucial factors bearing on outcomes. At the same time, these criteria create an unbridgeable gap between research and practice because findings cannot be generalized to the real world of practice.

## Flaw #7: Constructing Evidence

Literature reviews are key landscapes for situating a study within a larger body of prior work; earlier research is cited and constructs a rationale for the current investigation. Here, the track record of any given drug can be clouded in a scientific rhetorical fog, building an empirical case for solid backing of the drug even when the data say otherwise. In Reyes et al.'s (2006) study of Risperdal with youth diagnosed with disruptive behavior disorders, the literature review asserted that "Risperidone has consistently demonstrated efficacy and safety in both controlled short-term and open-label long-term studies" (p. 402). Five studies were cited to back this claim: two short term (Aman, De Smedt, Derivan, Lyons, & Findling, 2002; Snyder et al., 2002) and three longer term (Croonenberghs et al., 2005; Findling et al., 2004; Turgay, Binder, Snyder, & Fisman, 2002).

A review of these studies finds a consistent pattern. The two short-term trials both used a 1-week placebo washout, eliminating early placebo responders. Given that many participants were experienced with antipsychotic medications and their well-known sedative effects and that placebos were inactive, both participants and clinicians could likely distinguish the actual study groups, compromising the blind. Both of these trials showed significant differences between the Risperdal and placebo groups for key adverse events: somnolence (sedation), elevated serum prolactin (for boys), and weight increase. Aman et al. (2002) did not report adverse events in tabulated format for these key events, with the exception of prolactin elevation.

The three longer term studies were open-label extensions of the shorter term trials and examined the long-term efficacy and safety of Risperdal in children ages 5 to 12 with lower than average IQ scores. In all three trials, the top reported adverse event was somnolence, ranging from 20.6% to 51.9%. Weight gain was another frequently reported problem (from 17.3% to 36.4%). Only one study analyzed this effect in light of normative development, determining that 50% of the increased weight was above normal growth expectancies for the age group (Croonenberghs et al., 2002). The pattern of increased prolactin levels was observed across the three trials, and although EPSs were less common than other adverse events, they nonetheless occurred. Five participants in Croonenberghs et al.'s (2002) large study required anti-parkinsonan medications, 6 withdrew because of EPSs, and 2 developed tardive dyskinesia, whereas 26% of participants in Turgay et al. (2002) experienced EPSs. Overall, 76 of the 77 participants in Turgay et al. reported adverse events as did close to 92% in Croonenberghs et al. and nearly 91% in Findling et al. (2004).

Even with minimal safety data reported in these trials, it is not hard to discern a pattern of serious adverse effects. Yet, over and over, the authors of all five studies (cited in support of the drug in Reyes et al.'s, 2006, literature review) reveled in the drug's safety; "generally safe" and "well tolerated" are found in every abstract and conclusions section for all the studies. Efficacy findings of improved behavior across studies are virtually unanimous, though the authors failed to adequately account for the inevitable confounding of high rates of sedation with improvements on measures sensitive to this effect. In sum, the claim that "risperidone has consistently demonstrated efficacy and safety" (Reyes et al., 2006, p. 402), with the five studies reviewed here as evidence is at best misleading and at worst a rhetorical construction revealed only by examination of the data.

Janssen (or Johnson & Johnson, Janssen's parent company), manufacturer of the investigative drug, funded all five of the cited Risperdal studies, and they were authored by researchers financially entwined with this pharmaceutical company. Disclosures reveal that two lead authors were paid to participate in the study (see Turgay et al., 2002), and two authors were employees of Johnson & Johnson (see Croonenberghs et al., 2002). In both short-term studies, authors' financial disclosures were omitted, though each study revealed primary funding from Janssen. Disclosures in other publications authored by these studies' investigators, however, reveal that Aman and Findling have significant ties to this company, and De Smedt is an employee.

Meanwhile, with a presumed track record for safety and efficacy, Risperdal has become a drug of choice for children of subaverage IQ with disruptive behaviors and is widely used with young persons diagnosed with autism. Studies have also been conducted for nonautistic diagnosed youths whose IQs fall within normal ranges, indicating that it is increasingly viewed as a ready option for behaviorally difficult youth in general (Armeteros, Lewis, & Davalos, 2007; Reyes et al., 2006). The problems of sedation, weight gain, increased serum prolactin, and movement disorders have been effectively swept under the rhetorical rug, preventing a thorough scientific investigation of their import as well as funding and momentum for other forms of treatment that may prove effective and less toxic. Instead, the case for efficacy and safety, over time, becomes undisputed fact, its accuracy no longer in question.

## RISK–BENEFIT PROFILE FOR ALL AGE GROUPS

Psychiatric drugs clearly help some adults. An examination, however, of clinical trial research—especially in light of fatally flawed methodologies—fails to provide the definitive proof of efficacy so often cited in professional and lay press. On the basis of the FDA's meta-analytic review and without regard to methodological problems, the entire scientific case for antidepressants rests on the observation that in 189 clinical trials with 53,048 adult subjects, "50% of subjects who received active drug and 40% of subjects who received placebo were designated as responders" (Stone & Jones, 2006, p. 31)

For those who had hoped to show that persistence (trying more of the same or switching to a new drug) would overcome SSRI limitations, the STAR*D offers little support. Nor is there evidence for the widely accepted belief that a combination of drugs and therapy works best for most of those diagnosed with depression. Further, although comparable efficacy between drugs and psychotherapy is the rule in the short run, antidepressants (Shea et al., 1992) as well as other psychotropics fall short of psychotherapy in the long run (Holon, Stewart, & Strunk, 2006). Meanwhile, the extensive CATIE study reaffirms that antipsychotics present an unacceptable side effect profile with minimal efficacy beyond the temporary amelioration of psychotic symptoms. Both CATIE and STEP-BD highlight the limited results achieved with antipsychotics and the persistence of problems in social domains left untouched. In sum, based on a review of evidence supporting the efficacy and safety of psychiatric drugs with adults, a risk–benefit analysis suggests that psychotherapy be considered first, within the context of client preferences.

Pharmacotherapy helps some children and adolescents. However, the preponderance of empirical research indicates that the risk may not be worth it. The APA Working Group asked, "How many children should benefit from an antidepressant to justify one extra child harmed?" (APA Working Group, 2006, p. 114). They further noted that despite evidence for all ADHD treatments, the data indicate that the benefits of medication do not maintain over time, and the long-term adverse effects are unstudied and unknown. Given this, the group determined that "with regard to use over a period of 2 to 3 years, *the risk–benefit analysis of stimulant medication does not appear to be favorable* [italics added] because beneficial effects appear to dissipate while side effects (e.g., growth) do not" (p. 52). The APA Working Group's report omitted the controversy surrounding the risks for adverse cardiovascular events and mania associated with ADHD drugs (the report was in press before the FDA's analysis). Adding this to the equation, confidence in stimulants as best practice for childhood behavior problems further erodes, tilting the risk–benefit analysis toward more risk-free behavioral interventions.

Although pharmacotherapy involves considerable risk for young people, psychosocial interventions have a strong track record with virtually no adverse associated medical events (APA Working Group, 2006), which prompted the authors to conclude that

> for most of the disorders reviewed herein, there are psychosocial treatments that are solidly grounded in empirical support as stand-alone treatments. Moreover, the preponderance of available evidence indicates that psychosocial treatments are safer than psychoactive medications. Thus, *it is our recommendation that in most cases, psychosocial interventions be considered first* [italics added]. (p. 16)

In sum, the automatic prescription of psychotropic medications for adults and children, in light of the known risks and equivocal efficacy, is unwarranted. Where children are concerned, the stakes are higher. They are essentially mandated clients—most do not have a voice to say no to treatments or devise their own, and they depend on adults to safeguard their well-being (Sparks & Duncan, 2008). Clients, caretakers, and practitioners need to discern science from spin to arrive at an informed analysis of the evidence.

## COMMON FACTORS AND PSYCHIATRIC MEDICATIONS

Similar to psychotherapy, common factors loom large in medication effectiveness. As Greenberg (1999) pointed out, the argument that drugs work because of their active chemical properties (specific factors) rests on the ability to demonstrate the superiority of the drug over placebo in controlled randomized trials. However, despite study designs that actively favor the investigative drug, the placebo has shown, time and again, a robust potency. As we have seen, the difference in outcome between antidepressants and placebos is small at best, and the superiority of drugs over placebo across all classes loses ground under critical scrutiny. The case for medication efficacy due to specific, biochemical properties that target neural substrates of diagnosed disorders remains dubious (Moncrieff & Cohen, 2005). How, then, might the common factors provide an explanatory framework for the positive effects of psychiatric medications?

Wampold's (2001) meta-analysis assigns as much as 87% of the variance of psychotherapy outcome to extratherapeutic factors (including error and unexplained variance). These variables are incidental to the treatment and idiosyncratic to the specific client—part of the client and his or her environment that aid in recovery regardless of participation in therapy (Asay & Lambert, 1999). Extratherapeutic factors can explain the phenomenon known as *spontaneous remission*. Here, diagnosable conditions remit over time without treatment (Posternak & Miller, 2001)—even schizophrenia (de Girolamo, 1996; Harrow & Jobe, 2007). Whether attributed to biology, personal resources, or the result of inevitably changing life circumstances, clients tend to resolve difficulties that would be diagnosed and medicated in standard practice. Given that client factors comprise the largest portion of variance in outcome, it is reasonable to consider how clients use medications to their benefit. What is it about any given client's personal, social, and contextual resources that promote a favorable response to medication? How does asking this question shift the conversation to identify and amplify potent client attributes in the interest of not only immediate change but change over time? Here, the focus is on how clients take the offered intervention, whether medical or otherwise, and fashion unique solutions for even the most daunting dilemmas (Sparks, Duncan, & Miller, 2008).

Client factors intimately relate to other common factors: therapist effects, the alliance, and the treatment delivered (including placebo, expectancy, or allegiance effects). Who administers the medication (therapist effects) and the relationship he or she establishes with the client play determinant roles in whether the treatment is effective. The TDCRP revealed large psychiatrist effects: 7% to 9% of the variability in outcomes was due to the psychiatrist (McKay, Imel, & Wampold, 2006), up to triple the variance attributable to antidepressant treatment. The McKay et al. (2006) analysis revealed that clients of the most effective psychiatrists (top one third) who received a placebo had better outcomes that those of the least effective psychiatrists (bottom one third) receiving medication. In addition, the top psychiatrists in the placebo condition also had the best outcomes in the drug condition. Further highlighting the power of therapist effects, a study of 6,000 therapists (Wampold & Brown, 2005) found that when clients of more effective clinicians were medicated, the medication was more successful than for clients of less effective therapists. Medication was not helpful for the clients of the least effective psychotherapists.

Researchers in drug trials often view the alliance as a factor related to compliance rather than actual change (Greenberg, 1999). The TDCRP, however, upheld what researchers repeatedly have found: A positive alliance is one of the best predictors of outcome. Data from the TDCRP revealed that the alliance was predictive of success for all conditions (Krupnick et al., 1996), with no difference between drug and nondrug treatments. The alliance accounted for 21% of the variance across treatments.

The placebo response in psychiatric drug trials, as noted, has long been the bane of researchers, exhorting them to take extraordinary measures (largely unsuccessful) to counteract its effects. Expectancy accounts for significant portions of drug response and often matches the effects of the investigative drug (Kirsch et al., 2002). Any medication intervention, therefore, must be considered in concert with placebo and expectancy effects (i.e., the treatment delivered). The belief by clients that they are getting a powerful healing agent and the hope for improvement this engenders play powerful roles in outcome. In part, this class of therapeutic factors refers to the portion of improvement deriving from client's knowledge of being treated and assessment of the credibility of the therapy's rationale and related techniques. Outcome is enhanced when both client and therapist believe in the restorative power of the treatment (Frank & Frank, 1991).

For example, a clinical trial of antidepressants found that 90% of depressed participants who reported high expectancies for improvement responded to treatment compared with 33% of those who expected the medications to be "somewhat effective" (Krell, Leuchter, Morgan, Cook, & Abrams, 2004). TDCRP data also indicated that expectancies significantly predicted response across both the psychotherapy and pharmacotherapy conditions (Sotsky et al., 1991). Moreover, in the TDCRP, clients' perceptions of treatment fit with their beliefs about their depression and what would be helpful (psychotherapy or medication) contributed modestly to early engagement, continuation in therapy, and the development of a positive alliance (Elkin et al., 1999). Finally, a study of persons diagnosed with bipolar disorder who were treated with medication (Gaudiano & Miller, 2006) found that both expectancies and the alliance were predictive of outcome. The authors concluded that expectancy and alliance factors are not just important predictors in psychotherapy; prescribers should ask clients about expectations and attend to the alliance.

Understanding expectancy further contextualizes positive findings in drugs trials, especially when those treated with drugs receive greater attention and time. In the limitations section of the TADS study comparing combined Prozac and CBT, Prozac alone, CBT alone, and placebo for the treatment of adolescent depression, the authors acknowledged that variations in knowledge of treatment received as well as inequities in contact time with the clinicians existed across the four groups. A pharmacotherapist was assigned to each participant in the combined, medication alone, and placebo groups. This person monitored drug dosage and "offered general encouragement about the effectiveness of pharmacotherapy for MDD" (TADS Team, 2004, p. 809). The combined-group adolescents also received contact with a cognitive–behavioral therapist for 15 sessions. Parents in the combined group participated in psychoeducation groups about depression along with conjoint family sessions. Only the combined group received all of these "extra" components. The authors admitted that because of the inequality in conditions and lack of blinding, the "active ingredient" (p. 118) of improvement could not be determined.

Expectancy factors, including therapist allegiance, are fueled by media and advertising wooing consumers to view drugs as virtual guarantees of symptom relief and, even more, "the good life." At the same time, faith in psychiatric medications rests comfortably within a social context in which medical explanations and solutions hold great sway. When therapists have allegiance to medication, they likely reinforce expectancy for improvement. Similarly, the ritual of medicine—the diagnostic interview, the formal explanation (diagnosis), and the prescriptive treatment (medication)—holds all the allure of healing rituals that are part of the cultural scripts characteristic of human societies. In sum, medical "scripts," both from doctors' pads and the medical narrative, have the power to create potent placebo effects (evidenced by their prominence in the drug trial literature) that then can translate into improved outcomes.

Greenberg (1999) summarized the common elements in psychiatric drug therapy:

> Medication response can be readily altered by who delivers the drug, how its properties are described, the degree of familiarity with the setting in which it is presented, and the ethnic identity or socioeconomic status of the person ingesting it. (p. 301)

On the basis of the evidence, the specific ingredients of medication and their alleged biochemical impact are secondary to common factor effects in producing desired outcomes.

## CLINICAL IMPLICATIONS

> He is the best physician that know the worthlessness of the most medicines.
>
> —Benjamin Franklin

Two conclusions emerge from this chapter: First, when clinical trials are critically examined—does the study have a true double blind, are outcome measures clinician- or client-rated, how long did the study last, who funded the study and what are the authors' affiliations, are the groups representative of the general population and do they offer a fair contest, and does the study provide rhetoric or evidence—it is clear that psychiatric drug treatments should not be privileged over psychosocial options. And second, when effects to treatment are noted, who provides the treatment, the quality of the alliance, and the clinician and recipient's expectations for success provide a better explanation of the results than any presumed specific effects due to the medication.

These conclusions, however, do not eliminate medication as one choice among many, particularly when clients believe their problems to be biological and that drugs might be helpful. What is not supported is the automatic trigger to recommend medication without considering client preferences and a full range of options. The efficacy of psychotherapy has been irrefutably supported across all domains of symptom distress, with few if any instances indicating superior outcomes for medication, especially in the long run. Knowing that there is no irresistible scientific justification to medicate, therapists are free to put other options on the table and draw in the voices of their clients, to engage in an informed risk–benefit analysis to help clients choose treatments in concert with their values, preferences, and cultural contexts. Practitioners need not fear these conversations or feel timid in the face of medical opinion. The APA Working Group (2006) clearly defined the clinician's role: "A clinician's role is to provide the family with the most up-to-date evidence, as it becomes available, regarding short- and long-term risks and benefits of the treatments" (p. 174).

It is not outside the expertise of practitioners of all disciplines to critically examine and be informed about the evidence. Similarly, it is well within the scope of practice of mental health professionals to provide this information to clients in formats consistent with their language and preferred modes of learning and to make available unbiased sources where additional information can be obtained. Further, it is within clinicians' professional bounds to speak clearly about the pervasive conflicts of interest in many media outlets and press materials—not to take the medication option off the table but, as an ethical imperative, not to withhold any information that can help clients make the most informed decision possible. Such risk–benefit conversations seem supported by the APA Presidential Task Force on Evidence-Based Practice (2006) definition of *evidence-based practice:* "the integration of the best available research with clinical expertise in the context of patient characteristics, culture, and preferences" (p. 273). Risk–benefit discussions address the best available research and lean toward client preferences.

In the interest of empowering clients to make informed decisions about medications, we offer the following guidelines that honor client preferences as well as their central and heroic roles in the change endeavor, incorporate the evidence for drug efficacy and safety, and respect the right of all persons to be fully informed in critical treatment decisions:

1. Conduct a thorough and systematic assessment of the problem situation, combining information from all significantly involved persons and networks.
2. Develop a collaborative framework for understanding the problem with the client and significant others that includes

developmental, environmental, interactional, and sociocultural understandings.

3. Develop a plan that follows the assessment and framework of understanding and that is responsive to clients' view of the problem, strengths, cultural context, and preferences.

4. If medication is part of the plan, make sure all involved are aware of potential risks, known adverse events and withdrawal reactions; the meaning of off-label prescription; and the lack of studies supporting combining psychotropic medications. Suggest independent resources for obtaining additional information about risks and benefits, including physicians and unbiased sources.

5. Work collaboratively with clients and significant others to implement the plan, modifying as needed on the basis of systematic client feedback on progress. If medication is part of the plan, assist the client in viewing positive change as resulting from his or her efforts, and significant others as relevant in overcoming the problem, and include discussion of a time frame for discontinuation of medication.

The belief in the power of chemistry over social and psychological process—fueled by unprecedented promotion from the drug industry that targets all players in health care—forms the basis of pharmacology's growing centrality in psychotherapy research, training, and practice. Although some clients may be helped some of the time with this focus, it misdirects the field away from an empirically based understanding of what is responsible for change. Additionally, it promotes prescriptive treatments of questionable sustainability, fraught with potentially dangerous effects. We advocate that psychotherapists adopt a critical perspective of psychopharmacology, examine its impact on clients and the field, and realign themselves with known processes of change common across psychological and medical models.

## QUESTIONS FROM THE EDITORS

1. *You present a view of drug efficacy and safety that is not often, if ever, reported in the media. Why?*

It is hard not to sound like a conspiracy theorist when answering this question. Simply put, there is no mainstream media source that is not under the sway of pharmaceuticals. To appreciate this unnerving fact, one need only to examine primary sources—the actual clinical trial research—and compare it with descriptions in the popular press and Web sites providing "information" to the public. A good example is the STAR*D study. The pharmaceutical industry regularly releases write-ups announcing drug news (often reprinted without critique), and the STAR*D really hit the big time. The *Los Angeles Times* trumpeted "A Varied Assault on Depression Yields Gains" (Maugh, 2006) and described mythical results clearly at odds with STAR*D's findings. Moreover, the NIMH—a source most would assume to be beyond the reach of spin—misrepresented STAR*D findings even more grievously. The NIMH Web page omits the significant number of STAR*D dropouts and claims that roughly 50% achieved remission by taking two steps, either a single agent or an augment–switch choice. This figure could only be derived by cumulatively adding percentage rates across levels, a practice statistically meaningless and certainly misleading. Because the rates of effectiveness are calculated from the numbers of participants in each level, average, not cumulative, percentages correctly reflect overall improvement. For example, in the first two levels, out of a total of 4,168 participants, 1,114 achieved remission, a 27%, not 50%, rate. The STAR*D is but one example that demonstrates that primary sources must be consulted to distinguish science from science fiction.

2. *This is a thorny question, but what about prescriptive authority for psychologists?*

Considering APA's definition of evidence-based practice and the evidence presented in this chapter, what is ironic about psychology's push for prescriptive authority is the lack of empirical support for drug efficacy, surely not the "integration of the best available research" (APA Presidential Task Force on Evidence-Based Practice, p. 273). Furthermore, although some clients prefer using medications to address emotional problems, most do not, as demonstrated by the APA survey (Penn, Schoen, & Berland Associates, 2004) discussed in chapter 1 of this volume. Of potential consumers, 91% preferred a helper who would emphasize talk therapy, not drugs, as a first course of action. The longing for prescriptive authority, therefore, seems not to be "in the context of patient . . . preferences" (APA Presidential Task Force on Evidence-Based Practice, p. 273).

An oft-mentioned tagline by prescription proponents—the ability to prescribe carries with it the ability *not* to prescribe—seems satirical. Psychiatrists, at one time, were trained as psychotherapists. Despite the underwhelming data supporting drug efficacy, and under the intoxicating influence of massive marketing and increased personal income, psychiatrists have become the drug-focused practitioners they are today. Is psychology different? Consider a special feature on psychopharmacology in the February 2008 issue of the *Monitor on Psychology* that reported the following:

> Thinking about how being able to prescribe has improved patient care, he mentions a patient, a man in his 50s diagnosed with bipolar dis-

order. . . . [The psychologist] put him on a combination of medications no one had tried with him before. The medication brought relief from his manic symptoms for the first time. . . . "He tells me every time, he pats me on the shoulder and says, 'You saved me.' " (Munsey, 2008, p. 57).

Such multiple medication concoctions, the seeming standard of modern psychiatry, are not empirically supported and not FDA approved. The reported success of this one client (setting aside the savior aspects and the unfortunate assignment of credit for the relief to the psychologist instead of the client) will likely lead this psychologist to continue unsupported and unapproved polypharmaceutical solutions just like psychiatrists. The current fervor for prescriptive authority combined with a disturbing lack of awareness of the data does not inspire confidence in psychologist's abilities to swim upstream against the strong rapids of corporate influence and personal financial success.[7] The call for prescriptive authority seems more about self-interest than science and is far removed from the consumer base. Consequently, we believe the push for the prescription pad should be abandoned.

3. *Given your risk–benefit analyses, what are the implications for training programs?*

It is now standard practice that students not only know the *Diagnostic and Statistical Manual of Mental Disorders* (DSM) but also the latest compendium of psychotropics—and, like the *DSM*, without accompanying critique. When there is even the hint of depression, psychosis, or mood swings, trainees are taught to refer to physicians but forbidden to discuss risks and benefits. But the recommendations of the APA Working Group (2006) usher in a new day. Therapists can engage in critical analysis of the drug trial literature and the role it plays in professional guidelines, training mandates, and media. Such an analysis reveals the blemished underbelly of even the most sophisticated trials and effectively casts doubt on medication superiority and safety. On the basis of the evidence, a different training mandate emerges:

1. Teach students a critical perspective through an examination of primary research. A seven-flaws analysis as outlined in this chapter is a teachable tool to evaluate the science supporting medication prescription and privilege. Teach students that medication is an option not a mandate.

2. Provide students with opportunities to practice medication discussions with clients. Student facility with a range of options, as

---

[7]A recent exchange on an online psychology discussion forum with psychologists who had completed the coursework for prescriptive authority revealed little awareness of the major drug clinical trials as well as little appreciation of methodological problems or conflicts of interest. Rebuttal from these specially trained psychologists relied solely on information uncritically gleaned from secondary sources.

well as sources of unbiased information, increases the chances of more measured conversations and nonmedical alternatives.

3. Bolster student confidence in taking a view likely to be unpopular or discredited. Model respectful professional conversation while instilling a faith in the empirical evidence that justifies a far more conservative approach than currently practiced.

4. Teach students about the common factors—the known contributors to change—thereby increasing their reliance on clients, the therapy relationship, hope and expectancy, and their own abilities to resolve even the more severe life situations and problems.

5. Train students in outcome management. The proof of the pudding is in the taste. Teaching students to collaborate with clients to monitor the benefit of any intervention necessarily opens the door for frank conversations about what is working and what is not.

## REFERENCES

Aman, M. G., De Smedt, G., Derivan, A., Lyons, B., & Findling, R. (2002). Double-blind, placebo-controlled study of risperidone for the treatment of disruptive behaviors in children with subaverage intelligence. *American Journal of Psychiatry, 159,* 1337–1346.

American Psychological Association Presidential Task Force on Evidence-Based Practice. (2006). Evidence-based practice in psychology. *American Psychologist, 61,* 271–285.

American Psychological Association Working Group on Psychoactive Medications for Children and Adolescents. (2006). *Report of the Working Group on Psychoactive Medications for Children and Adolescents. Psychopharmacological, psychosocial, and combined interventions for childhood disorders: Evidence base, contextual factors, and future directions.* Washington, DC: American Psychological Association.

Angell, M. (2000). Is academic medicine for sale? *New England Journal of Medicine, 341,* 1516–1518.

Antonuccio, D. O., Danton, W. G., & DeNelsky, G. (1995). Psychotherapy vs. medication for depression: Challenging the conventional wisdom with data. *Professional Psychology: Research and Practice, 26,* 574–585.

Antonuccio. D. O., Danton, W. G., DeNelsky, G. Y., Greenberg, R. P., & Gordon, J. S. (1999). Raising questions about antidepressants. *Psychotherapy and Psychomatics, 68,* 3–14.

Antonuccio, D. O., Danton, W. G., & McClanahan, T. M. (2003). Psychology in the prescription era: Building a firewall between marketing and science. *American Psychologist, 58,* 1028–1043.

Aparasu, R., Bhatara, V., & Gupta, S. (2005). U.S. national trends in the use of anti-psychotics during office visits, 1998–2002. *Annals of Clinical Psychiatry, 17*(3), 147–152.

Asay, T. P., & Lambert, M. J. (1999). The empirical case for the common factors in therapy: Quantitative findings. In M. A. Hubble, B. L. Duncan, & S. D. Miller (Eds.), *The heart and soul of change: What works in therapy* (pp. 33–56). Washington, DC: American Psychological Association.

Armeteros, J. L., Lewis, J. E., & Davalos, M. (2007). Augmentation for treatment–resistant aggression in attention-deficit/hyperactivity disorder: A placebo-controlled pilot study. *Journal of the American Academy of Child & Adolescent Psychiatry, 46*, 558–565.

Bola, J. R., & Mosher, L. R. (2003). Treatment of acute psychosis with neuroleptics: Two-year outcomes from the Soteria Project. *Journal of Nervous and Mental Disease, 191*, 219–229.

Byrne, S. E., & Rothschild, A. J. (1998) Loss of antidepressant efficacy during maintenance therapy: Possible mechanisms and treatments. *Journal of Clinical Psychiatry, 59*, 279–288.

Case, B. G., Olfson, M., Marcus, S. C., & Siegel, C. (2007). Trends in the inpatient mental health treatment of children and adolescents in U.S. community hospitals between 1990 and 2000. *Archives of General Psychiatry, 64*, 89–96.

Choudhry, N. K., Stelfox, H. T., & Detsky, A. S. (2002). Relationships between authors of clinical practice guidelines and the pharmaceutical industry. *JAMA, 287*, 612–617.

Cooper, W. O., Arbogast, P. G., Ding, H., Hickson, G. B., Fuchs, C., & Ray, W. A. (2006). Trends in prescribing of antipsychotic medications for U.S. Children. *Ambulatory Pediatrics, 6*(2), 79–83.

Conners, C. K. (2002). Forty years of methylphenidate treatment in attention-deficit/hyperactivity disorder. *Journal of Attention Disorders, 6*(Suppl. 1), S17–S30.

Cosgrove, L, Krimsky, S., Vijayaraghavan, M., & Schneider, L. (2006). Financial ties between *DSM–IV* panel members and the pharmaceutical industry. *Psychotherapy Psychosomatics, 75*, 154–160.

Croonenberghs, J., Fegert, J. M., Findling, R. L., De Smedt, G., Van Dongen, S., & the Risperidone Disruptive Behavior Study Group. (2005). Risperidone in children with disruptive behavior disorders and subaverage intelligence: A 1-year, open-label study of 504 patients. *Journal of the American Academy of Child and Adolescent Psychiatry, 44*, 64–72.

Cuijpers, P., van Straten, A., Warmerdam, L., & Andersson, G. (2009). Psychotherapy versus the combination of psychotherapy and pharmacotherapy in the treatment of depression: A meta-analysis. *Depression and Anxiety, 26*, 279–288.

de Girolamo, G. (1996). WHO studies on schizophrenia: An overview of the results and their implications for the understanding of the disorder. *The Psychotherapy Patient, 9*, 213–231.

Elkin, I., Yamaguchi, J., Arnkoff, D., Glass, C., Sotsky, S., & Krupnick, J. (1999). "Patient–treatment fit" and early engagement in therapy. *Psychotherapy Research, 9*, 437–451.

Emslie, G. J., Heiligenstein, J. H., Wagner, K. D., Hoog, S. L., Ernest, D. E., Brown, E. et al. (2002). Fluoxetine for acute treatment of depression in children and adolescents: A placebo-controlled, randomized clinical trial. *Journal of the American Academy of Child & Adolescent Psychiatry, 41*, 1205–1215.

Emslie, G. J., Rush, A. J., Weinberg, W. A., Kowatch, R. A., Hughes, C. W., Carmody, T., et al. (1997). A double-blind, randomized, placebo-controlled trial of fluoxetine in children and adolescents with depression. *Archives of General Psychiatry, 54*, 1031–1037.

Fagiolini, A., Kupfer, D. J., Masalehdan, A., Scott, J. A., Houck, P. R., & Frank, E. (2005). Functional impairment in the remission phase of bipolar disorder. *Bipolar Disorders, 7*, 281–285.

Findling, R. L., Aman, M. G., Eerdekens, M., Derivan, A., Lyons, B., & the Risperidone Disruptive Behavior Study Group. (2004). Long-term, open-label study of risperidone in children with severe disruptive behaviors and below-average IQ. *American Journal of Psychiatry, 161*, 677–684.

Fisher, S., & Greenberg, R. P. (1997). *From placebo to panacea: Putting psychiatric drugs to the test.* New York: Wiley.

Frank, J. D., & Frank, J. B. (1991). *Persuasion and healing* (3rd ed.). Baltimore: John Hopkins University Press.

Greenberg, R. P. (1999). Common psychosocial factors in psychiatric drug therapy. In M. A. Hubble, B. L. Duncan, & S. D. Miller (Eds.), *The heart and soul of change: What works in therapy* (pp. 297–328). Washington, DC: American Psychological Association.

Greenberg, R. P., Bornstein, R. F., Greenberg, M. D., & Fisher, S. (1992) A meta-analysis of antidepressant outcome under "blinder" conditions. *Journal of Consulting and Clinical Psychology, 60*, 664–669

Greenberg, R. P., Bornstein, R. F., Zborowski, M. J., Fisher, S., & Greenberg, M. D. (1994). A meta-analysis of fluoxetine outcome in the treatment of depression. *Journal of Nervous and Mental Disease, 182*, 547–551.

Greenhill, L., Kollins, S., Abikoff, H., McCracken, J., Riddle, M., Swanson, J., et al. (2006). Efficacy and safety of immediate-release methylphenidate treatment for preschoolers with ADHD. *Journal of the American Academy of Child & Adolescent Psychiatry, 45*, 1284–1294.

Gaudiano, B. A., & Miller, I. W. (2006). Patients' expectancies, the alliance in pharmacotherapy, and treatment outcomes in bipolar disorder. *Journal of Consulting and Clinical Psychology, 74*, 671–676.

Haas, M., Unis, A. S., Copenhaver, M., et al. (2007, May). *Efficacy and safety of risperidone in adolescents with schizophrenia.* Poster session presented at the 160th Annual Meeting of the American Psychiatric Association, San Diego, CA.

Hammad T. A., Laughren, T., & Racoosin, J. (2006). Suicidality in pediatric patients treated with antidepressant drugs. *Archives of General Psychiatry, 63,* 332–339.

Harding, C., Zubin, R., & Strauss, D. (1987). Chronicity in schizophrenia: Fact, partial fact or artifact. *Hospital and Community Psychiatry, 38,* 477–484.

Harris, G. (2004, June 2). Antidepressants seen as effective for adolescents. *New York Times,* p. A1.

Harrow, M., & Jobe, T. H. (2007). Factors involved in outcome and recovery of schizophrenia patients not on antipsychotic medications: A 15-year multifollow-up study. *Journal of Nervous and Mental Disease, 195,* 406–414.

Healy, D. (2003). Lines of evidence on the risks of suicide with selective serotonin reuptake inhibitors. *Psychotherapy & Psychosomatics, 72*(2), 71–79

Heres, S., Davis, J., Maino, K., Jetzinger, E., Kissling, W., & Leucht, S. (2006). Why olanzapine beats risperidone, risperidone beats quetiapine, and quetiapine beats olanzapine: An exploratory analysis of head-to-head comparison studies of second-generation antipsychotics. *American Journal of Psychiatry, 163,* 185–194.

IMS Health (n.d.). *2008 U.S. sales and prescription information.* Retrieved April 2, 2009, from http://www.imshealth.com/portal/site/imshealth/menuitem

Jureidini, J. N., Doecke, C. J., Mansfield, P. R., Haby, M. M., Menkes, D. B., & Tonkin, A. I. (2004). Efficacy and safety of antidepressants for children and adolescents. *British Medical Journal, 328,* 879–883.

Jensen, P. S., Arnold, L. E., Swanson, J. M., Vitiello, B., Abikoff, H. B., Greenhill, L. L., et al. (2007). 3-year follow-up of the NIMH MTA study. *Journal of the American Academy of Child & Adolescent Psychiatry, 46,* 989–1002.

Keck, P. E., Calabrese, J. R., McQuade, R. D., Carlson, W. H., Carlson, B. X., Rollin, L. M., et al. (2006). A randomized, double-blind, placebo-controlled, 26-week trial of aripiprazole in recently manic patients with bipolar I disorder. *Journal of Clinical Psychiatry, 67,* 626–637.

Keller, M. B., McCullough, J. P., Klein, D. N., Arnow, B., Dunner, D. L., Gelenberg, A. J., et al. (2000). A comparison of nefazodone, the cognitive behavioral-analysis system of psychotherapy, and their combination for the treatment of chronic depression. *New England Journal of Medicine, 342,* 1462–1470.

Khan, A., Redding, N., & Brown, W. A. (2008). The persistence of placebo response in antidepressant trials. *Journal of Psychiatric Research, 42,* 791–796.

Kirsch, I., Deacon, B. J., Huedo-Medina, T. B., Scoboria, A., Moore, T. J., & Johnson, B. T. (2008). Initial severity and antidepressant benefits: A meta-analysis of data submitted to the Food and Drug Administration. *PLoS Medicine, 5*(2), e45.

Kirsch, I., Moore, T. J., Scoboria, A., Nicholls, S. N. (2002). The Emperor's new drugs: An analysis of antidepressant medication data submitted to the U.S. Food and Drug Administration. *Prevention & Treatment, 5,* Article 23. Retrieved October 2, 2002, from http://journals.apa.org/prevention/volume5/toc-jul15-02.htm

Kirsch, I., & Sapirstein, G. (1998, June 26). Listening to Prozac but hearing placebo: A meta-analysis of antidepressant medication. *Prevention & Treatment, 1,*

Article 0002a. Retrieved June 30, 1998, from http://journals.apa.org/prevention/volume1/pre0010002a.html

Krell, H. V., Leuchter, A. F., Morgan, M., Cook, I. A., & Abrams, M. (2004). Subject expectations of treatment effectiveness and outcome of treatment with an experimental antidepressant. *Journal of Clinical Psychiatry, 65,* 1174–1179.

Krupnick, J. L., Sotsky, S. M., Simmens, S., Moyher, J., Elkin, I., Watkins, J., & Pilkonis, P. A. (1996). The role of the therapeutic alliance in psychotherapy and pharmacotherapy outcome: Findings in the National Institute of Mental Health Treatment of Depression Collaborative Research Project. *Journal of Consulting and Clinical Psychology, 64,* 532–539.

Kushner, S., Unis, A., Copenhaver, et al. (2007, October). *Acute and continuous efficacy and safety of risperidone in adolescents with schizophrenia.* Poster session presented at the 54th Annual Meeting of the American Academy of Child and Adolescent Psychiatry, Boston.

Larson, M. J., Miller, K., & Fleming, K. J. (2007). Treatment with antidepressant medications in private health plans. *Administration Policy in Mental Health & Mental Health Services Research, 34,* 116–126.

Laughren, T. P. (1998, March 26). *Recommendations for approvable action for Celexa (citalopram) for the treatment of depression* [Memorandum]. Washington, DC: Department of Health and Human Services, Public Health Service, Food and Drug Administration, Center for Drug Evaluation and Research.

Laughren, T.P. (2004). *Background comments for February 2, 2004 meeting of Psychopharmacological Drugs Advisory Committee (PDAC) and Pediatric Subcommittee of the Antiinfective Drugs Advisory Committee (Peds AC)* [Memorandum]. Washington, DC: Department of Health and Human Services, Public Health Service, Food and Drug Administration, Center for Drug Evaluation and Research. Retrieved June 21, 2005, from http://www.fda.gov/ohrms/dockets/ac/04/briefing/4006B1_03_Background_Memo_01-05-04.htm

Lieberman, J. A. (2006). Comparative effectiveness of antipsychotic drugs. *Archives of General Psychiatry, 63,* 1069–1072.

Lieberman, J. A., Stroup, T. S., McEvoy, J. P., Swartz, M. S., Rosenheck, R. A., Perkins, D. O., et al. (2005). Effectiveness of antipsychotic drugs in patients with chronic schizophrenia. *New England Journal of Medicine, 353,* 1209–1223.

Lurie, P., Almeida, C. M., Stine, N., Stine, A., & Wolfe (2006). Financial conflict of interest disclosure and voting patterns at Food and Drug Administration Drug Advisory Committee meetings. *JAMA, 295, 26,* 1921–1928.

Maugh, T. H. (2006, March 23). A varied assault on depression yields gains; If one drug fails, a study finds, another often can be added or substituted with success. *Los Angeles Times,* p. A1.

Mathis, M. (2007, June 18). *Memorandum: Recommendation of approvable action for risperidone (Risperdal®) for the treatment of schizophrenia and bipolar I disorder in pediatric patients (response to PWR).* Retrieved November 1, 2007, from http://

www.fda.gov/cder/foi/esum/2007/020272s046s047,020588s006s037,021444s020 s021_rsperidone_clinical_BPCA.pdf

McClellan, J., Sikich, L., Findling, R. L., Frazier, J. A., Vitiello, B., Hlastala, S. A., et al. (2007). Treatment of early-onset schizophrenia spectrum disorders (TEOSS). *Journal of the American Academy of Child & Adolescent Psychiatry, 46*, 969–978.

McKay, K. M., Imel, Z., & Wampold, B. (2006). Psychiatrist effects in the psychopharmacological treatment of depression. *Journal of Affective Disorders, 92*(2–3), 287–90.

Medco Health Solutions, Inc. (2004, May 18). *Medco study reveals pediatric spending spike on drugs to treat behavioral problems.* Retrieved May 24, 2004, from http://www.drugtrend.com/medco/consumer/drugtrend/trends

Moncrieff, J. (2001). Are antidepressants overrated? A review of methodological problems in antidepressant trials. *Annals of Internal Medicine, 134*, 657–662.

Moncrieff, J. (2006). Why is it so difficult to stop psychiatric drug treatment? It may be nothing to do with the original problem. *Medical Hypotheses, 67*, 192–196.

Moncrieff, J., & Cohen, D. (2005). Rethinking models of psychotropic drug action. *Psychotherapy & Psychosomatics, 74*, 145–153.

Moncrieff, J., Wessely, S., & Hardy R. (2004) Active placebo versus antidepressants for depression. *Cochrane Data Base of Systematic Reviews,* Issue 1, Art No. CD003012. doi: 10.1002/14651858.CD003012.pub2)

Moreno, C., Laje, G., Blanco, C., Huiping, G., Schmidt, A. B., & Olfsen, M. (2007). National trends in the outpatient diagnosis and treatment of bipolar disorder in youth. *Archives of General Psychiatry, 64*, 1032–1039.

MTA Cooperative Group (1999). A 14-month randomized clinical trial of treatment strategies for attention-deficit/hyperactivity disorder. *Archives of General Psychiatry, 56*, 1073–1086.

MTA Cooperative Group. (2004) 24-month outcomes of treatment strategies for attention deficit/hyperactivity disorder (ADHD): The NIMH MTA follow-up. *Pediatrics, 113*, 754–761.

Munsey, C. (2008). Front-line psychopharmacology. *Monitor on Psychology, 39*(2), 56–57.

National Institute of Mental Health. (2008). *Depression* (NIH publication No. 08 3561). Retrieved March 10, 2008, from http://www.nimh.nih.gov/health/publications/depression/nimhdepression.pdf

National Institute of Mental Health. (n.d.). *Antidepressant medications for children and adolescents: Information for parents and caregivers.* Retrieved July 7, 2009, from http://www.nimh.nih.gov/health/topics/child-and-adolescent-mental-health/antidepressant-medications-for-children-and-adolescents-information-for-parents-and-caregivers.shtml

Nierenberg, A. A., Ostacher, M. J., Calabrese, J. R., Ketter, T. A., Marangell, L. B., Miklowitz, D. J., et al. (2006). Treatment-resistant bipolar depression: A STEP-BD equipoise randomized effectiveness trial of antidepressant augmentation with lamotrigine, inositol, or risperidone. *American Journal of Psychiatry, 163*, 210–216.

Pandina, G., DelBello, M., Kushner, S., et al. (2007, October). *Risperidone for the treatment of acute mania in bipolar youth.* Poster presented at the 54th Annual Meeting of the American Academy of Child and Adolescent Psychiatry, Boston.

Pandina, G., Kushner, S., Singer, J., et al. (2007, October). *Comparison of two risperidone dose ranges in adolescents with schizophrenia.* Poster presented at the 54th Annual Meeting of the American Academy of Child and Adolescent Psychiatry, Boston, MA.

Patten, S. B. (2004). The impact of antidepressant treatment on population health: Synthesis of data from two national data sources in Canada. *Population Health Metrics, 2*(9). Retrieved from http://www.pophealthmetrics.com

Pelham, W. (1999). The NIMH multimodal treatment study for attention-deficit hyperactivity disorder: Just say yes to drugs alone. *Canadian Journal of Psychiatry, 44,* 981–990.

Penn, Schoen, & Berland Associates. (2004). *Survey for the American Psychological Association.* Unpublished manuscript.

Perlis, R. H., Ostacher, M. J., Patel, J. K., Marangell, L. B., Zhang, H., Wisniewski, et al. (2006). Predictors of recurrence in bipolar disorder: Primary outcomes from the Systematic Treatment Enhancement Program for Bipolar Disorder (STEP-BD). *American Journal of Psychiatry, 163,* 217–224.

Posternak, M. A., & Miller, I. (2001). Untreated short-term course of major depression: A meta-analysis of outcomes from studies using wait-list control groups. *Journal of Affective Disorders, 66*(2–3), 139–146.

Preda, A., MacLean, R. W., Mazure, C. M., & Bowers, M. B. (2001). Antidepressant-associated mania and psychosis resulting in psychiatric admissions. *Journal of Clinical Psychiatry, 62,* 30–33.

Reyes, M., Buitelaar, J., Toren, P., Augustyns, I., & Eerdekens, M. (2006). A randomized, double-blind, placebo-controlled study of risperidone maintenance treatment in children and adolescents with disruptive behavior disorders. *American Journal of Psychiatry, 163,* 402–410.

Ross, R. G. (2008). New findings on antipsychotic use in children and adolescents with schizophrenia spectrum disorders. *American Journal of Psychiatry, 165,* 1369–1372.

Rush, A. J., Fava, M., Wisniewski, S. R., Lavori, P. W., Trivedi, M. H., Sackeim, H. A., et al. (2004). Sequenced treatment alternatives to relieve depression (STAR*D): Rationale and design. *Controlled Clinical Trials, 25*(1), 119–142.

Rush, A. J., Trivedi, M. H., Wisniewski, S. R., Nierenberg, A. A., Stewart, J. W., Warden, D., et al. (2006). Acute and longer-term outcomes in depressed outpatients requiring one or several treatment steps: A STAR*D report. *American Journal of Psychiatry, 163,* 1905–1917.

Rush, A. J., Trivedi, M. H., Wisniewski, S. R., Stewart, J. W., Nierenberg, A. A., Thase, M. E., et al. (2006). Bupropion-sr, sertraline, or venlafaxine-xr after failure of SSRIs for depression. *New England Journal of Medicine, 354,* 1231–1242.

Sachs, G. S., Thase, M. E., Otto, M. W., Bauer, M., Miklowitz, D., Wisniewski, S. R., et al. (2003). Rationale, design, and methods of the Systematic Treatment Enhancement Program for Bipolar Disorder (STEP-BD). *Biological Psychiatry, 53,* 1028–1042.

Safer, D. J. (2002). Design and reporting modifications in industry-sponsored comparative psychopharmacology trials. *Journal of Nervous and Mental Disease, 190,* 583–592.

Scheffler, R. M., Hinshaw, S. P., Modrek, S. & Levine, P. (2007). Trends: the global market for ADHD medications. *Health Affairs, 26,* 450.

Shea, M., Elkin, I., Imber, S., Sotsky, S., Watkins, J., Collins, J., et al. (1992). Course of depressive symptoms over follow-up: Findings from the National Institute of Mental Health Treatment of Depression Collaborative Research Program. *Archives of General Psychiatry, 49,* 782–787.

Sikich, L., Frazier, J. A., McClellan, A., Findling, R. L., Vitiello, B., Ritz, L., et al. (2008). Double-blind comparison of first- and second-generation in early-onset schizophrenia and schizoaffective disorder: Findings from the treatment of early-onset schizophrenia spectrum disorders (TEOSS) study. *American Journal of Psychiatry, 165,* 1420–1431.

Smith, R. (2003). Medical journals and pharmaceutical companies: Uneasy bedfellows. *British Medical Journal, 326,* 1202–1205.

Snyder, R., Turgay, A., Aman, M., Binder, C., Fisman, S., Carroll, A., et al. (2002). Effects of risperidone on conduct and disruptive behavior disorders in children with subaverage IQs. *Journal of the American Academy of Child & Adolescent Psychiatry, 41,* 1026–1036.

Sotsky, S. M., Glass, D. R., Shea, M. T., Pilkonis, P. A. Collins, J. F., Elkin, I., et al. (1991). Patient predictors of response to psychotherapy and pharmacotherapy: Findings in the NIMH Treatment of Depression Collaborative Research Program. *American Journal of Psychiatry, 148,* 997–1008.

Sparks, J., A. & Duncan, B. L. (2008). Do no harm: A critical risk/benefit analysis of child psychotropic medications. *Journal of Family Psychotherapy, 19,* 1–19.

Sparks, J. A., Duncan, B. L., & Miller, S. D. (2008). Common factors in psychotherapy. In J. Lebow (Ed.), *Twenty-first century psychotherapies: Contemporary approaches to theory and practice* (pp. 453–497). Hoboken, NJ: Wiley.

Stagnitti, M. N. (2007, February). *Trends in the use and expenditures for the therapeutic class prescribed psychotherapeutic agents and all subclasses, 1997 and 2004* (Statistical Brief #163). Rockville, MD: Agency for Healthcare Research and Quality. Retrieved July 10, 2007, from http://www.meps.ahrq.gov/mepsweb/ data_files/ publications/st163/stat163.pdf

Stone, M. B., & Jones, M. L. (2006, November). *Clinical review: Relationship between antidepressant drugs and suicidality in adults* (PowerPoint presentation). Silver Spring, MD: U.S. Food and Drug Administration, Center for Drug Evaluation and Research. Retrieved June 30, 2009, from http://www.fda.gov/ohrms/dockets/ac/06/ slides/2006-4272OPH1-11-sharav.ppt

Stroup, T. S., Lieberman, J. A., McEvoy, J. P., Swartz, M. S., Davis, S. M., Capuano, G. A., et al. (2007). Effectiveness of olanzapine, quetiapine, and risperidone in patients with chronic schizophrenia after discontinuing perphenazine: A CATIE study. *American Journal of Psychiatry, 164,* 415–427.

Swanson, J. M., Elliott, G. R., Greenhill, L. L., Wigal, T., Arnold, L. E., Vitiello B., et al. (2007). Effects of stimulant medication on growth rates across 3 years in the MTA follow-up. *Journal of the American Academy of Child & Adolescent Psychiatry, 46,* 1015–1027.

Swanson, J., Greenhill, L., Wigal, T., Kollins, S., Stehli, A., Davies, M. et al. (2006). Stimulant-related reductions of growth rates in the PATS. *Journal of the American Academy of Child & Adolescent Psychiatry, 45,* 1304–1313.

Swartz, M. S., Perkins, D. O., Stroup, T. S., Davis, S. M., Capuano, G., Rosenheck, R. A., et al. (2007). Effects of antipsychotic medications on psychosocial functioning in patients with chronic schizophrenia: Findings from the NIMH CATIE study. *American Journal of Psychiatry, 164,* 428–436.

Thase, M. E., Greenhouse, J. B., Frank, E., Reynolds, C. F., Pilkonis, P. A., Hurley, K., et al. (1997). Treatment of major depression with psychotherapy or psychotherapy–pharmacotherapy combinations. *Archives of General Psychiatry, 54,* 1009–1015.

Thase, M. E., & Jindal, R.D. (2004). Combining psychotherapy and psychopharmacology for treatment of mental disorders. In M. J. Lambert (Ed.), *Bergin and Garfield's handbook of psychotherapy and behavior change* (5th ed., pp. 743–766). New York: Wiley.

Treatment for Adolescents With Depression Study Team. (2004). Fluoxetine, cognitive–behavioral therapy, and their combination for adolescents with depression. *JAMA, 292,* 807–820.

Treatment for Adolescents With Depression Study Team. (2007). The Treatment for Adolescents With Depression Study (TADS): Long-term effectiveness and safety outcomes. *Archives of General Psychiatry, 64,* 1132–1144.

Trivedi, M. H., Fava, M., Wisniewski, S. R., Thase, M. E., Quitkin, F., Warden, D. et al. (2006). Medication augmentation after the failure of SSRIs for depression. *New England Journal of Medicine, 354,* 1243–1252.

Trivedi, M. H., Rush, A. J., Wisniewski, S. R., Nierenberg, A. A., Warden, D., Ritz, L., et al. (2006). Evaluation of outcomes with citalopram for depression using measurement-based care in STAR*D: Implications for clinical practice. *American Journal of Psychiatry, 163,* 28–40.

Turgay, L., Binder, C., Snyder, R., & Fisman, S. (2002). Long-term safety and efficacy of risperidone for the treatment of disruptive behavior disorders in children with subaverage IQs. *Pediatrics, 110.* Retrieved June 9, 2007, from http://www.pediatrics.org/cgi/content/full/110/3/e34

Turner, E. H., Matthews, A. M., Eftihia Linardatos, B. S., Tell, R. A., & Rosenthal, R. (2008). Selective publication of antidepressant trials and its influence on apparent efficacy. *New England Journal of Medicine, 358,* 252–260.

U.S. Food and Drug Administration (2003, January 3). *FDA approves Prozac for pediatric use to treat depression and OCD*. Retrieved January 25, 2003, from http://www.fda.gov/bbs/topics/ANSWERS/2003/ANS01187.html

U.S. Food and Drug Administration (2004, October 15). *FDA launches a multi-pronged strategy to strengthen safeguards for children treated with antidepressant medications*. Retrieved October 30, 2004, from http://www.fda.gov/bbs/topics/news/2004/NEW01124.html

U.S. Food and Drug Administration (2007a, May 2). *New warnings proposed for antidepressants*. Retrieved July 10, 2009, from http://www.fda.gov/ForConsumers/ConsumerUpdates/ucm048950.htm

U.S. Food and Drug Administration (2007b, August 22). *FDA approves Risperdal for two psychiatric conditions in children and adolescents*. Retrieved September 5, 2007, from http://www.fda.gov/bbs/topics/NEWS/2007/NEW01686.html

Wampold, B. E. (2001). *The great psychotherapy debate: Models, methods, and findings*. Hillsdale, NJ: Erlbaum.

Wampold, B. E., & Brown, G. (2005). Estimating therapist variability in outcomes attributable to therapists: A naturalistic study of outcomes in managed care. *Journal of Consulting and Clinical Psychology, 73*, 914–923.

Willman, D. (2003, December 7). Stealth merger: Drug companies and government medical research. *Los Angeles Times*, p. A1.

Zito, J. M., & Safer, S. J. (2005). Recent child pharmacoepidemiological findings. *Journal of Child & Adolescent Psychopharmacology, 15*, 5–9.

# II

# DELIVERING WHAT WORKS: PRACTICE-BASED EVIDENCE

# 8

# "YES, IT IS TIME FOR CLINICIANS TO ROUTINELY MONITOR TREATMENT OUTCOME"

MICHAEL J. LAMBERT

However beautiful the strategy, you should occasionally look at the results.

—Sir Winston Churchill

By the early 1970s, outcome research had established that various forms of psychotherapy had an overall positive effect on client outcomes. The same evidence showed that a small and consistent percentage of people deteriorated while in care (Bergin, 1971). Reported rates varied between 5% and 10%. The deterioration was mostly connected to client characteristics, but specific therapist behaviors were also implicated (e.g., forms of rejection; Lambert, Bergin, & Collins, 1977). It is unfortunate that the findings were almost entirely ignored by the field. At the time, research efforts were principally directed to studying brand name treatments and demonstrating the superiority of then-favored therapies in comparative outcome studies (Hubble, Duncan, & Miller, 1999; Lambert, Bergin & Garfield, 2004; Wampold, 2001).

Interest in the phenomenon of deterioration grew in the late 1980s with the emergence of cost containment efforts. Managed care entities, for example, scrambling to control or even cut costs had to show that reducing services did not diminish the effectiveness of treatments (see chap. 9, this volume). Assessing outcome was seen as a way of examining whether more could be accomplished with less, or at least proving that brief, efficient services could be as effective as intensive, long-term care. Managed care companies were slow to link the idea of preventing negative outcomes with outcome assessment and instead relied largely on implementing best practices of care. By the end of the decade, these companies were at least considering the value of using outcome assessment data to reduce negative effects.

Although it was seldom used systematically to enhance treatment, by the 1990s outcome measurement was being touted as an important aspect of clinical care (Stricker, Troy, & Shueman, 2000). In the same period, scientific and technological advances were enhancing methods for identifying and reducing negative client outcomes. One particularly important innovation was the development of statistical techniques that allowed researchers to examine change in individuals over time (Finch, Lambert, & Schaalje, 2001; Lutz et al., 2006). Massive amounts of data collected over many sessions across thousands of clients could be analyzed and used to model client recovery, a task that was impossible before the development of the new statistical procedures. Such methods, in turn, could be used to chart the course of change for the deteriorating, recovering, and average client. Eventually, a person's progress could be compared with that of similar clients, and probabilistic statements could be made about the likelihood of success and failure. A medical analogy illustrating this methodology is the routine use of growth charts for plotting infant head circumference by age and by that means identifying deviations from normal or average growth.

Surveys show that practitioners question the role of information technology in improving client care (with only 10% classified as "eager-adopters"; Meredith, Bair, & Ford, 2000). Even so, with the widespread availability and power of computers, it is now possible for providers to obtain outcome data about success with individual clients in real time. For two reasons, such practice-based evidence (Barkham et al., 2001; Duncan, Miller, & Sparks, 2004) is especially important. First, failure to improve and deterioration rates remain high in routine care (Hansen, Lambert, & Forman, 2002). Second, the available evidence indicates that therapists, despite their confidence in their clinical judgment, are not alert to treatment failure (e.g., Breslin, Sobell, Buchan, & Cunningham, 1997; Yalom & Lieberman, 1971).

Regarding the last point, consider findings from a study by Hannan et al. (2005) comparing therapist predictions of client deterioration with actuarial methods. Although therapists were aware of the study's purpose, familiar with the dependent measure, and informed that the base rate was likely to be 8%, they accurately predicted deterioration in only 1 out of 550 cases. In other words, therapists in the study did not identify 39 out of the 40 clients who deteriorated. In contrast, the actuarial method used by the computer correctly predicted 36 of the 40.

These and similar findings make clear that without timely feedback about client progress, practitioners grossly underestimate negative outcomes. Accordingly, they are less likely to make the adjustments necessary to forestall negative outcomes or, for that matter, improve positive outcomes. Owing to the extant research documenting the superiority of actuarial over clinical methods in making such predictions (Garb, 2005), there is little doubt that the greatest predictive success comes through real time, clinic-based application of computer-assisted actuarial methods. Indeed, in the future, such psychological lab test or vital sign data will be as important in behavioral health as in medicine.

In this chapter, I present additional evidence regarding the advantages of tracking progress, identifying at-risk clients, and providing real-time feedback. I then review outcome management systems currently used in routine care and discuss important, specific procedural aspects of monitoring and feedback. Here, I propose that the next step to advance the "heart and soul of change" in psychotherapy will come about through the formal monitoring of change and a willingness to enter frank and open discussions with clients about their progress. Additionally, I present an overview of data-based outcomes management, and I hope that readers will not only understand the context in which this work evolved but will also be motivated to avail themselves of recent research, studies that convincingly demonstrate the value of outcome management for promoting service delivery and client improvement.

## OUTCOMES MANAGEMENT

Over the past 10 years, much effort and attention have been directed toward identifying treatments that work in specific contexts and with different populations (e.g., disorders; Chambless et al., 1996, 1998). Such initiatives coincided with and were a response to demands coming from third-party payers (e.g., insurance agencies, government funding bodies) to improve accountability in health care service delivery. In both commercial and single payer systems, across medicine and other professions, those in charge of accounts, including those receiving services, wanted to know what they were getting for their investment (Bartlett & Cohen, 1993; G. S. Brown, Burlingame, Lambert, Jones, & Vaccaro, 2001).

Various groups—divisions of the American Psychological Association (APA), the National Institute of Mental Health, and the Substance Abuse and Mental Health Services Administration (SAMHSA) of the Department of Health and Human Services—have worked to identify and implement scientifically based practices (c.f., National Institutes of Health, 2002). As many practitioners and researchers feared, the creation of lists of empirically supported psychotherapies yielded several untoward consequences, chief among them restrictions on both the type and amount of care offered to clients. In fact, several states enacted legislation specifically aimed at limiting treatment options (e.g., Oregon, Washington, Arizona, Connecticut; for additional discussion, see chapter 6, this volume). Efforts to improve accountability, via lists and legislation, arguably are well intentioned. Nevertheless, the resulting limitations on clinical practice miss the proverbial point. No one needs an empirically supported psychotherapy that does not work for them (S. Miller, personal communication, May 2007).

In 2005, APA created a Presidential Task Force on Evidence-Based Practice. This body was charged with the responsibility of developing a more nuanced and scientifically valid definition of *evidence-based psychological practice* (EBPP; APA, 2006, p. 273). In a major move away from the position taken by APA Division 12 (Society of Clinical Psychology) nearly a decade earlier (Task Force on the Identification and Dissemination of Psychological Procedures; Chambless et al., 1996), the Task Force redefined EBPP as "the integration of the best available research with clinical expertise in the context of patient characteristics, culture, and preferences" (APA, 2006, p. 273). Regarding the phrase *clinical expertise*, moreover, the Task Force commented that

> clinical expertise also entails the monitoring of patient progress (and of changes in the patient's circumstances—e.g., job loss, major illness) that may suggest the need to adjust the treatment (Lambert, Bergin, & Garfield, 2004). If progress is not proceeding adequately, the psychologist alters or addresses problematic aspects of the treatment (e.g., problems in the therapeutic relationship or in the implementation of the goals of the treatment) as appropriate. (APA, 2006, p. 276–277)

Because the most recent APA Task Force has placed monitoring and altering treatment under the category of clinical expertise, it is reasonable to construe these activities as an EBPP. Additionally, as it turns out, monitoring and altering therapy are critical components of outcomes management. The term *outcomes management* encompasses two well-defined operations. It designates activities that use the client's actual response to treatment, the outcome, to improve the treatment response of individual clients. It also refers to administrators' collective use of summed data across clients to make decisions for the benefit of future clients. To enhance individual outcome, therapists are typically provided feedback about a client's progress in real time. In this management practice, the rapid delivery of progress information to therapists is essential. In turn, clinicians are counted on to use that data to enhance problem solving, with the client's participation, over the entire course of treatment.

The second operation of outcomes management practice allows administrators to judge the relative merits of treatment approaches through their examination of outcomes across many, often thousands, of clients. This procedure sharply contrasts with the widespread assumption that applying so-called best practices results in the best outcomes. Of course, both operations—

managing outcome for a particular client and for a large body of clients—are not mutually exclusive. Both can be achieved if client treatment response is routinely tracked.

In 2003, Lambert, Whipple, Hawkins, Vermeersch, Nielsen, and Smart published an article titled, "Is It Time for Clinicians to Routinely Track Patient Outcome?" It reported a meta-analysis of three studies that evaluated the consequences of giving progress information or feedback to therapists. Since that review, additional studies have been completed, providing strong empirical support for such methods. Given these findings, it is now possible, without the equivocation characteristic of most research reports, to answer affirmatively: "Yes, it *is* time for clinicians to routinely track client outcome."

In what follows, the evidence from clinical trials supporting the systematic collection and use of real-time outcome data is presented. The studies discussed rely on the use of a single set of measures (OQ Measures). At the end of the chapter, I highlight and review a variety of other measures and data collection systems implemented in clinical service delivery settings.

## Research on Ongoing Treatment Monitoring

Five large randomized controlled studies have been conducted evaluating the impact of using feedback on assessing and modifying treatment response (Harmon et al., 2007; Hawkins, Lambert, Vermeersch, Slade, & Tuttle, 2004; Lambert et al., 2001, 2002; Whipple et al., 2003). The studies share several features that in combination provide a strong empirical case for tracking client progress. The most important of these are the following: (a) random assignment of participants, (b) the use of the same therapist across treatment conditions (as a control for therapist effects), (c) a variety of treatment approaches or orientations, and (d) a high percentage of licensed clinicians (50%–100%) taking part in each study. Characteristics of the five studies are presented in Table 8.1. Four of the samples were equivalent (coming from the same clinic); participants in the 5th sample were older, more distressed, and treated in a hospital outpatient clinic.

Each study required approximately 1 year of data collection and included session-by-session measurement of outcome for more than 4,000 clients. The primary dependent variable in all studies was the Outcome Questionnaire, OQ-45 (described later). Further, in each, individual client response to treatment was compared with session-by-session normative data (i.e., *expected treatment response*; ETR) to identify clients not responding well to treatment. Poor responders were denoted as *signal-alarm* cases or as "Not-On-Track."

Progress data were supplied to therapists via a graph, along with color-coded warning messages when improvement was not occurring or not of the

TABLE 8.1
Summary of Design Characteristics of Controlled Outcome Studies
Aimed at Reducing Deterioration and Enhancing Positive Outcome

| Study | Clients (n) | Therapists (n) | TAU | Therapist feedback | Therapist and client feedback | Clinical support tools |
|---|---|---|---|---|---|---|
| Lambert et al. (2001) | 609 | 31 | X | X | | |
| Lambert et al. (2002) | 1,020 | 49 | X | X | | |
| Whipple et al. (2003) | 981 | 48 | X | X | | X |
| Hawkins et al. (2004) | 201 | 5 | X | X | X | |
| Harmon et al. (2007) | 1,374 | 47 | | X | X | X |

*Note.* TAU = treatment as usual (i.e., clients who were not on track and whose therapist was not given feedback). Data from Harmon et al. (2007), Hawkins et al. (2004), Lambert et al. (2001, 2002), and Whipple et al. (2003).

expected magnitude. Two studies assessed the impact of providing both therapists and clients with OQ-45 progress information. Two explored the impact of providing therapists with additional feedback regarding the client's assessment of the therapeutic relationship, motivation, and degree of social support, including a problem-solving decision tree with suggested interventions, a device called Clinical Support Tool (CST; Lambert, Whipple, et al., 2004). Assessments of the relationship, motivation, and social support (described more fully later) were given with the graph when it was observed that the client was not progressing as well as expected.

In current clinical applications, step-wise problem-solving procedures are administered, scored, and applied using an end user software program (OQ-Analyst; OQ Measures, 2004) running on a handheld computer. The use of such devices connected wirelessly to the clinician's desktop computer makes it possible to assess progress by the time a client walks into the therapist's office. Instantly, the therapist can determine whether the client is deviating significantly from the ETR. In brief, this commercially available software uses one of two different types of predictive algorithms: (a) statistical modeling of ETR on the basis of a nationwide sample of more than 11,000 cases and (b) a rational model based on clinician consensus ratings of satisfactory client progress.

Figure 8.1 presents a picture of the output from the OQ-Analyst software. This specific screen shot illustrates the progress of a fictional client, "Brad News," as measured over nine sessions. After a single visit, the program predicted that Brad was at significant risk of a negative outcome (R = red signal). At any given session, the therapist can look below the graph and read the message provided. Messages vary in urgency depending on the size of the difference among the current amount of progress, the ETR (indicated by the dark sloping line), and the amount of therapy.

What then are the consequences of providing feedback? The results of the five studies are clear: Providing therapists with feedback about client progress improves outcome for clients predicted to be at risk of deterioration. Providing therapists with additional feedback—including the client's assessment of the therapeutic alliance, readiness for change, and strength of existing extratherapeutic supports—increases the effect, doubling the number of clients who experience a clinically meaningful outcome.

In the studies, clients were divided into four groups: (a) treatment as usual (TAU; i.e., no feedback), (b) progress feedback to therapist, (c) progress feedback to therapist and client, and (d) progress feedback plus clinical support tools. Of particular note is the percentage of clients who deteriorated or ended treatment with reliable negative change. The data show that providing feedback regarding progress resulted in a decrease in the percentage of clients not on track who ended treatment with reliable negative change (from 20% to 13% or 15%, or an overall decrease of 25%–35%). Deterioration rates were further reduced when clinical support tools were added to progress feedback, with the percentage of deterioration falling to 8% (or an overall decrease of 60%).

When clients are not on track but meet criteria for reliable improvement and clinically significant change, additional benefits of feedback are realized. Percentages increased from 22% for TAU to 33%, when feedback regarding progress was provided to therapists, to 39% when feedback was shared with both clients and therapists, and to 45% when feedback was furnished in conjunction with the clinical support tools. These increasing rates of positive improvement, depending on the extent of decision-making information provided to therapists and clients, demonstrate that feedback prevents deterioration. They also show that feedback enhances positive outcomes in clinically meaningful ways. In short, the consequences of using feedback are not mere statistical changes, but real.

Beyond influencing the final treatment outcome, results of the five studies indicate that session utilization is affected by the provision of feedback. In four of the five studies, significant differences in treatment length were observed between experimental and control clients (Harmon et al., 2007; Lambert et al., 2001; Lambert et al., 2002; Whipple et al., 2003). Specifically, clients in the not-on-track feedback conditions received significantly more

| Name: | news, brad **ID:** | | Alert Status: | **Red** |
|---|---|---|---|---|
| **Session Date:** | 10/25/2005 **Session:** 8 | | **Most Recent Score:** | 106 |
| | | | **Initial Score:** | 85 |
| **Clinician:** | lambert, m **Clinic:** Clinic A | | **Change From Initial:** | Reliably Worse |
| **Diagnosis:** | Unknown Diagnosis | | **Current Distress Level:** High |
| **Algorithm:** | Empirical ▾ | | | |

**Most Recent Critical Item Status:**

8. **Suicide -** I have thoughts of **Frequently**
   ending my life.

11. **Substance Abuse -** After **Frequently**
   heavy drinking, I need a drink the
   next morning to get going.

26. **Substance Abuse -** I feel **Frequently**
   annoyed by people who criticize
   my drinking.

32. **Substance Abuse -** I have **Sometimes**
   trouble at work/school because of
   drinking or drug use.

44. **Work Violence -** I feel angry **Sometimes**
   enough at work/school to do
   something I might regret.

| Subscales | Current | Outpat. Norm | Comm. Norm |
|---|---|---|---|
| Symptom Distress: | 61 | 49 | 25 |
| Interpersonal Relations: | 26 | 20 | 10 |
| Social Role: | 19 | 14 | 10 |
| Total: | 106 | 83 | 45 |

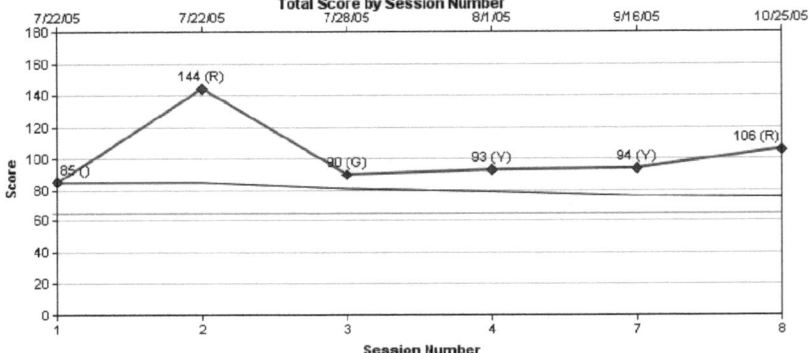

Total Score by Session Number

**Graph Label Legend:**
(R) = **Red**: High chance of negative outcome  (Y) = Yellow: Some chance of negative outcome
(G) = **Green**: Making expected progress  (W) = **White**: Functioning in normal range

**Feedback Message:**
The patient is deviating from the expected response to treatment. They are not on track to realize substantial benefit from treatment. Chances are they may drop out of treatment prematurely or have a negative treatment outcome. Steps should be taken to carefully review this case and identify reasons for poor progress. It is recommended that you be alert to the possible need to improve the therapeutic alliance, reconsider the client's readiness for change and the need to renegotiate the therapeutic contract, intervene to strengthen social supports, or possibly alter your treatment plan by intensifying treatment, shifting intervention strategies, or decide upon a new course of action, such as referral for medication. Continuous monitoring of future progress is highly recommended.

*Figure 8.1.* Output from Outcome Questionnaire Analyst software with the fictional client Brad News. Brad's scores are plotted with his score at the session of interest and include small single letters to indicate alarm status: (G) = Green, (Y) = Yellow, (R) = Red. The expected treatment response is indicated by the dark sloping line. The gray horizontal line at a score of 63 is the line demarcating normal functioning. Outpat. Norm = average score of outpatients; Comm. Norm = average score of nonpatients drawn from the community.

sessions than their TAU counterparts. Such findings indicate that increases in treatment length, along with retention of clients not progressing, may be an important mechanism of action through which feedback improves outcome.

In two of the five studies (Lambert et al., 2001; Whipple et al., 2003), clients identified as on track for a positive outcome and in the feedback condition received fewer sessions than those in the on-track group. Here again, feedback helped ensure an appropriate dose of services, with those most likely to benefit (about 25%) staying longer, and clients more likely to recover (75%) ending earlier. Taken together, these results have obvious implications for planning and maximizing the efficiency of service delivery.

## Beyond Progress Feedback: The Use of Clinical Support Tools

The data from the five randomized controlled clinical trials discussed previously make clear that providing feedback to therapists (and in one of two studies, directly to clients) is highly beneficial. As compelling as these results are, however, the same data show that a significant portion of clients do not derive benefit from treatment even when feedback is provided. To further bolster positive outcomes, Whipple et al. (2003) added a condition in which clinicians were provided with an organized problem-solving strategy for clients identified as not on track. After deciding on a hierarchy of variables that might account for the deterioration, an attempt was made to capture problematic aspects of the psychotherapy and other potential problems that could be directly influenced by therapist actions (Barber, 2007). These variables, in turn, were used to construct the CST, a structured method for identifying factors that could prompt effective actions by the therapist.

Because the empirical literature has shown that the quality of therapeutic alliance is consistently related to outcome, and other studies have indicated that client ratings of the alliance are more strongly correlated with outcome than therapist ratings (Horvath & Luborsky, 1993), the CST included a formal assessment of the clients' perceptions of the therapeutic relationship. The second variable included in the CST was motivation (e.g., Garfield, 1994). A review of the research suggested that motivation and dropout were significantly related. Instances were legion in which therapists moved ahead with treatment without securing the clients full commitment or without making sufficient efforts to foster more autonomous motivation (Zuroff et al., 2007). It was especially clear that substance abuse treatment had made inroads in boosting positive outcomes by measuring motivation and using motivational interviewing to increase positive participation (Miller & Rollnick, 2002).

Though often neglected because of therapists' near exclusive focus on in-session events, the literature strongly suggests that client-perceived social support moderates psychotherapy outcome (Cohen & Wills, 1985; Zimet,

Dahlem, Zimet, & Farley, 1988). Thus, social support was the third factor included in the CST. Measures of this important variable typically emphasize the degree to which clients have family and friends available for rendering assistance. Not only could perceived social support be measured, but many strategies were available for increasing these supports, including intervention in the client's social network, or use of group, family, couple, and self-help groups as adjuncts or replacements for individual treatment.

The fourth and final variable in the CST was errors in diagnostic and treatment planning. The basic point here is that clients who become signal-alarm cases are deteriorating in a preferred treatment that is not having its intended benefit. Some of these clients may merit a referral for medication evaluation or the addition of group work or self-help.

The CST package consisted of the decision tree, three measures with cutoff scores (indicating if the variable of interest was a problem), and a list of suggested interventions for each variable. For example, if the alliance was identified as problematic for a client, the therapist was directed to a list of interventions to consider for problem solving. Among the possible interventions, Safran and Muran's (2000) work on repairing ruptures in the therapeutic alliance was highlighted, quickly drawing the therapist's attention to these evidence-based interventions. Table 8.2, which summarizes the data from the original (Whipple et al., 2003) and replication study (Harmon et al., 2007), reveals a strong effect for this add-on intervention. In fact, not-on-track clients, randomly assigned to this intervention, left treatment (as a group) very close to the cutoff for normal functioning. At present, it is not possible to specify which, if any, of the CST feedback was most useful in reversing a negative course of change for not-on-track clients. The value of any information varies

TABLE 8.2
Percentage of Not-On-Track (Signal-Alarm) Cases Meeting Criteria for
Clinically Significant Change at Termination Summed Across Five Studies

| Outcome classification | TAU n (%) | T-Fb n (%) | T/C-Fb n (%) | T-Fb + CST n (%) |
|---|---|---|---|---|
| Deteriorated[a] | 64 (20) | 90 (15) | 19 (13) | 12 (8) |
| No change | 184 (58) | 316 (53) | 71 (48) | 73 (47) |
| Reliable or clinically significant change[b] | 70 (22) | 196 (33) | 57 (39) | 169 (45) |

Note. TAU = treatment as usual (i.e., clients who were not on track and whose therapist was not given feedback); T-Fb = clients who were not on track and whose therapist received feedback; T/C-Fb = therapist feedback plus written direct feedback to clients; T-Fb + CST = clients who were not on track and whose therapist received feedback and used clinical support tools. Data from Whipple et al. (2003) and Harmon et al. (2007).
[a]Worsened by at least 14 points on the Outcome Questionnaire from pretreatment to posttreatment.
[b]Improved by at least 14 points on the Outcome Questionnaire or improved and passed the cutoff between dysfunctional and functional populations.

widely on a case-by-case basis, and actual problem solving remains in the hands of the clinician.

Few research groups have published clinical trials replicating and extending the findings of the preceding studies. An exception is an investigation conducted by Berking, Orth, and Lutz (2006). They examined progress feedback in a Swiss inpatient population. Though their work used different methods and measures, they found a solid gain for the experimental group. In this condition, therapists received progress feedback compared with the TAU control group over a 30-day hospital stay. This is an important finding because it extends our research on outpatients to individuals who received care in a hospital setting in which clients received many treatments (rather than once weekly psychotherapy), and the effects of feedback were still clinically significant.

Another exception is a recent study conducted in Norway by Anker, Duncan, and Sparks (2009). Designed with the shared features of our research described earlier, this investigation of 205 couples is the only randomized clinical trial to date that compared feedback with TAU with couples. The Outcome Rating Scale (ORS; Miller, Duncan, Brown, Sparks, & Claud, 2003), Session Rating Scale (SRS; an alliance measure; Duncan et al., 2003), and the algorithms derived from a large normative sample designed to reflect a typical community mental health outpatient population were used to provide the feedback and measure outcome. Feedback significantly improved outcome: In the TAU condition, 22.6% of both individuals of a couple realized reliable or clinically significant change compared with 50.5% of the feedback group. The predicted score adjusted for severity of an average client in the feedback group was 4.89 points (the Reliable Change Index on the ORS is 5), higher than for an average client in the TAU. One hopes, as in this example, that future replications will continue to extend our research to other populations and modalities while using what we have come to consider the most important elements of feedback: that it is timely, includes warning signals, and is directed toward individuals whose positive outcome is in doubt.

Given the results of the present studies, it is fair to argue that such methods become a part of routine practice. In the individual studies themselves, the effect sizes for the difference between feedback and treatment as usual ranged from 0.34 to 0.92. Such large effect sizes are unusual when one considers the most generous estimates of the effect size of the difference between empirically supported and comparison treatments is 0.20 or less (Lambert & Ogles, 2004; Wampold, 2001). It is curious that those advocating the widespread adoption of empirically supported therapies do so on the basis of much smaller treatment effects than those associated with feedback. Because of the large sample sizes of the individual studies, the current findings are compelling. Of course, one need not choose between giving feedback and using empirically supported treatments. They can work in concert.

The use of feedback to improve outcome is both powerful and simple. Training is straightforward, and the procedures are easily mastered. The basic requirements include a measure of client functioning that changes as an effect of an intervention, estimation of an ETR, and markers of meaningful deviations from that response. Structured problem-solving strategies to facilitate an understanding of what is going wrong and the ability to apply this knowledge before a client terminates psychotherapy are also helpful and easy to develop and master. A significant advantage is that the process can be used regardless of theoretical orientation.

Finally, as seen, formal feedback has the advantages of informing clinicians about successes and failures as well as providing benchmarks for groups of treated individuals. Now, clinicians and administrators can choose from a variety of available outcome management systems. One hopes that the days in which clinical work and decision making rely only on informal assessments will soon come to an end. In the following section, I briefly summarize several widely used methods.

## OUTCOMES MANAGEMENT SYSTEMS

The first outcomes management system was developed by Howard and colleagues using an instrument known by the acronym COMPASS (Howard, Moras, Brill, Martinovitch, & Lutz, 1996). The COMPASS includes 68 items broken down into three scales: Current Well-Being, Current Symptoms, and Current Life Functioning. These scales are summed and the total score designated as the Mental Health Index. Instructions call for clients to rate items on a 5-point scale about their functioning in the preceding month. Supporting scales include a measure of the therapeutic bond, which presents problems and their significance to the client, including clinician ratings on the *Diagnostic and Statistical Manual of Mental Disorders* Global Assessment of Functioning Scale and Life Functioning. Clients and therapists are expected to complete the measure monthly throughout the course of treatment.

Using a variety of statistical modeling techniques, this feedback system provides an ETR. It is modeled for each client on the basis of the degree of initial disturbance and several client variables such as chronicity of problems. Significant negative deviations from the ETR are used as one aspect of alerting therapists to potential treatment failure. In addition, the ETR model uses several indicators of poor outcome. For instance, it monitors a discrepancy between client reported (good) health and clinician reported (poor) health and the failure to improve reliably by the 12th session. Lueger et al. (2001) provided ample data on the ability of this system to identify treatment failures.

As with any outcomes monitoring system, the COMPASS system has distinct advantages as well as limitations. On the plus side, it provides for the collection of data from both clinician and client, with extensive pretreatment examination of client functioning and a sophisticated method of predicting poor outcomes. Disadvantages of this system include the amount of time required of therapists and clients to complete forms, the need to submit assessments to a third party for scoring and interpretation, infrequency of data collection, and the likelihood of termination before feedback delivery. The latter drawback is especially important because in many clinical settings, 50% of clients will have terminated after 4 weeks.

The second major system to be developed and applied to outcomes management uses OQ measures. These consist of several adult and youth outcome questionnaires. The central measure within the system is the Outcome Questionnaire-45 (OQ-45; Lambert, Morton, et al., 2004). It is a self-report measure with 45 items targeting symptoms (mainly anxiety and depression), emotional states, interpersonal relationships, and social role performance. It was designed to monitor client functioning each week during routine care. Normative comparisons have been used to provide markers for individual client outcome derived from Jacobson and Truax's (1991) formulas for reliable and clinically significant change. Thus, the instrument can inform clinicians about the degree of success a specific client is experiencing in relation to a criterion for normal functioning. The OQ-45 has the advantage of being especially sensitive to treatment effects. It includes a large number of items that have been shown to change over the course of time in clients who are being treated but remaining stable in clients who are equally disturbed but not being treated (Vermeersch, Lambert, & Burlingame, 2002; Vermeersch et al., 2004).

As already described, identifying signal cases, or cases at risk of a poor result, is crucial for enhancing positive outcomes. Further, from a health care management perspective with a focus on containing costs and providing quality assurance, identifying signal cases is essential for efficient resource allocation. As with the COMPASS system, extensive research has been performed to develop ETR curves for the OQ system. Currently, ample evidence exists indicating that the measures can be successfully used to predict treatment failure (e.g., Ellsworth, Lambert, & Johnson, 2006) and enhance client outcomes (Harmon et al., 2007; Hawkins et al., 2004; Lambert et al., 2001; Lambert et al., 2002; Whipple et al., 2003).

Next, in Germany, Kordy, Hannöver, and Richard (2001) designed a computer-assisted, feedback-driven psychotherapy quality management system. Used in inpatient psychotherapy settings across Europe, it is available in a variety of languages. Rather than developing their own assessment tools, these researchers created a software product—AKQUASI—that administers, scores, and provides feedback on the basis of several standardized measures (e.g., Symptom Checklist-90, OQ-45). This flexible system was created to fulfill the World Health Organization's call for quality assurance in health care delivery. This appeal comprised four major goals: develop a monitoring system, detect failures and shortcomings in treatment, make the information available to all the parties who can act to improve the situation, and create a culture of learning and communication.

The AKQUASI product collects data on client characteristics, the helping alliance, and client satisfaction. Users receive a recommendation for using multiple measures of the same constructs and multiple viewpoints of clients' functioning to capture the complexity of change. The system is ideal for inpatient settings in which clients remain in treatment at least 30 days, and plenty of time is available for the assessments. It is less feasible in outpatient settings.

To improve quality of care, Kordy et al. (2001) placed special emphasis on detecting problems and providing feedback to therapists in case management meetings for 30-day inpatient stays. In this context, the researcher and clinicians discuss the findings together. Signal-alarm cases are selected if they are terminating therapy and in grave need of help or are suicidal, or if they show more negative than positive change across subscales of the measures.

At a second level of analysis, report cards are created for internal comparisons of grouped data over time, tied to external benchmarks. The main data of interest in these comparisons are the rate of detection of signal-alarm cases, with the expectation that they will decrease from benchmark data collected before the initiation of quality assurance initiatives. Limited validity data suggest that the majority (three fourths) of signal-alarm cases were accurately identified with the psychometric scales in comparison with use of other therapist- or client-provided information. The specificity (i.e., ability to identify clients who did not deteriorate) of the signal-alarm proved to be high, although it was not very sensitive (i.e., able to identify actual deteriorated cases).

The AKQUASI system has the advantage of offering multiple measures, in multiple languages, based on clinician as well as client ratings. As such, it is very ambitious in its assessment goals. In the end, it is mainly suitable for settings in which measurements can be repeated. In Europe, hospitalizations frequently last at least a month and extensive assessments at the onset of treatment are commonplace. As noted, extensive assessment is less feasible in outpatient care.

During a typical inpatient stay, retesting only takes place at the end of treatment or when a decision about the client is being made (e.g., the need for additional services). The general philosophy guiding assessment is that deterioration cannot be predicted in advance and that further treatment has a good chance of working, even if it is not altered, so long as the client remains in therapy. The decision rule for this system is uncomplicated: If the client is in the normal range of functioning, consider termination; if the client is functioning in the dysfunctional range, continue treatment.

Like all the monitoring systems reviewed here, this one is constantly evolving. Nevertheless, the delay between modification and research investigating the consequences of the changes presents a limitation. This system also requires a good deal of collaboration between researchers and clinicians. It creates a culture that blends science and clinical judgment, but it also takes considerable time and commitment on the part of both groups.

Barkham et al. (2001) created the Clinical Outcomes in Routine Evaluation (CORE) system. It is widely used in the United Kingdom to inform client care on the basis of information gathered from psychology services. The CORE consists of three independent tools. The CORE Outcome Measure (CORE-OM) is a 34-item client self-report questionnaire, administered before and after therapy (10- and 5-item versions are also commonly used for tracking). Ratings are rendered on a 5-point scale regarding how the person has been feeling over the past week. The CORE-OM provides a score indicating current global psychological distress. Pre- and posttreatment scores indicate how much change has occurred while a client has been in treatment. The second tool, the Therapy Assessment Form, is completed by practitioners to profile the client, presenting concerns and a pathway to treatment. Practitioners also complete the End of Therapy Form, which highlights the process during therapy, termination, and subjective impressions of outcome.

CORE-PC software and a CORE.net Web system are available to enhance data collection and benchmark feedback. The CORE now emphasizes both grouped data as well as individualized tracking reports on clients. Benchmark data are grouped and analyzed along specific categories. The CORE can assess whether cases are falling outside of service targets by monitoring time on waitlists, clinical deterioration, poor attendance, and early termination. Anytime the CORE-OM is readministered, the CORE-PC and CORE.net can show which cases have deteriorated, have remained unchanged, and have entered the ranks of normal functioning. Progress is monitored, and the information fed back to clinicians, if this is desired. Historically, the strength of this system resided principally in the data it provides to administrators and managers of service delivery systems. But now the CORE.net includes individual tracking features as depicted in Figure 8.2, which also includes a vignette description of the client portrayed on the graph.

Kraus and Horan (1997) developed the Treatment Outcome Package (TOP), which includes numerous evaluation tools covering child and adult functioning. Time of administration ranges from 2 to 25 min. TOP has primarily focused on administrative uses rather than feedback to therapists. Managers

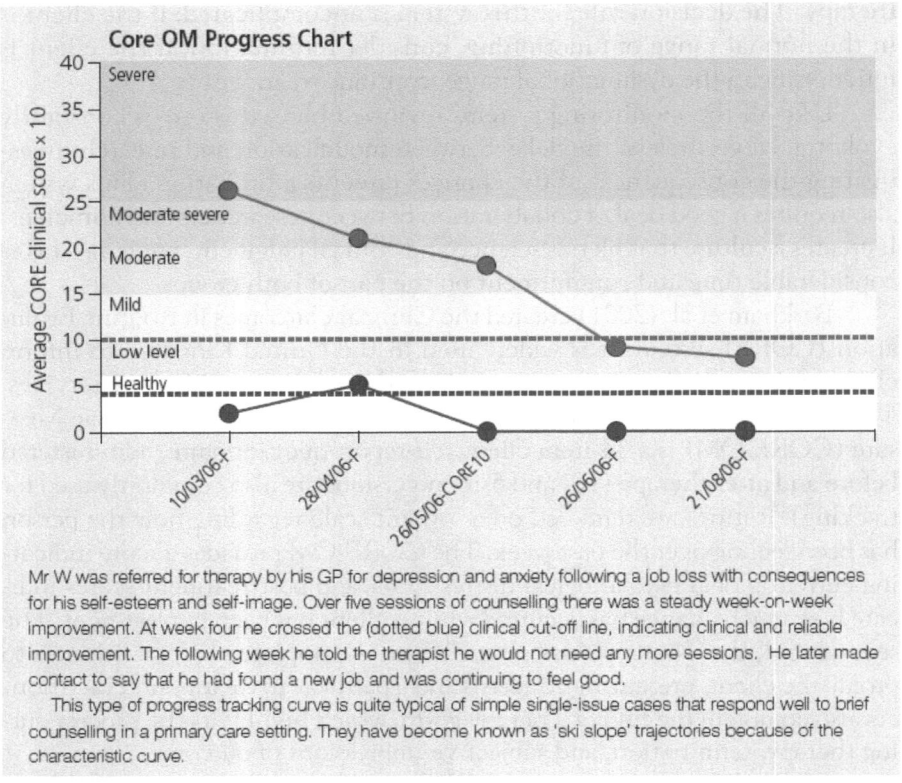

**Core OM Progress Chart**

Mr W was referred for therapy by his GP for depression and anxiety following a job loss with consequences for his self-esteem and self-image. Over five sessions of counselling there was a steady week-on-week improvement. At week four he crossed the (dotted blue) clinical cut-off line, indicating clinical and reliable improvement. The following week he told the therapist he would not need any more sessions. He later made contact to say that he had found a new job and was continuing to feel good.

This type of progress tracking curve is quite typical of simple single-issue cases that respond well to brief counselling in a primary care setting. They have become known as 'ski slope' trajectories because of the characteristic curve.

*Figure 8.2.* Output from the Clinical Outcomes Routine Evaluation Outcome Measure (CORE-OM) with the client Mr. W. The horizontal axis is the date the questionnaire was completed. "F" next to a session date indicates the five-item scale was used. "Core10" indicates the 10-item version was used on that date.

can examine progress throughout treatment and compare outcomes with appropriate benchmarks.

The functioning of adults and children is quantified across a variety of areas, and relevant measures include diagnostic aids, historical information, and written statements of treatment goals. The report for clinicians includes ratings on 23 high risk–related questions. Considerable emphasis is placed on the use of the report for treatment planning, the individualization of treatment goals, and the tracking of these goals. Client satisfaction, too, is measured and used as a quality assurance index.

As with the COMPASS system, TOP requires users to send off forms for scoring and reporting. This procedure limits rapid turnaround of feedback for clinicians and the frequency with which the response to treatment can be tracked. The adult symptom scale is long (around 85 items) and has considerable redundancy within each area of disturbance (e.g., sleep, anxiety, mood). For these reasons, TOP does provide reliable information for estimating degree of disturbance. The length of TOP, on the other hand, does not make it ideal for tracking treatment response on a weekly or even biweekly basis, unless tracking is limited to specific subscales. For clients whose subscales are elevated, the authors do recommend using their tracking system each week. Overall, this practice has the advantage of targeting specific problems for specific clients, but it also carries the disadvantage of leaving untracked many items measuring symptoms. More, the practice possibly overestimates the positive outcomes of treatment. It is also hard to compare different treatments when different targets are being tracked.

In contrast to the preceding methods, Miller, Duncan, Sorrell, and Brown (2005) created a very brief assessment package—the Partners for Change Outcome Management System (PCOMS). The PCOMS uses two 4-item (visual analogue) scales, one focusing on outcome (ORS) and the other aimed at assessing the therapeutic alliance (SRS). The measures are also available for use with children and adolescents (Duncan et al., 2006). Although brief, the ORS correlates modestly with other outcome measures, such as the OQ-45 (.58; Miller & Duncan, 2004). It has the advantage of directly involving both clinician and client in the process of measuring and discussing progress and the working relationship. At each session, the therapist provides the measures to the client. Because scoring takes place in the session, feedback is immediate. A commercially available Web-based system (see https://MyOutcomes.com) of administration, data collection, normative comparison, empirically based feedback messages as well as aggregate statistics addressing a variety of effectiveness and efficiency variables is available to enhance the benefits of paper-and-pencil use of PCOMS.

The PCOMS, using intake scores and progress at each session, provides information on anticipated treatment response. It also identifies clients whose improvement is falling short of expectations (Miller & Duncan, 2004). The authors have yet to examine accuracy of prediction of deterioration. Instead, they rely on sharing alliance and progress ratings with clients over the course of treatment. The goal is to ensure resolution of problems before they derail progress. The highly practical approach of PCOMS, with its general focus and brevity, makes it an attractive procedure for clinicians in private practice and larger systems of care. The authors have demonstrated that individualized markers of clinically significant change can be calculated and applied in routine practice.

Figure 8.3 provides a hypothetical example of feedback to both clinician and client for a client falling under benchmark predictions. ORS scores are graphically portrayed compared with the 50th percentile trajectory based on the client's intake score. Feedback messages interpret the scores, taking the

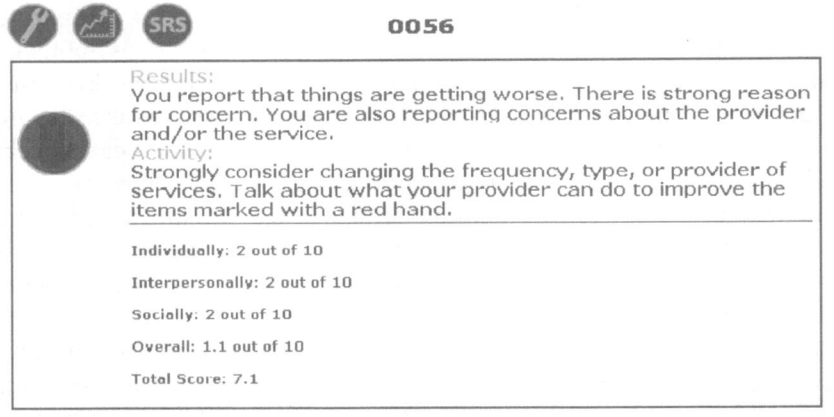

User Signed in: Provider1

SRS    0056

Results:
You report that things are getting worse. There is strong reason for concern. You are also reporting concerns about the provider and/or the service.
Activity:
Strongly consider changing the frequency, type, or provider of services. Talk about what your provider can do to improve the items marked with a red hand.

Individually: 2 out of 10

Interpersonally: 2 out of 10

Socially: 2 out of 10

Overall: 1.1 out of 10

Total Score: 7.1

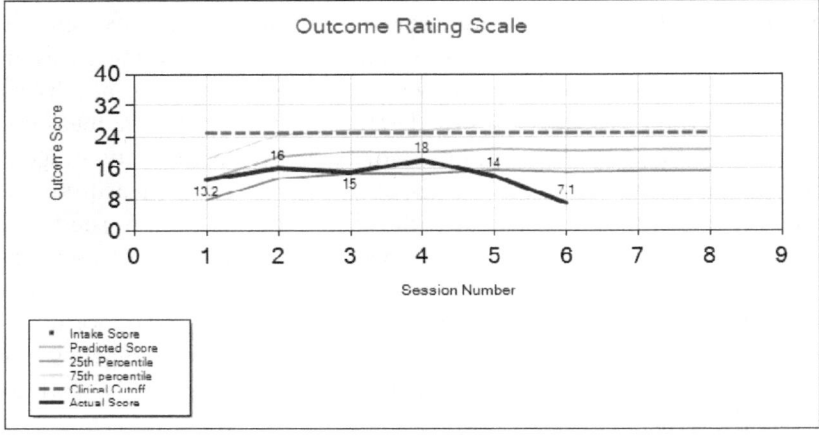

*Figure 8.3.* Output of the Partners for Change Outcome Management System.

alliance measure (SRS) into account, and encourage client and provider discussion about the next possible steps to avert a negative outcome.

In addition to Anker et al.'s (2009) feedback study described previously, the authors have examined tracking and feedback effects compared with preimplementation baseline figures (Miller, Duncan, Brown, Sorrell, & Chalk, 2006). In one applied setting, for instance, the authors reported that before implementation of feedback, 34% had reliably improved, whereas 19% had deteriorated. During the feedback phase, 47% improved, and 8% deteriorated. Because of the quasi-experimental nature of this study and changes in the treatment delivery system that accompanied the use of feedback, just how much feedback contributed to positive outcomes is a bit ambiguous. Nevertheless, these encouraging results support the notion that session-by-session feedback on progress and the therapeutic alliance can be used to promote client outcomes. In a soon-to-be-published study, Reese, Norsworthy, and Rowlands (in press) reported on the effects of PCOMS-based feedback compared with treatment as usual in a university-based training clinic and a university counseling center. Their findings were highly consistent with those reported by Lambert and colleagues. Despite small sample sizes, the differences between treatment-as-usual and feedback-assisted psychotherapy reached statistical significance, had medium effect sizes (Study 1, $d = 0.54$, and Study 2, $d = 0.49$, using Cohen's $d$ ), and reached reliable change on the ORS more frequently when compared with the no-feedback condition (80.0% vs. 54.2%, in Study 1; 66.67% vs. 41.40% in Study 2.). These researchers noted that feedback was helpful across clients, not just with off-track cases, and that feedback did not lengthen treatment in order to obtain its effects. As in Lambert and colleagues' research, trainees' clients improved as much as clients seen by professionals, but the clients of experienced clinicians accomplished the changes in a briefer time period. Other results from research conducted with PCOMS are reviewed in chapters 10 and 12 of this volume.

Each of the preceding systems has advantages and disadvantages. Each has achieved various levels of acceptance. All have accumulated treatment outcome data on thousands of clients, information that is being used to manage care based on treatment response. However, there is limited information about their comparative value on several major dimensions, including the accuracy of predicting treatment failure; the precision of cutoff scores for classifying reliable change and normal functioning, and most important, the degree to which different systems improve outcome. Although research on the consequence of providing OQ-45 feedback is considerable, it is possible that other methods may prove to be equally effective or superior. Comparative research is urgently needed but is a difficult challenge because of requirements for multiple assessments over the course of therapy.

All the systems have the advantage of facilitating outcome-informed care. The PCOMS and OQ Measures systems do this most directly by providing simple systems that involve client and therapist in weekly discussions on progress.

## Some Practical Issues for Implementation

The most significant problem encountered with outcomes management systems is clinician resistance. As noted earlier, only about 10% of clinicians are eager to adopt computer-based information technology. In addition, clinicians are very confident that they are more effective than the majority of their peers. They also believe they help most, if not all, of their clients. As a result, many see no need for the assistance provided by lab tests and formal monitoring. Finally, external evaluations of client outcomes are often regarded as a threat to clinicians' personal assessment of their effectiveness (Walfish, McAllister, O'Donnell, & Lambert, 2009).

When practitioners have chosen to monitor client change formally, implementation is much easier. Unfortunately, in most instances, outcome assessments have been imposed top down by external sources (e.g., management, insurance companies). Such rollouts are a serious impediment to success because they are perceived by line practitioners as benefiting management, giving scant attention to the real work. In such situations, neither clinician nor client feels that the formal assessment of treatment response is serving his or her interests.

Miller, Duncan, and colleagues (Duncan et al., 2004; Duncan & Sparks, 2002; Miller & Duncan, 2004) have presented step-by-step instructions for creating a culture that nurtures and sustains constructive feedback across clients, therapists, administrators, and payers. Their experience indicates that the use of formal measures of progress and alliance increases dramatically when everyone involved knows that the primary beneficiary of monitoring treatment response is the client.

From a practical perspective, the logistics of maintaining a treatment monitoring system are easier to manage when assessment becomes routine and information technologies are in place for administering and scoring measures. To be used, measures must be brief. Each of the systems reviewed reduces the burden of implementation to a bare minimum or attempts to do so (e.g., CORE's five-item scale, TOP's single subscale, PCOMS's four-item measures). J. Brown, Dreis, and Nace (1999) have argued that any measure or combination of measures that takes more than 5 minutes to complete result in lower compliance rates.

If monitoring does not occur at virtually every session, any system is limited by the unknown effects of client dropout or premature termination. It is uncommon for therapists to know when treatment is going to end. Therefore, expecting they will be ready with an assessment to obtain posttreatment data is unrealistic.

A central question in outcome management systems is, "Who is responsible for data collection?" Related questions include "When are assessments to be administered?" and "Who keeps track of this?" Should therapists manage questionnaires, and should they do so before or after the session? If assessment is intermittent, how does the therapist know when to give an assessment to Client A but not to Client B? Is the clinician expected to store data along with the client case file, or is this handled on the management side? If management is responsible for data collection and storage, how are therapists informed of the findings?

Experience implementing outcomes management in multiple settings indicates that the most efficient system has been to make administration of assessments routine. Clients complete a questionnaire before each appointment, thus affording the chance for immediate feedback before the session. Then the task of tracking who needs an assessment and who does not is eliminated. Assessments are simply administered by clinic receptionists or psychotherapists when clients check in for their appointments. An additional argument for frequent administration of assessments is that the algorithms used for identifying potential treatment failures provide better predictions when more data are collected.

As the reader can see, the choice of an outcomes management system has immediate practical considerations. These bear on the means of scoring assessments, managing the data, and receiving individual client feedback reports as well as the availability of monthly or quarterly summaries of outcome data for all or selected groups of clients. If all of these various tasks need to be managed by the therapist or an employee, a key element of monitoring, the provision of a signal-alarm to the practitioner, may be lost. Available evidence indicates that feedback helps only 25% to 30% of clients, those who are predicted to have a poor psychotherapy outcome. Little general benefit obtains for all clients except reductions in the number of sessions per client. The problem is that providers do not know whether and when a client will become a signal-alarm case. Therefore, tracking all clients is required. The development of various software programs for all the systems reviewed here enhances solutions to problems of implementation and speedy delivery of results to therapists. In the age of information technology, the future looks bright for using such advances for the benefit of clients.

The use of outcomes management systems is ushering in a significant change in how psychotherapy is conducted. This review underscores the value of monitoring treatment response, applying statistical algorithms for identifying problematic cases, providing timely feedback to therapists (and clients), and providing therapists with problem-solving strategies. It is becoming clear that such procedures are well substantiated, not just matters for debate or equivocation. When implemented, these procedures enhance client outcome and improve quality of care (Lambert, 2005).

## Implications

Substance Abuse and Mental Health Services Administration's National Registry of Evidence-Based Programs and Practices evaluated the OQ-Analyst as an evidence-based practice on two major criteria. The first criterion was the quality of empirical evidence supporting its effectiveness. The second was the availability of material making it ready for dissemination and widespread use, that is, implementation. The National Registry rates all submitted evidence-based practices on these two dimensions using a 5-point scale (0–4). The overall rating is a sum of separate ratings for implementation materials, training and support, and quality assurance. The OQ-Analyst was given a nearly perfect score of 3.9. Although all the available manuals and material that provided such a high rating cannot be presented here because of space limitations, they are available through the OQ Measures Web site (http://www.oqmeasures.com). The interventions are ready for implementation.

The following major points provide a good rationale for going forward with implementation:

- Yes, it is time to routinely track client outcome. Doing so consistently decreases deterioration rates and enhances positive outcomes for clients who go off track from a positive treatment response.
- Tracking client treatment response using standardized scales (mental health vital signs) is especially important given clinicians' tendency to be overly optimistic about the meaning of clients' lack of progress and their failure to judge when clients are headed toward a negative outcome.
- In addition to progress tracking, it appears that the use of decision support methods for these cases also substantially bolsters treatment effects. Clinical support tools that rely on a brief assessment, strategies for focusing clinicians' search for solutions, and provision of brief prompts to broaden therapist's interventions can be developed on the basis of common factor concepts such as the alliance, motivation, and social support difficulties, making them appealing regardless of therapist treatment orientation.
- Tracking client progress and alerting therapists to the potential of a negative outcome, along with assessing areas responsible for treatment failure, can be readily achieved with brief measures, computer-assisted technology, and little time expenditure on the part of clinicians. There is no excuse for failing to assist clients by using these methods. Certainly clients do not find being asked about their functioning inside and outside of psychotherapy to be a burden if the therapists discuss and use this information to make treatment more responsive to their needs.
- This new frontier for enhancing the effects of psychotherapy provides greater opportunities for clinicians to partner with clients in the collaborative efforts that are needed to maximize positive outcomes. One hopes that such methods find their way into mental health training programs and routine clinical care sooner rather than later.

# QUESTIONS FROM THE EDITORS

1. *What steps need to be taken to ensure that the measurement of outcome and provision of feedback do not fall prey to the same shortcomings as early definitions of* evidence-based practice *that ended up limiting rather than enhancing practice?*

Using the OQ Analyst to quantify treatment response and inform ongoing treatment is an "evidence-based practice." It does not impinge on the autonomy of providers and does not assume that providers are automatons that can provide dozens of different empirically supported psychotherapies. It would be unfortunate, however, at this early point the development of this practice for any system to be used exclusively. OQ-Analyst and other systems are evolving over time and will not remain fixed entities. All can be improved. In addition, new systems will likely develop and may prove to be even more helpful to clients than existing systems. It would not serve the interests of clients to have an existing system frozen in time. We are just at the threshold of understanding how client outcomes and assessment-based problem-solving strategies can be used in real time to ensure the best possible outcome for clients.

2. *Do clinicians provided with feedback learn? In other words, do they improve in their ability to detect and treat clients at risk of dropout or a negative or null outcome? If not, why not?*

No. Clinicians do not improve in their ability to detect the important signs of a negative outcome and thereby detect who is at risk of a negative outcome. In a way, this should not come as a surprise or be disappointing. Past research contrasting clinical versus actuarial prediction has consistently shown actuarial methods to be superior. Psychotherapists are optimistic about the clients' eventual improvement and remain determined in the face of slow and even negative progress. This optimism is an advantage to clients but at the cost of missing information that is essential for predicting a negative outcome.

In Hannan et al.'s (2006) study of therapist prediction, it was found that therapists did recognize that a portion of their clients had worsened from their status at intake. If they had used this information as a sign of an impending negative outcome, they would have dramatically improved their predictive accuracy. In contrast, the statistical method relies heavily on the information that clients worsen and can also assess how much worsening at a specific session is a negative indicator.

One cannot expect physicians to predict blood pressure or white blood cell counts; instead, they measure these vital signs and rely on cut scores and patterns of scores. Similarly, it is not necessary for psychotherapists to get better at tasks that can easily be accomplished through simple assessment procedures and the proper use of information technology.

3. *What are the implications of research on feedback for training and credentialing of behavioral health care professionals?*

It is important that training programs become familiar with the advantages of feedback for clients and that they encourage and assist students in learning to use such methods. It is unfortunate that few training programs are on the cutting edge of such practices and continue to supervise students in their therapy cases without the advantages of formally tracking client progress and using the predictive power of statistical modeling techniques and related actuarial methods. If speed of adoption of practices (on the basis of research evidence) in medicine, psychology, and business is any indicator, one can expect to wait 10 to 15 years for the field to make these methods routine. In the meantime, I hope that professional licensing boards do not play a role in forcing clinicians to adopt tracking methodology. I think this is most properly done by professional associations and administrators of clinical services.

## REFERENCES

American Psychological Association. (2006). Evidence-based practice in psychology. *American Psychologist, 61*, 271–285.

Anker, M., Duncan, B., & Sparks, J. (2009). Using client feedback to improve couple outcomes: A randomized clinical trial in a naturalistic setting. *Journal of Consulting and Clinical Psychology, 77*, 693–704.

Barber, J. P. (2007). Issues and findings in investigating predictors of psychotherapy outcome. Introduction to the special section. *Psychotherapy Research, 17*, 131–136.

Barkham, M., Margison, F., Leach, C., Lucock, M., Mellor-Clark, J., Evans, C., et al. (2001). Service profiling and outcomes benchmarking using the CORE-OM: Toward practice-based evidence in the psychological therapies. *Journal of Consulting and Clinical Psychology, 69*, 184–196.

Bartlett, J., & Cohen, J. (1993). Building an accountable, improvable delivery system. *Administration & Policy in Mental Health, 21*, 51–58.

Bergin, A. E. (1971). The evaluation of therapeutic outcomes. In A. E. Bergin & S. L. Garfield (Eds.), *Handbook of psychotherapy & behavior change* (pp. 217–270). New York: Wiley.

Berking, M., Orth, U., & Lutz, W. (2006). Wie effekiv sind systematische Rückmeldungen des Therapieverlaufs an den Therapeuten? Eine empirische Studie in einem stationär-verhaltenstherapeutischen Setting [How effective is systematic feedback during the course of therapy to the therapist? An empirical study of behavior in a hospital setting]. *Zeitschrift fur Klinische Psychologie und Psychotherapie, 35*, 21–29.

Breslin, F., Sobell, L.C., Buchan, G., & Cunningham, J. (1997). Toward a stepped-care approach to treating problem drinkers: The predictive validity of within-treatment variables and therapist prognostic ratings. *Addiction, 92*, 1479–1489.

Brown, J., Dreis, S., & Nace, D. (1999). What really makes a difference in psychotherapy outcome? Why does managed care want to know? In M. A. Hubble, B. L. Duncan, & S. D. Miller (Eds.), *The heart and soul of change: What works in therapy* (pp. 389–406). Washington, DC: American Psychological Association.

Brown, G. S., Burlingame, G. M., Lambert, M. J., Jones, E. & Vaccaro, J. (2001). Pushing the quality envelope: A new outcomes management system. *Psychiatric Services, 52*, 925–934.

Chambless, D. L., Baker, M. J., Baucom, D. H., Beutler, L. E., Calhoun, K. S., Crits-Cristoph, P., et al. (1998). Update on empirically validated therapies, II. *The Clinical Psychologist, 51*(1), 3–16.

Chambless, D. L., Sanderson, W. C., Shoham, V., Bennett Johnson, S., Pope, K. S., Crits-Cristoph, P., et al. (1996). An update on empirically validated therapies. *The Clinical Psychologist, 49*(2), 5–18.

Cohen, S., & Wills, T. A. (1985). Stress, social support and the buffering hypothesis. *Psychological Bulletin, 98*, 310–357.

Duncan, B. L., Miller, S., & Sparks, J. (2004). *The heroic client: A revolutionary way to improve effectiveness through client-directed, outcome-informed therapy.* San Francisco: Jossey-Bass.

Duncan, B. L., Miller, S. D., Sparks, J. A., Claud, D. A., Reynolds, L. R., Brown, J., & Johnson, L. D. (2003). The Session Rating Scale: Preliminary psychometric properties of a "working" alliance measure. *Journal of Brief Therapy, 3*(1), 3–12.

Duncan, B. L., & Sparks, J. (2002). *Heroic clients, heroic agencies: Partners for change.* Ft. Lauderdale, FL: Author.

Duncan, B. L., Sparks, J., Miller, S., Bohanske, R., & Claud, D. (2006). Giving youth a voice: A preliminary study of the reliability and validity of a brief outcome measure for children. *Journal of Brief Therapy, 5*(2), 66–82.

Ellsworth, J. R., Lambert, M. J., & Johnson, J. (2006). A comparison of the Outcome Questionnaire-45 and Outcome Questionnaire-30 in classification and prediction of treatment outcome. *Clinical Psychology and Psychotherapy, 13*, 380–391.

Finch, A. E., Lambert, M. J., & Schaalje, B. G. (2001). Psychotherapy quality control: The statistical generation of expected recovery curves for integration into an early warning system. *Clinical Psychology and Psychotherapy, 8*, 231–242.

Garb, H. N. (2005). Clinical judgment and decision making. *Annual Review of Clinical Psychology, 55*, 13–23.

Garfield, S. L. (1994). Research on client variables in psychotherapy. In S. L. Garfield & A. E. Bergin (Eds.), *Handbook of psychotherapy and behavior change* (4th ed., pp. 72–113). New York: Wiley.

Hannan, C., Lambert, M. J., Harmon, C., Nielsen, S. L., Smart, D. W., Shimokawa, K., et al. (2005). A lab test and algorithms for identifying clients at risk for treatment failure. *Journal of Clinical Psychology: In Session, 61*, 155–63.

Hansen, N. B., Lambert, M. J., & Forman, E. V. (2002). The psychotherapy dose–response effect and its implications for treatment delivery services. *Clinical Psychology: Science and Practice, 9*, 329–343.

Harmon, S. C., Lambert, M. J., Smart, D. W., Hawkins, E. J., Nielsen, S. L., Slade, K., et al. (2007). Enhancing outcome for potential treatment failures: Therapist/client feedback and clinical support tools. *Psychotherapy Research, 17*, 379–392.

Hawkins, E. J., Lambert, M. J., Vermeersch, D. A., Slade, K., & Tuttle, K. (2004). The effects of providing patient progress information to therapists and patients. *Psychotherapy Research, 14*, 308–327.

Horvath, A. O., & Luborsky, L. (1993). The role of the therapeutic alliance in psychotherapy. *Journal of Consulting and Clinical Psychology, 61*, 561–573.

Howard, K. I., Moras, K., Brill, P. L., Martinovich, Z., & Lutz, W. (1996). Evaluation of psychotherapy: Efficacy, effectiveness, and patient progress. *American Psychologist, 51*, 1059–1064.

Hubble, M. A., Duncan, B. L., & Miller, S. D. (1999). *The heart and soul of change: What works in therapy.* Washington, DC: American Psychological Association.

Jacobson, N. S., & Truax, P. (1991). Clinical significance: A statistical approach to defining meaningful change in psychotherapy research. *Journal of Consulting and Clinical Psychology, 59*, 12–19.

Kordy, H., Hannöver, W., & Richard, M. (2001). Computer-assisted feedback-driven quality management for psychotherapy: The Stuttgart–Heidelberg model. *Journal of Consulting and Clinical Psychology, 69*, 173–183.

Kraus, D. R., & Horan, F. P. (1997). Outcomes roadblocks: Problems and solutions. *Behavioral Health Management, 17*(5), 22–26.

Lambert, M. J. (2005, Spring). Enhancing psychotherapy through feedback to clinicians. *The Register Report, 31*, 15–19.

Lambert, M. J., Bergin, A. E., & Collins, J. L. (1977). Therapist induced deterioration in psychotherapy patients. In A. S. Gurman, & A. M. Razin (Eds.), *Effective psychotherapy: A handbook of research* (pp. 452–481). New York: Pergamon Press.

Lambert, M. J., Bergin, A. E., Garfield, S. L. (2004). Introduction and overview. In M. J. Lambert (Ed.), *Bergin & Garfield's handbook of psychotherapy & behavior change* (5th ed., pp. 3–15). New York: Wiley.

Lambert, M. J., Morton, J. J., Hatfield, D., Harmon, C., Hamilton, S., Reid, R. C., et al. (2004). *Administration and scoring manual for the Outcome Questionnaire-45.* Salt Lake City, UT: OQ Measures.

Lambert, M. J., & Ogles, B. M. (2004). The efficacy and effectiveness of psychotherapy. In M. J. Lambert (Ed.), *Bergin & Garfield's handbook of psychotherapy and behavior change.* (5th ed., pp. 139–193). New York: Wiley.

Lambert, M. J., Whipple, J. L., Harmon, C., Shimokawa, K., Slade, K., Christopherson, C. (2004). *Clinical support tools manual.* Provo, UT: Department of Psychology, Brigham Young University.

Lambert, M. J., Whipple, J. L., Hawkins, E. J., Vermeersch, D. A., Nielsen, S. L., & Smart, D. W. (2003). Is it time for clinicians to routinely track patient outcome?: A meta-analysis. *Clinical Psychology: Science & Practice, 10*, 288–301.

Lambert, M. J., Whipple, J. L., Smart, D. W., Vermeersch, D. A., Nielsen, S. L., & Hawkins, E. J. (2001). The effects of providing therapists with feedback on client progress during psychotherapy: Are outcomes enhanced? *Psychotherapy Research, 11*, 49–68.

Lambert, M. J., Whipple, J. L., Vermeersch, D. A., Smart, D. W., Hawkins, E. J., Nielsen, S. L., & Goates, M. K. (2002). Enhancing psychotherapy outcomes via providing feedback on client progress: A replication. *Clinical Psychology and Psychotherapy, 9*, 91–103.

Lueger, R. J., Howard, K. I., Martinovich Z., Lutz, W., Anderson, E. E., & Grissom, G. (2001). Assessing treatment progress of individual clients using expected treatment response models. *Journal of Consulting and Clinical Psychology, 69*, 150–158.

Lutz, W., Lambert, M. J., Harmon, S. C., Stulz, N., Tschitsaz, A., & Schürch, E. (2006). The probability of treatment success, failure and duration—What can be learned from empirical data to support decision making in clinical practice? *Clinical Psychology & Psychotherapy, 13*, 223–232.

Meredith, R. L., Bair, S. L., & Ford, G. R. (2000). Information management for clinical decision making. In G. Stricker, W. G. Troy, & S. A. Shueman (Eds.), *Handbook of quality management in behavioral health* (pp. 53–94). New York: Kluwer/Plenum Press.

Miller, S. D. & Duncan, B. L. (2004). *The Outcome and Session Rating Scales: Administration and scoring manual*. Chicago: Institute for the Study of Therapeutic Change.

Miller, S. D., Duncan, B. L., Brown, J., Sorrell, R., & Chalk, M. B. (2006). Using formal client feedback to improve retention and outcome: Making ongoing real-time assessment feasible. *Journal of Brief Therapy, 5*(1), 5–22.

Miller, S. D., Duncan, B. L., Brown, J., Sparks, J., & Claud, D. (2003). The outcome rating scale: A preliminary study of the reliability, validity, and feasibility of a brief visual analog measure. *Journal of Brief Therapy, 2*(2), 91–100.

Miller, S. D., Duncan, B. L., Sorrell, R., & Brown, G.S. (2005). The Partners for Change Outcome System. *Journal of Clinical Psychology: In Session, 61*, 199–208.

Miller, W. R. & Rollnick, S. (2002). *Motivational interviewing: Preparing people for change* (2nd ed.). New York: Guilford Press.

National Institutes of Health. (2002). State implementation of evidence-based practices: Bridging science and service (National Institute of Mental Health and Substance Abuse and Mental Health Services Administration Request for Application MH-03-007). Retrieved December 19, 2006, from http://grants.nih.gov/grants/guide/rfa-files/RFA-MH-03-007.html

OQ Measures. (2004). *OQ-Analyst user's guide* [Computer software and manual]. Available at http://www.oqmeasures.com

Reese, R. J., Norsworthy, L. A., & Rowlands, S. (in press). Does a continuous feedback system improve psychotherapy outcome? *Psychotherapy: Theory, Research, Practice, Training.*

Safran, J. D. & Muran, J. C. (2000). *Negotiating the therapeutic alliance: A relational treatment guide*. New York: Guilford Press.

Stricker, G., Troy, W. G., & Shueman, S. A. (2000). *Handbook of quality management in behavioral health*. New York: Kluwer/Plenum Press.

Vermeersch, D. A., Lambert, M. J., & Burlingame, G. M. (2002). Outcome questionnaire: Item sensitivity to change. *Journal of Personality Assessment, 74*, 242–261.

Vermeersch, D. A., Whipple, J. L., Lambert, M. J., Hawkins, E. J., Burchfield, C. M., & Okiishi, J. C. (2004). Outcome Questionnaire: Is it sensitive to changes in counseling center clients? *Journal of Counseling Psychology, 51*, 38–49.

Wampold, B. (2001). *The great psychotherapy debate*. Mahwah, NJ: Erlbaum.

Walfish, S., McAlister, B., O'Donnell, P., & Lambert, M. J. (2009). *Are all therapists from Lake Wobegon? An investigation of self-assessment bias in mental health providers*. Manuscript under review.

Whipple, J. L., Lambert, M. J., Vermeersch, D. A., Smart, D. W., Nielsen, S. L., & Hawkins, E. J. (2003). Improving the effects of psychotherapy: The use of early identification of treatment failure and problem solving strategies in routine practice. *Journal of Counseling Psychology, 58*, 59–68.

Yalom, I. D., & Lieberman, M. A. (1971). A study of encounter group casualties. *Archives of General Psychiatry, 25*, 16–30.

Zimet, G. D., Dahlem, N. W., Zimet, S. G., & Farley, G. K. (1988). The multidimensional scale of perceived social support. *Journal of Personality Assessment, 52*, 30–41.

Zuroff, D. C., Koestner, R., Moskowitz, D. S., McBride, C., Marshall, M., & Bagby, M. R. (2007). Autonomous motivation for therapy: A new common factor in brief treatments for depression. *Psychotherapy Research, 17*, 137–147.

# 9

# OUTCOMES MANAGEMENT, REIMBURSEMENT, AND THE FUTURE OF PSYCHOTHERAPY

G. S. (JEB) BROWN AND TAKUYA MINAMI

Lack of money is no obstacle. Lack of an idea is an obstacle.
—Ken Hakuda

First, let us state the obvious: Psychotherapy is a business. It is a purchased service—whoever pays for it believes that its benefits are worth the price. Revenues to support the business of psychotherapy come from multiple sources; for a typical client, they are likely a combination of out-of-pocket expense and a subsidy provided by an employer, health plan, governmental entity, or other organization or institution (e.g., employer-sponsored employee assistance program).

Psychotherapy, as a service, is believed by many in the public—as well as employers, insurance companies, health care plans, and various governmental entities—to successfully reduce disabling psychological symptoms. Psychotherapy is also thought to improve day-to-day functioning and relationships with family and others and even to offset medical costs. Among practicing therapists, all of these benefits are so self-evident that it is almost an article of faith. It is obvious, however, that faith alone does not determine the value of psychotherapy for society as a whole (and, in particular, for those who fund the services).

If the trend in reimbursement rates for psychotherapy services is any indication of the strength of society's faith in psychotherapy, the future looks bleak in comparison with other forms of treatments for psychological distress (e.g., medication). A recent survey of the public's perception of psycho-therapy is instructive. In 2004, a large managed behavioral health care company (PacifiCare Behavioral Health [PBH]) and *Psychology Today* sponsored a telephone survey conducted by Harris International to gauge the public's beliefs regarding the value of mental health services in general and psychotherapy in particular. In general, respondents who knew of someone who had been in psychotherapy perceived that it had been helpful (with 67% in agreement). However, when asked if they could imagine a situation in which they themselves might seek out a psychotherapist, 65% responded no.

An inspection of Table 9.1 reveals two additional results from the survey that speak directly to the public's perception of the value of psycho-therapy. First, the majority of respondents agreed that treatment works. At the same time, however, most believed that it takes too long and costs too much. Such results could have devastating long-term consequences for the field, especially when compared with claims that competing forms of treatment (e.g., medication) provide needed relief more quickly—typically within 2 to 3 months.

Fortunately, existing evidence strongly contradicts widespread public perception about real-world clinical practice. For example, in one of the largest consumer surveys ever conducted about psychotherapy (Drugs vs. Talk Therapy, 2004; Mental Health: Does Therapy Help?, 1995; Seligman, 1995), researchers showed that on average, people received 10 sessions of psycho-therapy, a duration of slightly more than 2 months if therapy is delivered on a weekly basis. Moreover, 80% of those in the study who received *short-term therapy*, defined as lasting 6 months or less, reported that it helped. In regard to cost, a study of mental health coverage with employer-sponsored health insurance found that 98% and 96% of covered workers had outpatient and inpatient mental health coverage, respectively (Barry et al., 2003), indicating psychotherapy is subsidized for many people.

TABLE 9.1
Public Perceptions of Psychotherapy

| Question | Response | Percentage |
|---|---|---|
| How long is the average person in therapy? | 3 months or less | 14 |
| | 3 to 6 months | 26 |
| | 6 months or more | 45 |
| | Not sure | 15 |
| Cost–benefit[a] | Costs outweigh the benefits | 43 |
| | Cost–benefit about right | 29 |
| | Benefits outweigh the cost | 11 |

*Note.* Data from Harris International (2004).
[a]Complete question: "In your opinion, do the benefits generally outweigh the costs, do the costs usually outweigh the benefits, or do you think the costs are usually about right for what people get?"

The evidence cited here contradicting popular notions about the cost and duration of psychological intervention may be taken by some practitioners to mean that the field has a marketing problem. In other words, everything will be fine if we actively inform the general public about the true effectiveness of psychotherapy. Unfortunately, efforts to improve the image of psychotherapy are rarely seen. However, as with everything else in the marketplace, provision of clinical service is not impervious to commodity pricing.

According to a report by the Substance Abuse and Mental Health Services Administration (SAMHSA), the number of mental health practitioners in the United States continues to be on the rise (U.S. Department of Health and Human Services, 2004). In a previous estimate in 1999, it was assumed that there were approximately 400,000 mental health providers in the United States, which had a population of roughly 260 million at the time (Brown, Dreis, & Nace, 1999). Using a very liberal estimate of utilization (10%), this meant that there were approximately 65 clients per practitioner. The same assumption applied today shows that the number of clients per practitioner has dropped to 35 (836,000 practitioners, 293 million U.S. citizens). In other words, in the past decade, the increased supply of therapists means that the demand for services for an average therapist has dropped by more than 45%. The imbalance between supply and demand should be a major concern for professional organizations representing therapists. It is curious, however, that instead of pursuing ways to regulate supply, the efforts of the various professional organizations seem targeted to pursuing privileges held by medical doctors (e.g., prescribing medication) and increasing access to health care panels and reimbursement rates (American Psychological Association Practice Directorate, 2009). Few appear to have considered the consequences of such actions: As more therapists seek to enter the business, the greater the downward pressure on reimbursement—unless, of course, demand grows at a pace that supports the supply, a scenario that hardly seems likely. Arguments for basing reimbursement rates on freedom of choice for consumers and the right of any willing provider (or, at least for those who belong to a particular professional organization) fail to consider the current imbalance between supply and demand and threaten to leave clinicians with the ability to bill but at rates incapable of sustaining a professional career. Estimates show that reimbursement rates from managed care companies have failed to keep up with the increase in cost of living over the past 10 years. As just one example, the Consumer Price Index increased more than 20% between 1997 and 2005, whereas reimbursement rates for psychologists remained essentially unchanged at around $75 per session (Fee, Practice and Managed Care Survey, 2006).

In this chapter, we present a historical overview of psychotherapy reimbursement, examine the current of the market forces that are eroding the value of psychotherapy services, and argue that outcomes management offers a pathway out of our current predicament. Addressing the serious financial and marketing problems facing future clinical practice, the content of this chapter may feel removed from the warm and fuzzy world of psychotherapy, and perhaps, unlike the rest of the book, even heartless and soulless by conceptualizing psychotherapy as a commodity. To put it bluntly, however, there will be no future if the field fails to face the harsh realities of the business world. The absence of marketing by professional organizations makes naive the assumption that there will be any growth in demand for the services therapists offer (other than keeping up with population growth). Indeed, studies have found psychotherapy utilization rates have remained relatively flat over the years (less than 4%; Weissman et al., 2006). We explore strategies for sustaining psychotherapy as a business under these challenging circumstances in the context of the field's history, overall health care trends, and research on what in fact is the commodity we call psychotherapy.

## POLITICAL AND ECONOMIC FACTORS AFFECTING MENTAL HEALTH SERVICES REIMBURSEMENT

Psychotherapy has its origins in various medical treatments applied in the 19th century to a common and mysterious ailment known as *neurasthenia*, or *nervous exhaustion*. Because medical practitioners of that era saw medicine as a profession based on the scientific study of physiochemical (i.e., somatic) processes, mental illness—and in fact all mental states—were considered byproducts of some yet unknown physiochemical process. Thus, whereas popular culture was becoming increasingly interested in "mind cures" (including those espoused by Christian Science and the New Thought movements), organized medicine continued to ignore the psyche (Caplan, 1998).

At the turn of the last century, American psychologist William James, along with a small group of colleagues in the United States, France, Italy, and Switzerland, pioneered the field of experimental psychopathology. From 1880 to 1910, their efforts helped make Boston the center of scientific psychotherapy for the English-speaking world. The organization known as the Boston School of Psychopathology—which included James and his student G. Stanley Hall as well as neurologists and psychiatrists—did much to help establish the legitimacy of psychotherapy as a form of medical treatment for psychic distress. By the time Freud gave his lectures at Clark University in 1909, psychotherapy was already established as a valid medical practice in the United States. Naturally, professional medicine was happy to assert that physicians were the only ones capable of administering the new (and lucrative) form of treatment.

World War II changed matters dramatically, in particular increasing the demand for mental health services. The shortage of psychiatrists opened the door for psychology as a profession. With support and funding from the federal government, psychology rapidly transitioned from a mostly experimental to a professional field intent on providing clinical services. The rapid increase in new schools of humanistic and behavioral therapies during the postwar years further eroded organized medicine's hold on psychotherapy. By 1960, clinical psychology grew to become the largest area in psychology. Psychotherapy services were increasingly provided not only by physicians and psychologists with doctoral level training but also by a growing number of less expensive professionals, including those trained at a master's level with as little as 18 months of postgraduate study.

During this period of rapid expansion, reimbursement for psychotherapy, where it existed, was in the form of payment of fees for services rendered. The fee-for-service indemnity plan was the dominant form of employer-provided health insurance. Providers were paid their customary and usual fees and granted broad latitude to determine the method and length (dose) of treatment. During the decades immediately following World War II, mental health practitioners of various disciplines successfully lobbied and were litigated to become eligible for reimbursement for services. There were few cost controls, and individuals had broad latitude to choose the provider of their choice (Hayes, Barlow, & Nelson-Grey, 1999). At this time, only a small number of prepaid health plans existed. These forerunners of today's health maintenance organizations (HMOs) provided access to health services for a small monthly premium. Members could access health care services for preventive care as well as treatment for injuries and illness. Despite their relative lower cost at the time, such plans remained small, serving no more than a few thousand members.

In 1963, the Community Mental Health Centers Act provided federal grants to states for the establishment of local mental health centers throughout the United States with the goal of fostering the transfer of care for the mentally ill away from state hospitals and back to the community. Funding for psychological services was diversifying. Medicare and Medicaid in short order were providing government-funded coverage (albeit limited) for treatment of mental disorders. Medicaid was particularly important because it funded the treatment for the severely mentally ill in nursing homes and psychiatric wards of community hospitals. On the other hand, Medicare made private insurance for individuals over 65 virtually obsolete and also unleashed a frenzy of spending by doctors, patients, and hospitals.

As medical costs increased during the 1960s, private insurance became increasingly expensive. This, in turn, led to a call from liberal politicians—such as the young senator from Massachusetts Edward Kennedy—for government-funded health care for all citizens. Although many professional organizations applauded expanding government funding for mental health services, other forces were forming to promote free enterprise–based solutions.

In particular, Paul Ellwood, a Minnesota physician who left the practice of medicine to devote his time to health care reform, began having discussions with what is now the U.S. Department of Health and Human Services. He and his colleagues were convinced that Medicare represented the beginning of a slippery slope toward socialized medicine. His goal was to create an alternate model for funding health care in which costs would be contained by providing preventive care services: Doctors would be paid to keep people healthy. In his mind, HMOs were the perfect free enterprise solution, using the profit motive to contain costs (Ellwood et al., 1971). The Nixon administration, concerned with the rapidly escalating cost of health care and wishing to fend off calls from liberals for further health care funding from the government, bought into Ellwood's plan. When signing the Health Maintenance Organization Act of 1973 (S-14), Nixon stated:

> S-14 represents one response to the challenge of finding new and better ways to improve health care for the people of this country. It will build on the partnership that exists between the Federal and private sector by allowing both the provider and the consumer of health services to exercise the widest possible freedom of choice. (Woolley & Peters, n.d.)

The act had three main provisions: (a) grants and loans to start or expand an HMO, (b) removal of any state-imposed restrictions on HMOs as long as the HMOs were federally certified, and (c) a requirement for employers with 25 or more employees to offer federally certified HMO options alongside traditional indemnity-style insurance. To qualify for federal subsidies, HMOs were required to provide a specified minimal set of services, including outpatient mental health and substance abuse treatment services. The federal government was slow to certify HMOs until amendments to the HMO act were made in 1976 and 1978 that provided additional financial and administrative incentives. The result was a rapid growth in HMOs: Whereas fewer than 40 HMOs were certified by 1970, more than 236 were in business by 1980 (Gruber, Shadle, & Polich, 1988).

Although one of the main arguments for HMOs was that they would keep patients healthy by offering low-cost preventive care, the primary motivation for their creation was to manage costs. HMOs were granted carte blanche to determine which services and treatments were covered for any individual patient without incurring liability for medical malpractice. At the same time, the plans provided financial incentives to physicians for containing costs. Such arrangements were considered necessary for HMOs to curtail spending.

Through a process known as *utilization review*, HMOs determined the appropriateness of requests for treatment procedures by comparing the rationale for the requests against established treatment guidelines. In turn, procedures would either be approved or denied, or less expensive (but presumably equally effective) alternatives would be authorized. The medical and ethical rationale for the use of such intensive inspect-and-control methods for approval of physician-recommended medical care was to ensure that the recommended treatment was medically necessary, that is, consistent with commonly recognized standards of care. In reality, however, the rewards associated with denying or decreasing care inevitably came into conflict with providers, whose income was dependent on providing a rationale that higher levels of spending on patient care was appropriate patient care. This was particularly true for inpatient treatment programs.

The impact of HMOs (and other related health plan entities collectively referred to as *managed care*) on providers of services related to mental health and substance abuse was not immediately apparent. In fact, during the same period in which most medical treatments were being targeted for cost containment, behavioral health care continued to grow. A number of factors drove increased spending on behavioral health care: increased insurance coverage, growing social acceptance of mental health care, introduction of new medications, and increase in use of inpatient treatment.

In particular, the number of free-standing, specialty inpatient psychiatric hospitals soared during this period, as for-profit hospital corporations found such institutions to be handsome sources of profit (Sharkey, 1994; U.S. House of Representatives, 1992). Eventually, as with any market, supply outpaced demand, leading to tough competition among hospitals. Many used practices that appeared to exploit the patient's insurance coverage in pursuit of profit. As a result, during the 1980s and early 1990s, the cost of behavioral health care services increased at a rate double that of other health care services (Strosahl, 1994).

The widespread perception of clinically inappropriate overuse of inpatient services led large employers to conclude that the cost of care could be reduced by shifting behavioral health care to outpatient settings. And, in fact, studies later showed that decreasing use of inpatient services resulted in an overall increase in mental health services in general while simultaneously decreasing costs to employees and employers (Goldman, McCulloch, Cuffel, & Kozma, 1999; Sturm, 1997). However, although adept at managing medical costs, HMOs lacked expertise in overseeing costs associated with behavioral health services. Specialty companies thought to have the expertise necessary to determine the medical necessity of mental health care arose to fill the gap, giving birth to the managed care revolution. Mental health services were carved out from other medical services, and managed behavioral health care organizations (MBHOs) competed for contracts to manage mental health and substance abuse services. The number of individuals in the United States covered through an MBHO increased from 78 million in 1992 to more than 150 million in 1998

(Scheffler, 1999). By the end of the century, 88% of people were enrolled in a carved-out MBHO plan (Kiesler, 2000).

In the early days of managed care, most MBHOs used the same inspect-and-control methods that had been applied to medical services, in particular working to contain inpatient utilization by shifting treatment to outpatient psychotherapy. In many instances, containment efforts were drastic, with some organizations authorizing as few as three or four sessions of psychotherapy at a time and then requiring clinicians to reapply for additional services. The rationale given for such micromanagement was "quality assurance." In practice, however, the process only served to burden clinicians and MBHOs with costly oversight procedures (e.g., paperwork and telephone management). In time, the trend shifted, and the intense monitoring decreased. Most MBHOs concluded that the overly stringent utilization review process was neither necessary nor cost effective for outpatient psychotherapy. They also found that consumer demand for psychotherapy was relatively flat, with the majority of people completing treatment in 10 sessions or fewer, regardless of the number of sessions authorized (Olfson, Marcus, Druss, & Pincus, 2002).

## CURRENT TRENDS IN MENTAL HEALTH SERVICES REIMBURSEMENT

Although exact figures are difficult to come by, available evidence indicates that spending for mental health and substance abuse treatment decreased as a percentage of total health care throughout the 1990s. One study (HayGroup, 1999) commissioned by the National Association of Psychiatric Health Systems and Association of Behavioral Group Practices found that behavioral health spending by medium and large employers decreased nearly 50% (from 6.1% to 3.2%) as a percentage of overall health benefits during the 10-year period ending in 1998. The primary reason given by the authors of the report for the decrease was the steep reduction in inpatient utilization.

More recently, SAMHSA published a report estimating the amount spent on mental health treatment services (Mark et al., 2005). This report, unlike the previous study, included the cost of medications. Although the total national expenditure for mental health and substance abuse services rose from $60 billion in 1991 to $104 billion in 2001, the average annual increase of 5.6% is less than the annual growth of 6.5% for all health care–related spending. As a result, even when the cost of medications is included, spending for mental health as a percentage of all health care spending decreased from 8.2% in 1991 to 7.6% in 2001. The decrease becomes more alarming when one considers that spending on psychotropic medications grew at an annual rate of 17% during the same period (Mark et al., 2005)!

Spending by private health insurers was also being transformed. Mark and Coffey (2003) pointed out that between 1992 and 1999, the percentage of services reimbursed on a fee-for-service basis dropped from 90% to 25%. As a result, the annual cost per insured life fell, from $115 in 1992 to $95 in 1999, a decrease of 17%. In 1992, inpatient treatment accounted for 48% of all expenditures for mental health and substance abuse treatment, whereas spending on psychotropic drugs and outpatient services accounted for 20% and 31%, respectively. However, by 1999, medications and inpatient treatment had essentially switched places, with drugs claiming 48% of all monies spent and inpatient treatment reduced to 18%. Meanwhile, the percentage of dollars going to outpatient treatment remained virtually unchanged, at 34%. Recall, however, that this is 34% of a pie already made smaller by the 17% decrease in funding noted earlier.

The financial status of psychotherapy is further threatened by the historical dearth of growth in use of outpatient services. Using household sections of the 1987 National Medical Expenditure Survey and the 1997 Medical Expenditure Panel Survey, Olfson et al. (2002) showed that the percentage of respondents reporting use of psychotherapy services did not change significantly over a 10-year period beginning in 1987 (3.2% and 3.6%, respectively). To be sure, people did not stop seeking help; rather, they simply chose other avenues. Indeed, the percentage of respondents reporting use of psychiatric medications increased nearly fourfold during the same period. Therapists are free to explain away such findings by citing, for example, the ease and no-fault nature of pharmacotherapy, but the bottom line is clear: Psychotherapy is losing market share to medications.

## SUPPLY, DEMAND, AND THE VALUE OF BEHAVIORAL HEALTH SERVICES AS A COMMODITY

If current trends continue, and there is little reason to suspect otherwise, it is very unlikely that demand for mental health services will increase. The paucity of efforts aimed at altering public perception regarding the benefits of psychotherapy suggests that the field is not even aware a problem exists. Given flat utilization rates, the best the field can hope for is that the number of potential consumers of mental health services keeps pace with overall population growth. According to data generated from the U.S. Census, this means there has been a mere 1.24% increase in the number of people seeking mental health services per year (U.S. Census Bureau, 2004).

Table 9.2 presents the sobering picture that emerges when the ratio of existing mental health professionals to expected population growth is considered. According to a recent SAMHSA report (U.S. Department of Health and

## TABLE 9.2
### Estimated Number of Mental Health Professionals

| Profession | Year | | | | | | | | | | Yearly increase (%) |
|---|---|---|---|---|---|---|---|---|---|---|---|
| | 1983 | 1984 | 1988 | 1989 | 1992 | 1995 | 1996 | 2002 | 2003 | 2004 | |
| Psychiatry | 29,853 | | | | | | | 41,145 | | | 1.70 |
| Psychology | 44,680 | | | | | | | | | 84,883 | 3.10 |
| Social work | | | | 81,737 | | | | | | 103,128 | 1.56 |
| Psychiatric nursing | | 10,034 | | | | | | | 8,751 | | −0.72 |
| Counseling | | | | | | | 61,100 | | | 100,533 | 6.42 |
| Marriage and family therapy | | | | | | 46,227 | | | | 50,158 | 0.91 |
| Psychosocial rehabilitation | | | 20,909 | | | | 100,000 | | | | 21.61 |
| School psychology | | | | | 21,012 | | | | | 37,893 | 5.04 |

*Note.* The estimated number of mental health providers in each discipline is from U.S. Department of Health and Human Services (2004). Only the earliest and latest estimates for each profession were included. Empty cells indicate no specific data for that year.

Human Services, 2004), the number of psychologists (excluding those who work in schools) increased from 44,680 to 84,883 between the years 1983 and 2004, which is a growth of 3.1% per annum and therefore more than double the estimated growth in demand. Even more alarming, master's level counselors and psychosocial rehabilitation providers grew at annual rates of 6.42% and 21.61%, respectively. The same may be said of social workers, whose numbers have swelled to more than 400,000. By contrast, the number of psychiatrists grew at a rate of 1.7%, a figure commensurate with population growth that in part explains the disproportionately higher rates of reimbursement received by these practitioners.

In 2004, the total number of mental health professionals in the United States was estimated to be roughly 836,000. Given a population of approximately 293 million (U.S. Census Bureau, 2004), this means that one mental health provider exists for every 350 U.S. residents (men, women, and children). If approximately 10% (i.e., 35) choose to seek the help of a therapist (a figure of more than double the historic utilization rates) and meet an average of 10 sessions per year (a figure double national averages) the average clinician would be able to bill for 350 hours of services annually. At $100 per hour, that would mean an income of $35,000 before expenses, assuming no clients drop out and all pay their bill in full. If such figures are not sufficiently frightening, add to the mix 400,000+ primary care physicians (Biola, Green, Phillips, Guirguis-Blake, & Fryer, 2003a), most of whom prescribe psychotropic medications. The simple reality is that there are nowhere near enough clients to sustain the current or future livelihoods of all clinicians.

What is more, available evidence makes clear that the perceived value of psychotherapy has fallen in the eyes of consumers. The decrease in utilization of psychotherapy relative to medications combined with decreased spending on behavioral health care proves this to be the case. That reimbursement rates have remained flat while the cost of living has increased by 20% shows that the value of the commodity has also fallen in the eyes of the payers. In a marketplace environment, the simple reality is that low demand and high supply increase competition. In short, behavioral health care providers must compete with one another as well as against the larger pool of health care providers and products.

Classical economics (e.g., Keynes, 1936) are sufficient to illustrate the implications of such trends for the individual practitioner. Consumers (i.e., clients) prefer having access to large provider networks provided by MBHOs. At the same time, customers (i.e., employers and other health care purchasers) also expect MBHOs to contain costs, which often leads to limiting provider reimbursement. Professional organizations, with the intent of good will for their members, appear motivated to keep MBHOs open to any willing licensed provider. Individual providers, on the other hand, obviously feel compelled to join the MBHOs' provider networks to have access to clients who have insurance coverage. Consequently, providers are forced to accept the MBHOs' fee schedules with little or no room for negotiation. In sum, large MBHO provider networks are competing for a limited pool of referrals, which in turn, ensures that reimbursement rates to the providers remain minimal. This is a happy scenario for both the MBHOs and their consumers: Abundant choices in providers willing to provide behavioral health services at a low cost.

Obviously, for providers, the current environment is a disaster: The individual clinician is but one of many in a market full of other therapists (with more and cheaper versions entering the field every year). As noted in the January 2006 issue of *Psychotherapy Finances*, it is becoming harder and harder to make a living accepting clients from MBHOs. The same issue points out that developing a boutique practice and only accepting cash for services rendered may work for some clinicians, but overall there are not enough customers paying the full and customary fees out of pocket to offset the lost revenue from managed care. As recently as 2000, self-pay customers accounted for 44% of income for all private practitioners combined, whereas managed care contributed 30%. However, in 2006, the ratio had reversed, with managed care contributing 44% and self-pay accounting for only 27% of practitioners' income. To put it bluntly, the current economic picture for the average psychotherapist is quite pessimistic.

## THE TRUE "COMMODITY" IN PSYCHOTHERAPY

Given the foregoing, there is little doubt about the future of clinical practice. First, spending in mental health services has steadily decreased in comparison with physical health care, even though the utilization rate has been fairly stable over the recent years. Second, even within mental health spending, psychotherapy is clearly losing out to psychotropic medications. Psychotherapists are, in effect, in competition with the pharmaceutical industry for insurance dollars. Under the current trends in insurance, out-of-pocket expenses for seeking psychotherapy are likely higher than those associated with filling a prescription written by a family physician. Third, and finally, the supply of therapists currently outstrips demand. Lack of regulation in supply has clearly accelerated the decrease in the perceived value of psychotherapy.

It is clear that providers need an edge. But what? There are two possible ways for clinicians to get a leg up in the increasingly competitive world of behavioral health. The first follows the path chosen by many in the field of medicine: specialization. Among physicians, evidence indicates that generalists are the most undervalued (Biola, Green, Phillips, Guirguis-Blake, & Fryer, 2003b). Despite their often greater workload, for example, primary care physicians are paid significantly less than are specialists. A trend in specialization is already being seen in some areas of professional psychology, particularly in child clinical psychology and neuropsychology. Given the oversupply noted earlier, however, specialization in and of itself will soon prove insufficient to maintain income disparities favoring specialists. Unless one chooses an area not already saturated with other mental health providers, the struggle to make a living will likely continue.

The other route for increasing the competitiveness of mental health providers requires some explanation because it involves a fundamental shift in the paradigm that has guided much if not most of the development and practice of psychotherapy. As Wampold (chap. 2, this volume) points out, medicine has played a significant role in determining how psychotherapy has been conceptualized and practiced. Over the past century, it has also seriously hindered understanding of how psychotherapy actually works.

In contemporary medicine, there is very little doubt about the potency of specific treatments. For example, chemotherapy and radiation are specific procedures to treat cancer, both of which have been tested empirically and verified as efficacious. As such, whether a patient recovers from cancer is determined primarily by the type and amount of chemotherapy and radiation. Who delivers the treatment does not (or should not, within the reigning medical paradigm) affect the efficacy of both therapies. The end goal in medicine is, in fact, the identification of specific treatment procedures for given illnesses.

It should come as little surprise that pioneers in the field of psychotherapy applied the concept of specificity to the "talking cure." After all, many were physicians themselves. The attribution of clinical effects to the specific techniques associated with a given theory of psychotherapy has continued to the present. In fact, all major schools posit that their specific techniques target the underlying etiology responsible for psychopathology. For example, in their now classic work *Cognitive Therapy for Depression*, Beck, Rush, Shaw, and Emery (1979) clearly stated the role of specific factors in the treatment of depression:

> The specific therapeutic techniques . . . are designed to identify, reality-test, and correct distorted conceptualizations and the dysfunctional beliefs (schemas) underlying these cognitions. The patient learns to master problems and situations which he previously considered insuperable by reevaluating and correcting his thinking. The cognitive therapist helps the patient to think and act more realistically and adaptively about his psychological problems and thus reduces symptoms. (p. 4)

As the evidence reviewed throughout this volume reveals, however, numerous investigations to confirm the efficacy of specific techniques as postulated by theories of psychotherapy have ended in failure (e.g., Ahn & Wampold, 2001; Jacobson et al., 1996). Moreover, meta-analytic investigations have repeatedly shown that psychological treatments for most disorders and populations are roughly equivalent in their efficacy despite critical differences in theory and associated techniques (e.g., Robinson, Berman, & Neimeyer, 1990; Smith & Glass, 1977; Wampold, 2001; Wampold et al., 1997). As a result, the field finds itself facing the same question asked of medicine in 1885:

> How was it, certain physicians asked, that so many different modalities of somatic therapies ranging from electricity and hydrotherapy to diet, rest, nutrition, and medication could achieve identical results? Might they not share a common ground? Deducing from the variegated experiences of a wide array of somatic treatments, the Boston neurologist Morton Prince declared, "I think if these treatments are carefully analyzed it will be found that there is one factor that is common in them all, namely, the psychical element." (Caplan, 1998, p. 45)

It is possible that a day will come in the future when specific psychotherapies will prove differentially effective for specific diagnoses. Until that time, one must follow in the footsteps of Prince and ask, "What then, is this 'psychical element?'"

## Therapists' Impact on Clinical Outcomes

The strongest evidence regarding the psychical element points to the person providing the treatment, that is, the therapist. Simply put, some therapists are more effective than others. As surprising as this may seem to some, it is not a new finding. In fact, empirical evidence regarding the variability in outcome among treatment providers dates back to the earliest days of the field (e.g., Luborsky, 1952; Rosenzweig, 1936). Rosenzweig (1936), in his classic article (see Prologue, this volume) explained this point clearly:

> In conclusion, it may be said that given a therapist who has an effective personality and who consistently adheres in his treatment to a system of concepts which he has mastered and which is in one significant way or another adapted to the problems of the sick personality, then it is of comparatively little consequence what particular method that therapist uses. (p. 414)

Taking advantage of the currently available statistical techniques, studies have confirmed that therapists' clinical ability is indeed far from uniform. This phenomenon is commonly referred to as *therapist effects*. During the past 2 decades, data from clinical trials have been reanalyzed to see what percentage of the treatment outcome could be attributed to the therapists providing the treatment rather than to the treatment itself (e.g., Blatt, Sanislow, Zuroff, & Pilkonis, 1996; Crits-Christoph et al., 1991; Crits-Christoph & Mintz, 1991; Elkin, 1999; Huppert et al., 2001; Kim, Wampold, & Bolt, 2006).

These studies consistently show that therapists are likely far more responsible for the effect of treatment than the method of psychotherapy used, even when the use of a particular approach is carefully controlled via treatment manuals and adherence tests.

Research indicates that the impact of the provider on outcome extends to psychotropic medication, as well. In a reanalysis of data from the National Institute of Mental Health Treatment of Depression Collaborative Research Project, the largest and most sophisticated study on the treatment of depression ever conducted, McKay, Imel, and Wampold (2006) found that the prescriber of the drug was much more important than the drug itself! It is interesting that psychiatrists with the best outcomes when prescribing medication also had the best outcomes when a placebo was used. In fact, the three most effective psychiatrists in the study achieved better outcomes using a placebo than the three poorest performing prescribers using an antidepressant. This finding is consistent with results of the analysis of the therapist effects in a managed care network, which likewise indicated the effectiveness of medications was highly dependent on the psychotherapist (Wampold & Brown, 2005).

**Evaluating the Commodity**

The fact that psychotherapists, the commodity in psychotherapy, are not equally effective has different implications under different market conditions. As an analogy, consider housing. In a market in which demand is significantly greater than supply, a seller's market is said to exist. Under such circumstances, buyers looking for a home will have to lower their expectations and pay more than they initially intended. On the other hand, when supply is greater than demand, buyers have the upper hand. Real estate agents, dependent on home sales for their livelihood, will demand that sellers reduce their prices and spruce up their homes. To appeal to potential buyers, real estate agents will also seek the best houses available on the market.

The same dynamics unfortunately apply to psychotherapy. Available evidence makes clear that a buyer's market exists for psychotherapy. Under these conditions, employers seeking behavioral health plans look around for the best offer they can get for their money. In turn, MBHOs, dependent on sales of health care plans for their livelihood, will demand that practitioners reduce their prices. To appeal to potential employers seeking health care plans, MBHOs will also seek the most effective psychotherapy available in the market. Given that the quality of psychotherapy ultimately depends on the therapist, it is thus inevitable that MBHOs will attempt to identify the best therapists.

# OUTCOMES MANAGEMENT IN
# THE MANAGED CARE ENVIRONMENT

Several MBHOs have already launched initiatives to measure treatment outcomes within their networks. The Human Affairs International Outcomes Clinical Information System Project (1995–1998), the PacifiCare Behavioral Health (PBH) ALERT project (1998–2006), and Resources for Living SIGNAL system are three well-documented prototypes of outcomes-informed care initiatives (Brown, Burlingame, Lambert, Jones, & Vacarro, 2001; Brown et al., 1999; Brown, Fraser, & Bendoraitis, 1995; Brown, Lambert, Jones, & Minami, 2005; Miller, Duncan, Sorrell, & Brown, 2005). All of these projects included the following goals: (a) to encourage frequent administration of a client self-report outcome questionnaire, (b) to set up a centralized database for all outcome data, (c) to provide feedback to practitioners in the form of individual case alerts as well as outcomes across all clients on caseload, (d) to use information on provider outcomes to identify highly effective providers for purposes of steering referrals,[1] and (e) to involve independent researchers and encourage publication of results.

By 2006, more than 10,000 clinicians were participating in the PBH project. The company hired independent consultants and academic researchers to develop a system for tracking outcomes and alerting therapists about at risk cases. It is important to note that data generated by the resulting ALERT system were made available for analyses and publications in peer-reviewed journals without editorial oversight. Because the outcome data were stored in a single location, it was easy to merge treatment outcome data with databases on network providers, service and pharmacy claims databases, and with data on benefit design, copayments, and so on. The creation of this data warehouse permitted researchers to explore the relationship between provider effectiveness, treatment methods, cost of care, and outcomes.

The publications that resulted from this collaboration between PBH and independent researchers provided a rich source of information. For example, it was demonstrated that psychotherapy provided under the PBH coverage was likely as effective as the most rigorous clinical trials in psychotherapy (Minami et al., 2008). The study further showed that the average number of weeks in treatment to obtain clinically significant results was less than 9, with a median of 6 weeks, clearly demonstrating that the length of treatment necessary to benefit from psychotherapy was significantly shorter than perceived by the general public.

---

[1]This goal is controversial. See chapter 14, this volume, for potential downsides, as well as footnote 7 in chapter 12 of this volume about incentives for therapist performance.

Data from PBH also showed that therapists differed in their overall effectiveness and that the variability was much greater when clients were on medication (Wampold & Brown, 2005). Specifically, the positive impact of psychotropic medications was more pronounced for clients who were treated by therapists who had above-average treatment outcomes. The clients of therapists with below-average treatment outcomes fared no better when treated with medication than when receiving psychotherapy alone. In addition, the results indicated that the therapists with above-average outcomes achieved better results with psychotherapy alone than their less effective peers achieved with the combination of psychotherapy and medications!

Findings from the PBH project have obvious and significant financial implications. Take, for example, the result that the effectiveness of medication is impacted by the clinician. If so, depending on who the clinician is, money spent on medications may or may not result in substantial improvement. Factoring in the cost of medication greatly magnifies the value of effective clinicians.

Subsequent analyses, including cross-validations of clinicians' results from one sample to another, have confirmed the above findings with both adults and children. For example, after adjusting for differences in case mix (e.g., initial symptom severity, client demographics), Brown (2006) found that clinicians with above-average outcomes during one period of time were likely to have above-average outcomes at future points in time. The differences in effectiveness during the cross-validation phase remained large enough to suggest that increasing the flow of new referrals to the most effective providers in the network would still result in significantly lower overall costs while improving client outcomes (Brown & Jones, 2005; Brown et al., 2005; Wampold & Brown, 2005).

The results of analyses reported in these peer-reviewed journal articles provide a unique picture of the sources of variance in the cost and outcomes of outpatient mental health care as it is generally practiced in the United States. After controlling for differences in case mix using variables commonly available (e.g., diagnosis, age, sex, intake scores, prior treatment history), one cannot explain most of the variance, presumably because of factors beyond the control of clinicians or health plans. However, the evidence clearly points to the individual clinician being the single largest source of explained variance that is within control.

It is not surprising that the evidence gathered by researchers led PBH to conclude that the most effective pathway to improving outcomes and increasing the value of treatment was to increase the number of referrals sent to the most effective clinicians. In 2006, PBH announced the Honors for Outcomes initiative. Clinicians with above-average outcomes and consistency of data collection were included on a list for preferential steerage of new referrals. These

Honors providers were also listed on a web site so that potential consumers could make an informed choice about providers within the PBH network.

## Determining the "Value" of Psychotherapy

The *value index,* which is a simplification of a more complex commodity index often used in business, is simply the benefit divided by the cost of the service. To illustrate, assume that the average cost to treat depression in an outpatient setting is $1,000. This estimate is given for purposes of illustration only, and actual costs vary depending on the benefit design, area of service delivery, and type of practitioner, among other factors. Many plans, for example, reimburse practitioners with a doctorate at higher rates than those with master's degrees. For the sake of this example, assume that outpatient psychotherapy for depression results in an average improvement of 0.80 in effect size units. With this effect size, the value index, which is again the magnitude of benefit divided by the cost, is 0.0008 for every $1 in costs (i.e., 0.80 for every $1,000).

When the value index is used as a cost–benefit benchmark for clinicians in the PBH data, the implications are nothing short of staggering. Honors clinicians, for example, average 1.0 in effect size units per $1,000 in costs (i.e., 0.001). By contrast, non-Honors clinicians average 0.4 in effect size units per $1,000 in costs (i.e., 0.0004). In other words, services provided by Honors clinicians have more than twice the value of those in the non-Honors group. Moreover, although the reasons are unknown at present, clinicians practicing in multidisciplinary group practices average 15% to 25% fewer sessions per case than clinicians in solo practice. At the same time, clients treated in these settings average significantly larger effect sizes than those treated by solo practitioners (Brown & Jones, 2005). Group practices in the PBH network that qualified for the Honors for Outcomes listing averaged an improvement of 1.5 effect size units for every $1,000 in cost. The value of services at these group practices was therefore almost 4 times greater than for solo non-Honors clinicians (Brown, 2007).

From the perspective of employers purchasing health care plans, one persuasive rationale for measuring treatment outcomes is that money spent on psychotherapy services results in improved productivity in the workplace and reduction in other medical costs. The evidence is clear: Behavioral health problems result in significant loss of productivity costs (Greenberg et al., 2003; Kessler et al., 2006; Stewart, Ricci, Chee, Hahn, & Morganstein, 2003). If expected improvement in productivity and reduction in medical costs is dependent on the individual clinician, then employers have a significant financial stake in ensuring that their employees have access to the most effective provider available. In other words, paying for treatment services provided by highly effective clinicians will result in a significant return on investment. As such, employers have considerable interest in giving preferential referrals and reimbursement to clinicians who have evidence of effectiveness: Every dollar spent on services provided by these clinicians is likely to result in significant benefit to the client, which in turn will benefit the employer.

However, because differences in effectiveness among providers are currently not taken into account, it is very hard for those purchasing services to determine their potential return on investment. Given the current oversupply of psychotherapists, such lack of differentiation has a disproportionately negative impact on the most effective therapists. Although it is understandable that therapists, regardless of their effectiveness, may find the prospect of measuring outcomes uncomfortable, continuing with business as usual will simply ensure that the interests of the least effective practitioners are protected at the expense of employers; effective psychotherapists; and most important, the clients.

## Being Competitive in the Current Psychotherapy Market

Current trends do not bode well for the future of psychotherapy reimbursement. Large MBHOs are driven to provide what the market demands: Maximum choice to consumers via large networks of providers. With no shortage of licensed mental health practitioners vying for inclusion on provider panels at cut-rate reimbursement rates, market forces will continue to drive down the relative value of psychotherapy services. The buyer's market gripping the field since the mid-1990s will continue and intensify.

There are certainly some bright spots. As this chapter was being prepared in early 2009, it appeared that the Paul Wellstone and Pete Domenici Mental Health Parity and Addiction Equity Act of 2008 will assure that behavioral health will be given equal footing with medical and surgical benefits. It is interesting that some MBHOs have also argued convincingly that expanding benefits for behavioral health care need not result in significant escalation in overall health care costs (Goldman et al., 1999; Savitz, Grace, & Brown, 1993; Sturm, 1997). In addition, the Surgeon General's report on mental health care concluded that the cost to society to provide parity coverage for serious psychiatric disorders is modest (U.S. Department of Health and Human Services, 1999).

Unfortunately, although the passage of parity legislation may result in an increase in demand for mental health services, it is unlikely that the increase will ever exceed the current supply of mental health services providers. As a result, it is likely that interest in outcomes will continue to increase among MBHOs and employer groups. For example, United Behavioral Health (UBH), which provides mental health services to more than 22 million subscribers, is currently promoting outcomes-informed care throughout its network of more than 60,000 practitioners. Other MBHOs are also reported to be considering various outcomes initiatives. In the state of Arizona, Magellan is using the Partners for Change Outcome Management System (Duncan, Miller, & Sparks, 2004; Miller et al., 2005) to track the outcomes of all public sector clients (for a discussion of outcome tracking systems, see chap. 8, this volume; for a specific example of implementation, see chap. 10, this volume). Some companies are using incentives to promote the use of outcome questionnaires by their network providers. For example, Azocar et al. (2007), using data from UBH, found that the clinicians' use of client outcome data was associated with greater improvement at 6 months from baseline compared with the outcomes of clinicians not using the outcome information. Although clinicians currently receive no direct benefit for measuring outcomes regardless of their effectiveness, results from this study and others are more than sufficient for UBH to use incentives to have clinicians implement outcome questionnaires.

Incentives aside, after being licensed to practice independently, why would any therapist want to use formal measures of client progress in their clinical work? For practitioners who are not alarmed by the aforementioned factors, there is not much reason. This is because those who are not alarmed either have well-established practices (or are nearing retirement) or are practicing in an organization that is insulated from market trends (e.g., state- or federal-funded agencies, university and college counseling centers). For everyone else, however, the motivation is survival.

As discussed earlier, under conditions in which the odds of being able to make a reasonable living by providing psychotherapy are low, participating in outcomes-informed care is a viable alternative. Imagine for a moment that a significant percentage of therapists embraced outcomes-informed care and began using some formal measure of progress with all of their clients. Further, assume that these therapists had access to the same kinds of technology and data analytic capabilities available to large MBHOs, enabling them to pool their data, evaluate their outcomes, and compare their effectiveness with credible benchmarks, thereby providing evidence of their effectiveness of treatment to consumers, other payers, and clients. Therapists with superior outcomes could use the data for marketing purposes. Those falling short would be able to work at improving their outcomes. What would happen if 10% to 15% of practitioners in a large metropolitan area pooled their data, subjected it to external, independent analyses, and were able to show collectively that their results matched or exceeded benchmarks obtained from clinical trials? Could these practitioners then make the case to employers and local health plans to give preferential treatment in terms of reimbursement and referrals? Could these practitioners also appeal to the minority of clients who are willing to pay out of pocket?

Currently, technical and financial barriers against outcomes-informed practice are virtually nonexistent. Without a doubt, such questions will be answered prior to the publication of a third edition of *The Heart and Soul of Change*. Indeed, self-selected, motivated, and outcomes-informed clinicians are already taking such steps in various parts around the globe.

An outcomes-informed care initiative unfolding in the states of Washington and Oregon is an example of recent developments. In this case, a unique set of circumstances brought together clinicians, employers, and a regional health plan (i.e., Regence). Briefly, a major employer in the Pacific Northwest encouraged Regence to evaluate the effectiveness of behavioral health care services. At the same time, one of the largest behavioral health group practices serving Regence members urged the company to implement an outcomes-informed care initiative.

The initiative differed from previous outcomes-informed care initiatives in that rather than using standardized and copyrighted questionnaires, it used an innovative measurement methodology advocated by the nonprofit organization known as ACORN (A Collaborative Outcomes Resource Network). The methodology focuses on testing the psychometric properties of individual items and then selecting the best items for a specific measurement purpose. Items are first tested in a community sample of individuals not receiving any treatment, and then they are pilot tested in clinical settings. Then, all of the items go through a well-established psychometric evaluation known as the *item torture test* (e.g., Greco, Lambert, & Baer, 2008). Once the psychometric properties of the items are known, different organizations are then able to choose from the item pool to create brief outcome questionnaires uniquely tailored to the needs of that organization. If the existing item pool lacks a needed item, new items can be developed and tested.

Because all of the ACORN questionnaires share a core set of items with established psychometric properties, it is a relatively easy matter to equate the scores from the various alternative forms of the ACORN outcome measures. The number of items on the questionnaires could vary from fewer than 10 to more than 20 depending on the purpose of the measure and the degree of measurement precision needed. Measurement precision is dependent on the reliability of the questionnaire, which is in turn a function of both the content and number of items. Field-testing of the ACORN items in clinical settings revealed that questionnaires consisting of 12 to 16 well-established items assessing the most common complaints among individuals seeking psychotherapy offered an optimal trade-off between reliability and questionnaire length.

Within a few months of the initial pilot testing of the new questionnaires, several other large health plans began to pilot the questionnaires across a wide variety of treatment settings. The result was that within 9 months of testing the first versions of the questionnaires, the collaborative data repository shared by all of the organizations contained data for thousands of clients receiving treatment in the real world.

In addition, a work group of researchers and practitioners worked collaboratively to establish benchmarks for clinician effectiveness. This effort has expanded to include a number of representatives from various insurance, managed behavioral health care, disease management, and employee assistance companies as well as professional organizations. This collaboration resulted in a white paper describing an explicit methodology for calculating criteria-based estimates of clinician effectiveness to be implemented across the various organizations and shared openly with clinicians. The coauthors of this white paper represent a diverse group of academic researchers and health plan executives who share a common vision for improving client outcomes.

The long-term success of ACORN, which evolved from the Regence project, is far from certain. Although the initial response of large practices and clinics has been very positive, the continued success is dependent on individual clinicians using the outcome questionnaires consistently over a long period of time.

The trends are encouraging. Other national and regional managed behavioral health care organizations are stepping up efforts to recruit clinicians who are willing to participate in outcomes-informed care initiatives. For example, as this book is going to press, two of the nation's largest MBHOs (ValueOptions and UBH) are dramatically stepping up their efforts to involve therapists in outcomes-informed care initiatives.

## CONCLUSIONS: WHAT THE INDEPENDENT PRACTITIONER CAN DO

Frankly, the odds of effective clinicians being able to increase psychotherapy reimbursement from third-party payers without providing evidence of their outcomes are slim to none. Effective clinicians will need to act collectively to take advantage of outcomes-informed care. Without producing evidence of their clinical effectiveness and distinguishing themselves from the rest of the mental health providers, it is hard to imagine any other scenario but succumbing to the overall downward pressure on psychotherapy reimbursement as a result of a saturated market.

With the foregoing in mind, we end this chapter with some suggestions for clinicians who are motivated to implement outcomes-informed care to demonstrate their value and increase their reimbursement:

- Get in the habit of collecting outcome data on all clients. Do not wait for someone else to do it. You can choose from a variety of existing outcome measures because there are now outcome measures that are not proprietary or are free for individual use and have solid psychometric properties. See http://www.psychoutcomes.org and http://www.centerforclinicalexcellence.com for more information.

- If an MBHO offers to collect outcome data on your clients, accept the offer, but ask (a) if the MBHO will let you use their questionnaire with all of your clients regardless of their referral sources, (b) if they will accept evidence of your effectiveness and give you preferential referrals if you are above average as compared with other providers in their network, and (c) if they are willing to provide some small compensation to offset the cost of collecting such valuable data. If nothing else, this will get their attention.

- Look for opportunities to collaborate with other outcomes-informed care providers in the area, or online. There is strength in numbers; your data combined with that of your colleagues is much more powerful and attractive than your data by itself.

- Create or download and use a software product for tracking outcomes. To keep costs down, think about forming a data cooperative with other practices in your community. Bargain collectively to contract with a company that can provide state-of-the-art outcomes measurement services along with sophisticated data analytic, reporting, and benchmarking services. Drive a hard bargain; it's a competitive business.

- Take advantage of any opportunity to benchmark your outcomes against regional and national norms. Know where you stand, and make use of that information to improve your outcomes—or even better, use them to actively market yourself!

- Educate your clients about the evidence for outcomes-informed care and the importance of providing feedback to you, the clinician. Model humility, humanity, and openness. It is okay to let them know that your outcomes appear to be pretty good (if they are) but that you are always looking for ways to improve.

- Collaborate with other clinicians in your community to educate local employers and health plans about the importance of using practitioners who can provide evidence of effectiveness. Show them how to get the best possible return on their investment in behavioral health care dollars.

- Lobby individually and collectively to payers and referral sources to give preferential treatment to outcomes-informed care providers who have evidence of effectiveness.

It is an unfortunate reality that not all mental health practitioners will survive the current market conditions. Clinicians wanting to survive and thrive in this market will need to prove themselves to the demanding market. Consequently, those who cannot do so will have to leave the market. No, there is nothing warm and fuzzy about it, and it sounds heartless and soulless. There are perhaps many to blame for the current reality—government, MBHOs, professional organizations, academic institutions, and so on. On the other hand, if market pressure is forcing clinicians to be better at what they do, they are then simply in competition with each other on the basis of the rules of the so-called free market. And one supposes—and hopes—that this will all lead to the clients' benefit. Ultimately, this is where our hearts and souls as clinicians lie.

## QUESTIONS FROM THE EDITORS

1. *What do you believe accounts for the dramatic differences in effectiveness among practicing clinicians?*

As a general rule, things vary. In addition, the harder the task is, the more variability becomes apparent. Therefore, it should come as no surprise that clinicians also vary in their effectiveness of psychological treatments, much as does with anything requiring a high level of skill. It is often suggested that if we cannot explain this variability and use it to guide clinicians to improve their outcomes, then the finding is of little practical use. We could not disagree more, and ultimately, in a capital market, no consumer actually cares how the superior results are obtained (as long as the method is legal and ethical). Consumers will pay for demonstrated outcomes. Although the exact sources of the variability in treatment effectiveness are unknown, we assume that a number of hard-to-define (much less quantify) variables may come into play, including personality, emotional intelligence, therapist beliefs and expectations, and technical proficiency as well as the ability to put all of the foregoing together in an artistic form.

It is tempting to introduce the concept of *talent*, which is currently considered something that can be coached but not taught. One often uses the word in a complimentary manner, as in "Dr. So and So is a talented clinician," without having a clear idea of what this means. The concept of talent invokes ideas of innate abilities that can be honed and culminated but also suggesting that if you lack this innate magic no amount of practice will take you to an elite level. However, research on how "stars" in different fields differ from their "less talented" peers suggests a very different picture.

Miller, Hubble, and Duncan's (2007) article "Supershrinks"—therapists whose outcomes are a cut above the rest—provides a provocative fresh look at the question of talent versus practice and hard work in achieving superior psychotherapy results. Research on top performers in many different fields of endeavor reveals that they have two things in common: They practice more than their peers, and they constantly seek performance feedback. They know what their results are, and they work hard to get better.

Michael Jordan, arguably the greatest basketball player of all time, is legendary in his commitment to hard work and constant practice with incredible focus and commitment to improving his game. Whatever his native abilities are, it is also true that he simply has worked harder than everyone else around him. One thing is certain, though. If Michael Jordan had had to learn the game of basketball without ever getting feedback on whether the ball went into the hoop, virtually any 12-year-old who had spent time shooting hoops in the school yard could have outscored Michael in a real game.

2. *Former American Psychological Association President Nicholas Cummings made similar predictions regarding reimbursement rates in late 1970s. Like now, clinicians failed to heed or take any constructive steps (other than litigation and legislation) to deal with pressing market changes. What accounts for the field's continuing inertia?*

Many factors contribute to the field's inability to mount a constructive response to the economic realities facing psychotherapists. Two collective decisions loom large, however. First, as noted in the body of the chapter, professional organizations expended all their time and energy advocating for the collective interests of all of their members. Rather than looking at the effects of oversupply and encouraging members to compete more effectively, an adversarial position was assumed toward managed care. This is akin to criticizing the real estate agent about the housing market.

The second critical failure is that many clinicians are not interested in measuring outcomes, thereby making it extremely difficult for any payer or employer to determine the value of their services, much less appreciate the importance of the individual clinician. Again, the various professional organizations have done very little to encourage their membership to collect outcome data in an effort to demonstrate the value of their services.

3. *In your opinion, what coursework is missing from graduate school programs regarding business practices and market economics?*

We believe that basic understanding of introductory classes in economics is sufficient to evaluate market trends, and therefore, if students have been exposed to introductory economics during their undergraduate education (and have comprehended the material), then additional courses are perhaps unnecessary for the majority of clinicians. Of course, additional courses in business accounting and marketing may indeed help those who are motivated to establish and expand their private practices or are interested in assuming managerial positions in mental health agencies.

As explained throughout our chapter, what students need to learn along with business practices and market economics is what to sell—their competence. Thus, students need to learn (a) how to measure their clinical outcomes and (b) how to interpret their outcomes. Their instructors, on the other hand, must (c) know how to incorporate outcome assessments in all of their clinical courses and (d) provide clinical guidance (e.g., supervision, practicum, internship) on the basis of outcomes. Therefore, we suggest a complete overhaul of current graduate training.

First of all, courses in professional issues must include the current market trend and inform the students that they are going into a profession with fierce competition. Obviously, this is not the kind of information that academic departments would like to share with their students because of the possible impact on recruitment and retention. However, we believe that informing students about the reality along with what they could do to be competitive would in fact provide an edge over graduates from other programs.

Second, coursework in theory and skills of psychotherapy or training in empirically supported and manualized treatments must clearly include information regarding their outcomes and the context in which they were measured (and equally important, the context in which they have not been measured). Incorporation of this information primes the students to view treatments with the emphasis on their outcomes rather than what the theories are supposed to do. Currently, as reviewed above, there is hardly any evidence for specificity.

Third, courses in research design, psychometrics, and analysis should emphasize those practices that are crucial for outcome measurement, including pre- and poststandardized change scores, crucial covariates (e.g., initial severity, treatment length), instrument characteristics (e.g., specificity and reactivity), and outcomes data management. Although other group and correlational designs are important to conduct research, primary importance for clinicians would be to comprehend what exactly they are measuring about the treatment they provide. Coursework should also explain how data from clinical trials could potentially inform the obtained magnitude of their own treatment (i.e., benchmarking).

Fourth, given the above prerequisites, all practice courses (e.g., practicum, internship) should measure treatment outcomes from the outset of training (see the Questions From the Editors in chap. 12, this volume, for an example). In addition, students will likely benefit if common process factors that are known to impact treatment outcomes (e.g., working alliance) are also assessed. Both process and outcome data obtained from their clients should then be actively used in their clinical supervision. Therefore, supervisors must also understand how to incorporate them into their work.

Last, all other coursework should also speak to how it impacts outcomes. For example, what are outcomes obtained for career interventions and for multicultural counseling competence? What is the effect of diagnosis and psychological assessment on treatment outcomes? In other words, courses should be revamped so that outcomes, that is, evidence of efficacy and effectiveness, come first. In total, we believe that these modifications are a necessity for students to be able to fully claim their training is evidence-based practice in psychology.

## REFERENCES

Ahn, H., & Wampold, B. E. (2001). Where oh where are the specific ingredients? A meta-analysis of component studies in counseling and psychotherapy. *Journal of Counseling Psychology, 48,* 251–257.

American Psychological Association Practice Directorate. (2009). *Keynote speech to 2007 State Leadership Conference.* Retrieved July 7, 2009, from http://www.apa.org/practice/slc_2007_speech.html

Azocar, F., Cuffel, B., McCulloch, J., McCabe, J. F., Tani, S., & Brodey, B. B. (2007). Monitoring patient improvement and treatment outcomes in managed behavioral health. *Journal of Healthcare Quality, 29,* 4–12.

Barry, C. L., Gabel, J. R., Frank, R. G., Hawkins, S., Whitmore, H. H., & Pickreign, J. D. (2003). Design of mental health benefits: Still unequal after all these years. *Health Affairs, 22,* 127–137.

Beck, A. T., Rush, A. J., Shaw, B. F., & Emery, G. (1979). *Cognitive therapy of depression.* New York: Guilford Press.

Biola, H., Green, L. A., Phillips, R. L., Guirguis-Blake, J., & Fryer, G. E. (2003a, October 15). The U.S. primary care physician workforce: Minimal growth 1980–1999. *American Family Physician, 68,* 1483.

Biola, H., Green, L. A., Phillips, R. L., Guirguis-Blake, J., & Fryer, G. E. (2003b, October 15). The U.S. primary care physician workforce: Undervalued service. *American Family Physician, 68,* 1486.

Blatt, S. J., Sanislow, C. A., Zuroff, D. C., & Pilkonis, P. A. (1996). Characteristics of effective therapists: Further analyses of data from the National Institute of Mental Health treatment of depression collaborative research program. *Journal of Consulting and Clinical Psychology, 64,* 1276–1284.

Brown, G. S. (2006, June). *The importance of therapist effects in the treatment of children and adolescents.* Paper presented at the 2006 Joint National Conference on Mental Health Block Grant and National Conference on Mental Health Statistics, Washington, DC.

Brown, G. S. (2007, August). *Implications of therapist effects for employers and health plans.* Paper presented at the 115th Annual Convention of the American Psychological Association, San Francisco, CA.

Brown, G. S., Burlingame, G. M., Lambert, M. J., Jones, E., & Vacarro, J. (2001). Pushing the quality envelope: A new outcomes management system. *Psychiatric Services, 52,* 925–934.

Brown, G. S., Dreis, S., & Nace, D. K. (1999). What really makes a difference in psychotherapy outcomes? Why does managed care want to know? In M. A. Hubble, B. L. Duncan, & S. D. Miller (Eds.), *The heart and soul of change: What works in therapy* (pp. 389–406). Washington, DC: American Psychological Association.

Brown G. S., Fraser J. B., & Bendoraitis T. M. (1995). Transforming the future—The coming impact of clinical information systems. *Behavioral Health Management, 14*, 8–12.

Brown, G. S., & Jones, E. (2005). Implementation of a feedback system in a managed care environment: What are patients teaching us? *Journal of Clinical Psychology: In Session, 61*, 187–198.

Brown, G. S., Lambert, M. J., Jones, E., & Minami, T. (2005). Identifying highly effective psychotherapists in a managed care environment. *American Journal of Managed Care, 11*, 513–520.

Caplan, E. (1998). *Mind games: American culture and the birth of psychotherapy*. Berkeley: University of California Press.

Crits-Christoph, P., Baranackie, K., Kurcias, J. S., Carroll, K., Luborsky, L., McLellan, T., et al. (1991). Meta-analysis of therapist effects in psychotherapy outcome studies. *Psychotherapy Research, 1*, 81–91.

Crits-Christoph, P., & Mintz, J. (1991). Implications of therapist effects for the design and analysis of comparative studies of psychotherapies. *Journal of Consulting and Clinical Psychology, 59*, 20–26.

Drugs vs. talk therapy: 3,079 readers rate their care for depression and anxiety. (2004, October). *Consumer Reports*. Available from http://www.consumerreports.org

Duncan, B. L., Miller. S. D., & Sparks, J. A. (2004). *The heroic client: Principles of client-directed, outcome-informed therapy* (Rev. ed.). San Francisco: Jossey-Bass.

Elkin, I. (1999). A major dilemma in psychotherapy outcome research: Disentangling therapists from therapies. *Clinical Psychology: Science and Practice, 6*, 10–32.

Ellwood, P. M., Jr., Anderson, N. N., Billings, J. E., Carlson, R. J., Hoagberg, E. G., & McClure, W. (1971). Health maintenance strategy. *Medical Care, 9*, 292–298.

Fee, practice and managed care survey. (2006, January). *Psychotherapy Finances, 32*, 1–5.

Goldman, W., McCulloch, J., Cuffel, B., & Kozma, D. (1999). More evidence for the insurability of managed behavioral health care. *Health Affairs, 18*, 172–181.

Greco, L. A., Lambert, W., & Baer, R. A. (2008). Psychological inflexibility in childhood and adolescence: Development and evaluation of the Avoidance and Fusion Questionnaire for Youth. *Psychological Assessment, 20*, 93–102.

Greenberg, P. E., Kessler, R. C., Birnbaum, H. G., Leong, S. A., Lowe, S. W., Berglund, P. A., & Corey-Lisle, P. K. (2003). The economic burden of depression in the United States: How did it change between 1990 and 2000? *Journal of Clinical Psychiatry, 64*, 1465–1475.

Gruber, L. R., Shadle, M., & Polich, C. L. (1988). From movement to industry: The growth of HMOs. *Health Affairs, 7*, 197–208.

Harris International. (2004). [Report prepared for PacifiCare Behavioral Health, Inc.]. Unpublished data.

Hayes, S. C., Barlow, D. H., & Nelson-Grey, R. O. (1999). *The scientist practitioner: Research and accountability in the age of managed care*. Boston: Allyn & Bacon.

HayGroup. (1999). *Health care plan design and cost trends: 1988 to 1999*. Retrieved July 1, 2009, from http://www.naphs.org/News/hay99/hay99.pdf

Huppert, J. D., Bufka, L. F., Barlow, D. H., Gorman, J. M., Shear, M. K., & Woods, S. W. (2001). Therapists, therapist variables, and cognitive–behavioral therapy outcomes in a multicenter trial for panic disorder. *Journal of Consulting and Clinical Psychology, 69*, 747–755.

Jacobson, N. S., Dobson, K. S., Truax, P. A., Addis, M. E., Koerner, K., Gollan, J. K., et al. (1996). A component analysis of cognitive–behavioral treatment for depression. *Journal of Consulting and Clinical Psychology, 64*, 295–304.

Kessler, R. C., Akiskal, H. S., Ames, M., Birnbaum, H., Greenberg, P., Hirschfeld, R. M. A., et al. (2006). Prevalence and effects of mood disorders on work performance in a nationally representative sample of U.S. workers. *American Journal of Psychiatry, 163*, 1561–1568.

Keynes, J. M. (1936). *The general theory of employment, interest and money*. London: McMillan.

Kiesler, C. A. (2000). The next wave of change in psychology and mental health services in the health care revolution. *American Psychologist, 55*, 481–487.

Kim, D., Wampold, B. E., & Bolt, D. M. (2006). Therapist effects in psychotherapy: A random-effects modeling of the National Institute of Mental Health Treatment of Depression Collaborative Research Program data. *Psychotherapy Research, 16*, 161–172.

Luborsky, L. (1952). The personality of the psychotherapist. *Menninger Quarterly, 6*(4), 1–6.

Mark, T. L., & Coffey, R. M. (2003). What drove private health insurance spending on mental health and substance abuse care, 1992–1999? *Health Affairs, 22*, 165–172.

Mark, T. L., Coffey, R. M., McKusick, D. R., Harwood, H., King, E., Bouchery, E., et al. (2005). *National estimates of expenditures for mental health services and substance abuse treatment, 1991–2001* (SAMHSA Publication No. SMA 05-3999). Rockville, MD: Substance Abuse and Mental Health Services Administration.

McKay, K. M., Imel, Z. E., & Wampold, B. E. (2006). Psychiatrist effects in the psychopharmacological treatment of depression. *Journal of Affective Disorders, 92*, 287–290.

Mental health: Does therapy help? (1995, November). *Consumer Reports*, pp. 734–739.

Miller, S. D., Duncan, B. L., Sorrell R., Brown, G. S. (2005). The partners for change outcome management system. *Journal of Clinical Psychology, 61*, 199–208.

Miller, S. D., Hubble, M., & Duncan, B. L. (2007, November/December) Super-shrinks: What's the secret of their success? *Psychotherapy Networker*. Retrieved

July 1, 2009, from http://www.psychotherapynetworker.org/magazine/recent issues/175-supershrinks

Minami, T., Wampold, B. E., Serlin, R. C., Hamilton, E. G., Brown, G. S., & Kircher, J. C. (2008). Benchmarking the effectiveness of psychotherapy treatment for adult depression in a managed care environment: A preliminary study. *Journal of Consulting and Clinical Psychology, 76*, 116–124.

Olfson, M., Marcus, S. C., Druss, B., & Pincus, H. A. (2002). National trends in the use of outpatient psychotherapy. *American Journal of Psychiatry, 159*, 1914–1920.

Robinson, L. A., Berman, J. S., & Neimeyer, R. A. (1990). Psychotherapy for the treatment of depression: A comprehensive review of controlled outcome research. *Psychological Bulletin, 108*, 30–49.

Rosenzweig, S. (1936). Some implicit common factors in diverse methods of psychotherapy. *American Journal of Orthopsychiatry, 6*, 412–415.

Savitz, A. S., Grace, J. G., & Brown, G. S. (1993). "Parity" for mental health: Can it be achieved? *Administration and Policy in Mental Health and Mental Health Services Research, 21*, 7–13.

Scheffler, R. M. (1999). Managed behavioral health care and supply-side economics. *Journal of Mental Health Policy and Economics, 2*, 21–28.

Seligman, M. E. P. (1995). The effectiveness of psychotherapy: The *Consumer Reports* study. *American Psychologist, 50*, 965–974.

Sharkey, J. (1994). *Bedlam: Greed, profiteering, and fraud in a mental health system gone crazy*. New York: St. Martin's Press.

Smith, M. L., & Glass, G. V. (1977). Meta-analysis of psychotherapy outcome studies. *American Psychologist, 32*, 752–760.

Stewart, W. F., Ricci, J. A., Chee, E., Hahn, S. R., & Morganstein, D. (2003). Cost of lost productive work time among U.S. workers with depression. *JAMA, 289*, 3135–3144.

Strosahl, K. (1994). Entering the new frontier of managed mental health care: Gold mines and land mines. *Cognitive and Behavioral Practice, 1*, 5–23.

Sturm, R. (1997). How expensive is unlimited mental health coverage under managed care? *JAMA, 278*, 1533–1537.

U.S. Census Bureau. (2004). *U.S. interim projections by age, sex, race, and Hispanic origin*. Retrieved September 21, 2007, from http://www.census.gov/ipc/www/usinterimproj/

U.S. Department of Health and Human Services. (1999). *Mental health: A report of the surgeon general*. Rockville, MD: Author. Retrieved September 23, 2007, from http://www.surgeongeneral.gov/library/mentalhealth/home.html

U.S. Department of Health and Human Services. (2004). *Mental health, United States, 2004* (DHHS Pub No. SMA-06-4195). Rockville, MD: Author.

U.S. House of Representatives. (1992). *The profits of misery: How inpatient psychiatric treatment bilks the system and betrays our trust*. Washington, DC: U.S. Government Printing Office.

Wampold, B. E. (2001). *The great psychotherapy debate: Model, methods, and findings.* Mahwah, NJ: Erlbaum.

Wampold, B. E. & Brown, G. S. (2005). Estimating variability in outcomes attributable to therapists: A naturalistic study of outcomes in managed care. *Journal of Consulting and Clinical Psychology, 73*, 914–923.

Wampold, B. E., Mondin, G. W., Moody, M., Stich, F., Benson, K., & Ahn, H. (1997). A meta-analysis of outcome studies comparing bona fide psychotherapies: Empirically, "all must have prizes." *Psychological Bulletin, 122*, 203–215.

Weissman, M. M., Verdeli, H., Gameroff, M. J., Bledsoe, S. E., Betts, K., Mufson, L., et al. (2006). National survey of psychotherapy training in psychiatry, psychology, and social work. *Archives of General Psychiatry, 63*, 925–934.

Woolley, J. T., & Peters, G. (n.d.). *The American presidency project.* Santa Barbara, CA: University of California (hosted), G. Peters (database). Retrieved September 19, 2007, from http://www.presidency.ucsb.edu/ws/index.php?pid=4092#

# 10

# TRANSFORMING PUBLIC BEHAVIORAL HEALTH CARE: A CASE EXAMPLE OF CONSUMER-DIRECTED SERVICES, RECOVERY, AND THE COMMON FACTORS

ROBERT T. BOHANSKE AND MICHAEL FRANCZAK

> Nobody can go back and start a new beginning, but anyone can start today and make a new ending.
>
> —Maria Robinson

Behavioral or mental health disorders rank first among the causes of disability in the United States and Western Europe. In the United Kingdom, for example, 38% of individuals receiving disability benefits have a mental health diagnosis, nearly twice the next highest reason for receipt of government subsidy (i.e., unemployment; Layard, 2006). Disability rates in the United States have soared. In 2003, there were nearly 6 million people who were either disabled by mental illness (Social Security Disability statistics) or diagnosed as mentally ill (Social Security Income statistics), a disability rate of about 20 people per 100,000 population, nearly 6 times what it was in 1955 (Whitaker, 2005).

According to a Substance Abuse Mental Health Services Administration report, $104 billion goes each year to mental health and substance abuse treatment services (Mark et al., 2005). It is surprising that more public funds are spent on behavioral than physical health care (57% vs. 46%; President's New Freedom Commission on Mental Health [PNFCMH], 2003). Despite the staggering costs, the very system set up to help those in need is seriously fragmented, in disarray, and in need of major reform.

This is, in point of fact, the conclusion reached by the PNFCMH Interim Report: "America's mental health service delivery system is in shambles [and] . . . incapable of efficiently delivering . . . effective treatments," said Chairperson Michael F. Hogan. "There are so many programs operating under such different rules that it is often impossible for families and consumers to find the care that they urgently need" (PNFCMH, 2002, p. ii). The commission also determined that mental health delivery systems are not oriented to the single most important goal of the people they serve: the hope of recovery.

Public behavioral health care (PBH) is a singular example of the problems identified by the PNFCMH. To be sure, the troubles are not of recent origin. Nineteen years ago, Ann Johnson, author of *Out of Bedlam: The Truth about Deinstitutionalization*, decried the deplorable state of PBH. On the basis of her own experience and examination of state and national surveys dating back to 1978, she described a well-established pattern of short-term solutions, piecemeal and after-the-fact programming, and inadequate organizational oversight. "Mental health funding," she wrote, "is a product of politics, expediency, and fads" (Johnson, 1990, p. 219). She went on to say, "The mental health system is not coherent, nor is it highly suggestive of mental health" (p. 234).

Since Johnson made her indictment, many attempts have been made to fix the system. More often than not, however, PBH has been crippled by the very procedures instituted for improving care. Here is an illustration. On arrival to a clinic or facility, would-be clients are confronted with a series of forms, consents, and policies. In the State of Arizona, for example, a minimum of 44 forms are required for enrolling a person in care and initiating treatment. Further, managed care companies are frequently retained to handle the distribution of public funds and ensure accountability. Add more forms. Then, each agency has its own policies and procedures necessitated by national regulatory and accrediting bodies (e.g., NCQA, COA, JCAHO, CARF). Add still more paperwork. Every group has its own forms that often contain the same information but are rarely if ever integrated into a single, streamlined record.

The complicated and time-consuming authorization process was graphically illustrated in a recent meeting of the Arizona Department of Health, Division of Behavioral Health Services, Best Practices Committee (2007). The forms needed to obtain a marriage certificate, buy a new home, lease an automobile, apply for a passport, open a bank account, and die of natural causes were assembled. Altogether, the various documents weighed 1.4 ounces. By contrast, the paperwork required for enrolling a single mother in counseling to talk about difficulties her child was experiencing at school came in at 1.25 pounds. In short, as the sheer weight and volume of paperwork attest, the delivery of behavioral health services is regulated from more levels than clinicians or consumers could ever anticipate or imagine. That consumers are served at all seems almost a sidebar, an unintended outcome, to the prerogatives of the various players.

If that were not enough, in the past decade *fiscal consciousness, treatment accountability, outcomes,* and *empirically supported therapies* have emerged as the latest bywords of PBH. Regarding the latter, the rush to adopt, if not restrict service provision, to evidence-based treatments has added new layers of management, policies, and procedures. Regulatory bodies and funding entities are demanding proof of compliance to mandated protocols. Along the way, therapeutic choice and consumer freedom have been pushed to the back seat.

A clear expression and immediate repercussion of the frustrations and inefficiencies encountered by consumers navigating the PBH system is seen in the number who discontinue service. Although studies vary in both the definition and prevalence, available evidence indicates that 20% to 57% of consumers fail to return following the first visit (Pekarik, 1985). Wierzbicki and Pekarik (1993), in a meta-analysis of 125 studies, reported a mean dropout rate of nearly 47%. Furthermore, between 30% and 50% of those in need of services fail to make it to their first visit (Arizona Department of Health, Division of Behavioral Health Services, 2007; Issakidis & Andrews, 2004). These troubling statistics perhaps make sense from a consumer's point of view: They want treatments that work for them and not to "get the treatment" from the very people to whom they turn for help. Indeed, in this context, dropping out could be viewed as healthy, even self-affirming, a refusal to put up with service that is both unresponsive and insensitive.

Clearly, the time has come for new thinking. Picking up on the centrality of the client to treatment success advanced in chapter 3 of this volume and the boon to outcome brought about by client feedback highlighted in chapter 8, we argue in this chapter that providing consumer-directed, outcome-informed services is PBH's greatest hope for transformation. We assert that finding out what consumers want and what works in their unique situations offers a better formula for change than more regulations, additional process measures, or the imposition of the latest fads or prescriptive treatments. The chapter begins with an examination of the call for transformation outlined by the PNFCMH and related bodies. Rounding out the historical backdrop of PBH change, the emergence of the recovery movement and its fundamental components, as developed in a national consensus statement, are reviewed. With that context set, this chapter describes how transformation was achieved in two behavioral health agencies in Arizona and presents the advantages in both effectiveness and efficiency attained. Finally, the implications for transformation on a larger scale are offered.

## THE CALL FOR TRANSFORMATION

At the beginning of this decade, three major collaborative efforts aimed at reforming the behavioral health care system were undertaken. All three published similar findings. In 2000, the Annapolis Coalition on the Behavioral

Health Workforce, an interdisciplinary group sponsored by the American College of Mental Health Administration and Academic Behavioral Health Consortium, was formed to address concerns about the quality of education and training of behavioral health providers. The group made extensive recommendations in their 2007 report titled "An Action Plan for Behavioral Health Workforce Development."

In 2005, the Campaign for Mental Health Reform (CMHR), a group of 16 national health organizations, released its report, "Roadmap for Federal Action on America's Mental Health Crisis." During the same time period, the PNFCMH was established and produced a number of reports identifying problems and making recommendations for improving mental health services (PNFCMH, 2002, 2003). The resulting documents contained far-reaching and comprehensive proposals for reforming mental health services. Among the most important were those bearing on (a) consumer-centered services, (b) recovery of real-life functioning versus the cure of illness, and (c) common curative factors in behavioral care.

## Consumer-Centered Services

The final report of the PNFCMH echoed the recommendations of both the Annapolis Coalition and the CMHR when it boldly asserted that transformation must begin by placing consumers "at the *center* of the system of care" (PNFCMH, 2003, p. 27). Too often, the report pointed out, service delivery is oriented toward the requirements of bureaucracies and stakeholders. In short, meeting administrative, process, and quality assurance measures and procedures takes precedence. Along the way, the consumers—their choices, opinions, and options—are lost. According to the PNFCMH, "achieving the promise," as the report was aptly titled, means

> a consumer- and family-driven system, [in which] consumers choose their own programs and the providers that will help them most. Their needs and preferences drive the policy and financing decisions that affect them. Care is consumer-centered, with providers working in full partnership with the consumers they serve to develop individualized plans of care. (p. 28)

Similar pronouncements from the various commissions indicate that consumers are being heard. Changes, however, have been slow in the making, often hamstrung by sheer inertia, or worse, political agendas to keep the system as it is. As a result, in the brief period between the PNFCMH's final report and CMHR's "Roadmap," the latter group issued an emergency response, asking Congress to "direct CMS [Centers for Medicare and Medicaid Services] to identify barriers to the application of consumer self-direction initiatives to people with mental illnesses and make recommendations for eliminating them" (CMHR, 2005, p. 16). In terms of time frames, the Annapolis Coalition on the Behavioral Health Workforce (2007) has suggested that it may take up to 10 years for the necessary changes to be implemented across all levels of service delivery.

## Recovery

"Successfully transforming the mental health service delivery system," the final PNFCMH report indicated, "rests on two principles" (PNFCMH, 2003, p. 4). The first principle, as discussed above, was the development of consumer-centered services. The second guiding principle for transformation was that the emphasis in care needed to shift away from treating illness and toward facilitating and supporting recovery. In a dramatic departure from tradition and precedent, the report concluded that the mental health system "must focus on increasing consumers' ability to successfully cope with life's challenges . . . and on building resilience, *not just on managing symptoms*" (PNFCMH, 2003, p. 5).

Historically, in the field of behavioral health, recovery was a term reserved for substance abuse treatment programs. Individuals in treatment or posttreatment phases were said to be in recovery. Similar uses of the term are found in 12-step programs, often referring to the avoidance or abstinence from some behavior or chemical. To provide both clarity and guidance, SAMHSA and the Interagency Committee on Disability Research, in partnership with six other federal agencies, convened the National Consensus Conference on Mental Health Recovery and Mental Health Systems Transformation in December 2004. With the participation of consumers, advocates, family members, providers, academicians, and researchers the *National Consensus Statement on Mental Health Recovery* (NCSMHR) was tendered:

> Mental health recovery is a journey of healing and transformation enabling a person with a mental health problem to live a meaningful life in a community of his or her choice while striving to achieve his or her full potential. (National Consensus Conference on Mental Health Recovery and Mental Health Systems Transformation, 2004a, p. 1).

A sharp departure from customary discourse on mental illness, the language of the consensus statement was decidedly upbeat and positive. For its part, the recovery movement challenges all providers, no matter the setting, to reject the practices of reductionism and objectification. It tells all that change does not come about by focusing on what is wrong with clients, but instead, on what is right about them. A recovery-driven service shifts away from professional-directed treatment based on diagnostic labels and prescriptive treatments to individually tailored, consumer-authored plans. Together with consumer-directed services, the radical shift away from illness toward recovery means that mental health professionals must be both responsible and responsive to their customer base and directly involve clients in decision making.

## Common Factors

In addition to defining recovery, the NCSMHR identified the fundamental components of recovery. A natural fit with the idea of attaining systematic client feedback about the fit and benefit of services (see chap. 8, this volume), the NCSMHR emphasized the importance of client involvement in service planning and delivery, as well as individualized services tailored to the consumer. It was as though the consensus statement was based on a review of the common factors literature. An inspection of Exhibit 10.1 reveals several statements that could have been lifted from this book. For example, the statement "Recovery focuses on valuing and building on the multiple capacities, resiliencies, talents, coping abilities, and inherent worth of individuals" (National Consensus Conference on Mental Health Recovery and Mental Health Systems Transformation, 2004a, p. 2) would have surely found a home in chapter 3 of this volume. Similarly, chapter 4 of this volume would likely embrace "The process of recovery moves forward through interaction with others in supportive, trust-based relationships. . . . Respect ensures the inclusion and full participation of consumers in all aspects of their lives" (National Consensus Conference on Mental Health Recovery and Mental Health Systems Transformation, 2004a, p. 2). And finally, this statement, "Recovery provides the essential and motivating message of a better future—that people can and do overcome the barriers and obstacles that confront them. . . . Hope is the catalyst of the recovery process," sounds like an excerpt torn from Frank's concept of remoralization (see chap. 5, this volume). In short, the NCSMHR is calling for services based on the common factors: services that recognize clients as the primary movers of change, that require the unique tailoring of intervention to their preferences, and that call for relationships that are collaborative and respectful.

The NCSMHR makes good empirical sense. Multiple studies in every aspect of PBH care, from dropouts to medication adherence, demonstrate that the alliance and client preferences are major factors in the outcome that clients achieve (Barber, Connolly, Crits-Christoph, Gladis, & Siqueland, 2000). More than 20 years ago, for example, Pekarik (1985) found that high dropout rates were attributable, in large part, to incompatibility between therapist treatment approaches and client preferences. Dropouts could be curtailed significantly, the study indicated, by delivering a treatment more in sync with the desires of those being served. Similar findings were reported by Baekeland and Lundwall (1975), who identified three major factors responsible for attrition from therapy: the client's favorable or unfavorable orientation to the

EXHIBIT 10.1
National Consensus Statement on Mental Health Recovery:
The 10 Fundamental Components

**Self-Direction:** Consumers lead, control, exercise choice over, and determine their own path of recovery by optimizing autonomy, independence, and control of resources to achieve a self-determined life. By definition, the recovery process must be self-directed by the individual, who defines his or her own life goals and designs a unique path towards those goals.

**Individualized and Person Centered:** There are multiple pathways to recovery based on an individual's unique strengths and resiliencies as well as his or her needs, preferences, experiences (including past trauma), and cultural background in all of its diverse representations. Individuals also identify recovery as being an ongoing journey and an end result as well as an overall paradigm for achieving wellness and optimal mental health.

**Empowerment:** Consumers have the authority to choose from a range of options and to participate in all decisions—including the allocation of resources—that will affect their lives, and are educated and supported in so doing. They have the ability to join with other consumers to collectively and effectively speak for themselves about their needs, wants, desires, and aspirations. Through empowerment, an individual gains control of his or her own destiny and influences the organizational and societal structures in his or her life.

**Holistic:** Recovery encompasses an individual's whole life, including mind, body, spirit, and community. Recovery embraces all aspects of life, including housing, employment, education, mental health and healthcare treatment and services, complementary and naturalistic services, addictions treatment, spirituality, creativity, social networks, community participation, and family supports as determined by the person. Families, providers, organizations, systems, communities, and society play crucial roles in creating and maintaining meaningful opportunities for consumer access to these supports.

**Non-Linear:** Recovery is not a step-by-step process but one based on continual growth, occasional setbacks, and learning from experience. Recovery begins with an initial stage of awareness in which a person recognizes that positive change is possible. This awareness enables the consumer to move on to fully engage in the work of recovery.

**Strengths-Based:** Recovery focuses on valuing and building on the multiple capacities, resiliencies, talents, coping abilities, and inherent worth of individuals. By building on these strengths, consumers leave stymied life roles behind and engage in new life roles (e.g., partner, caregiver, friend, student, employee). The process of recovery moves forward through interaction with others in supportive, trust-based relationships.

**Peer Support:** Mutual support—including the sharing of experiential knowledge and skills and social learning—plays an invaluable role in recovery. Consumers encourage and engage other consumers in recovery and provide each other with a sense of belonging, supportive relationships, valued roles, and community.

**Respect:** Community, systems, and societal acceptance and appreciation of consumers —including protecting their rights and eliminating discrimination and stigma—are crucial in achieving recovery. Self-acceptance and regaining belief in one's self are particularly vital. Respect ensures the inclusion and full participation of consumers in all aspects of their lives.

**Responsibility:** Consumers have a personal responsibility for their own self-care and journeys of recovery. Taking steps towards their goals may require great courage. Consumers must strive to understand and give meaning to their experiences and identify coping strategies and healing processes to promote their own wellness.

*(continues)*

---

**Hope:** Recovery provides the essential and motivating message of a better future—that people can and do overcome the barriers and obstacles that confront them. Hope is internalized; but can be fostered by peers, families, friends, providers, and others. Hope is the catalyst of the recovery process. Mental health recovery not only benefits individuals with mental health disabilities by focusing on their abilities to live, work, learn, and fully participate in our society, but also enriches the texture of American community life. America reaps the benefits of the contributions individuals with mental disabilities can make, ultimately becoming a stronger and healthier nation.

---

*Note.* From National Consensus Conference on Mental Health Recovery and Mental Health Systems Transformation (2004b).

treatment setting and therapist; the therapist's personality, attitude toward clients, and therapy style; and environmental factors. More recently, Osterberg and Blaschke (2005) confirmed and extended the findings to the arena of medication, noting that noncompliance was largely attributable to the consumer's lack of belief in the benefit of the treatment and a poor provider–patient relationship. Like others before them, these researchers found that honoring client treatment preferences and goals clearly impacted clinical adherence, involvement, and outcome.

## Summary

Public behavioral health is gearing up for transformation. All involved agree change is necessary. The makings for a more effective and humane system of care have been identified. The overwhelming consensus is that consumers, with their attendant hopes, expectations, strengths, and resources, in combination with a positive therapeutic alliance, account for the largest share of outcome in recovery. To succeed, such factors must be courted and the focus of care shifted away from managing illness and toward facilitating recovery.

What remains to be stated is that no list of consensus statements, first-step action agendas, or mental health campaigns, no matter how commendable, will lead to system transformation. Moreover, as is the case with any broad and comprehensive initiative, there is a significant risk of adopting yet another model of service that fails to deliver service to the individual. In other words, consumer-driven, recovery-oriented services can become as dictatorial and heavy-handed as the paradigm they are designed to replace: a Procrustean bed into which all consumers are forced regardless of fit.

The key to ensuring that PBH avoids the mistakes of the past and remains responsive to the individual is to have a fail-safe mechanism in place that assures the consumer's voice is not lost. As chapter 8 of this volume demonstrates, research and experience to date indicate that the means are already available. At every opportunity, from clients' first session to their last and from the identification of their strengths to the development and execution of the service delivery plan, the clinical interaction can be monitored to assure both a good fit and measurable progress. As reviewed in chapter 8, available empirical evidence shows dramatic improvements in both retention and outcome when consumer feedback is sought and then used to structure and refine behavioral health services. In sum, the field has, like no other time in history, both the will and means for successful transformation.

## IMPROVED EFFICIENCY AND OUTCOMES: IMPLEMENTING CLIENT-DIRECTED, OUTCOME-INFORMED CARE IN PUBLIC BEHAVIORAL HEALTH

Southwest Behavioral Health Services (SBHS) and Marc Center (MC) are large, nonprofit, multidisciplinary community behavioral health organizations providing services to people living in the Phoenix metropolitan area, rural western Maricopa County, and Northern Gila County in the State of Arizona. Both agencies employ more than 500 direct care staff. SBHS has an annual budget of $36 million. In a typical year, SBHS provides clinical services to a diverse group of clients through a wide variety of programs, including psychotherapy, prevention, and homeless outreach. MC serves both behavioral health and developmentally disabled populations with a $23 million annual budget. MC is a leader in community-based employment and residential (community living) and in-home services. Despite rapid growth and perennial shortages in funding, SBHS has always labored to accomplish the company's core purpose; their mission statement reads in part: "We *inspire* people to *feel better* and reach their *potential*" (SBHS, 2007).

Like every other PBH agency in the country, SBHS was under the gun to adopt and implement various *best practices*, specific treatments widely believed to result in better outcomes for specific disorders. Administration and staff were doing their absolute level best to meet the latest unfunded mandates issued by various governmental and accrediting bodies. However, rising levels of paperwork, oversight, and process control procedures combined to increase workload, decrease clinical flexibility, and undermine responsiveness to the client base. Rather than simply surrender to these external pressures, another path was taken: The codirector of the Institute for the Study of Therapeutic Change, Scott D. Miller, was invited to SBHS in 2003 to speak about client-directed, outcome-informed (CDOI) work, a way of thinking and practicing that seemed to fit the emerging consumer–recovery zeitgeist. Duncan and Sparks (2007) stated that CDOI

> contains no fixed techniques and no causal theory regarding the concerns that bring people to therapy or substance abuse treatment. Any interaction with a client can be client-directed and outcome-informed when the consumer's voice is privileged, recovery is expected, and helpers purposefully form strong partnerships with clients: (1) to enhance the factors across theories that account for successful outcome; (2) to use the client's ideas and preferences (theory of change) to guide choice of technique and model; and (3) to inform the work with reliable and valid measures of the consumer's experience of the alliance and outcome. (p. 14)

The 2-day training conducted by Miller stimulated several staff to attend the second Heart and Soul of Change conference held in Austin, Texas, in May 2004. This biennial conference, dedicated to translating the latest empirical evidence about the common factors and feedback into everyday clinical practice, featured many contributors to this volume, including editors Barry L. Duncan, Scott D. Miller, and Bruce E. Wampold. Consistent with the recommendations of the PNFCMH, the philosophy and related practices explicated at the conference placed consumers and their recovery at the very heart of service delivery. Accountability, too, was built in to the process. Simple and valid measures of progress and engagement were offered that replaced time-consuming and irrelevant paperwork. In addition, the conference provided a practical guide for implementation of the ideas called *Heroic Clients, Heroic Agencies: Partners for Change* (Duncan & Sparks, 2002).

The SBHS team was particularly impressed with data presented by David Claud (Claud et al., 2004), the director of a community behavioral health program in Palm Beach County, Florida. Like SBHS, the staff at the Center for Family Services (CFS) struggled to cope with limited resources, seemingly endless requests for services, competing demands from various stakeholders, lengthy episodes of care, and high no-show and attrition rates. After implementing the principles and practices taught at the conference, CFS not only achieved a dramatic turnaround in clinical outcomes but also solved many of the problems that cripple PBH agencies nationwide. For example, average length of stay decreased more than 40%. Cancellation and no-show rates dropped by 40% and 25%, respectively. Most impressive of all, the percentage of clients in long-term treatment that experienced little or no measured improvement fell by 80%! In 1 year, CFS saved nearly $500,000, funds that were used to hire additional staff and provide more services.

Hard to ignore and bordering on impossible to believe, here was a way of working that appeared to give everyone everything they wanted. When a change, such as demonstrated in Florida, can result in nearly a half million dollar in savings, services expanded, waiting lists reduced, and contract pro-ductivity increased, even the most rigid administrator cannot help take notice. Simply put, those served are better off, sooner.

Despite the obvious benefits, Claud et al. (2004) reported that such a transformation was not without challenges. For all the legitimate complaints raised by therapists about paperwork, oversight and accountability procedures, administrators are not in a position to ignore or dismiss the "imperial whims" of the stakeholders—the people who pay the bills. The paperwork burden remained. For all of the talk about client "voice and choice," the process of put-ting clients in charge requires a revision of therapists' professional identity, the extent of which cannot be fully appreciated beforehand. To illustrate, clinicians in one program at CFS strenuously objected to the idea of being "graded" by their clients. Others challenged the validity of ratings given by people compro-mised by psychopathology. Still others cited the potentially detrimental con-sequences of expecting clients who may be fragile or damaged to guide their own care. And finally, clients, accustomed to agency-centric services, were rightly suspicious about promises of the new and improved brand of care. Nevertheless, CFS and their consumers prevailed.

Mindful of the hard work ahead, the momentum of the conference car-ried the team back to Phoenix. Immediately on return, a clinic at the MC was selected as a site to conduct a pilot study. Services at this particular facility were directed toward the dually diagnosed, that is, people with both a diagnosis of severe mental illness and a substance abuse or dependence problem. No-show rates there ranged between 30% and 50%, with fewer than 16% attending all scheduled visits. Staff morale and productivity were poor.

Although all staff had been trained via intra-agency training in CDOI, few had managed to fully implement it in their day-to-day clinical work. Without the infrastructure to support change, it is unlikely to happen. Con-sequently, work was begun to transform the agency's culture from top to bot-tom. Paperwork, staff meetings, clinical language, and the intake process were targeted for change. A language focused on wellness and strength replaced the traditional deficit- and illness-based lexicon. Formal consumer feedback regarding progress and the quality of the therapeutic alliance was integrated into every staff meeting and all clinical documentation. In short, one could not escape the consumer's experience of their service.

Change was afoot. Yet, the system still was organized to fulfill adminis-trative needs and prerogatives. For instance, to meet mandated requirements regarding accessibility of care, an elaborate intake system had been estab-lished in which intake specialists first met with clients to tender a diagnosis, establish medical necessity, and then determine the level of care. Eliminat-ing this middleman, while simultaneously adhering to compulsory rules and regulations, was no small feat. Ultimately, the system was abolished. Clinical staff and clients were matched at intake and services initiated at the first interview.

By the end of the first month of the pilot, the number of clients attending all scheduled visits had increased from 16% to 63%. Four months later, 92% of clients entering service after the pilot started were attending all scheduled appointments ($n = 140$). Meanwhile, perfect attendance rates for those in services prior to the formal initiation of the pilot had increased to 70% ($n = 367$). In fact, the lower attrition rates were now a source of frustration. Staff reported no longer having the free time they once had for completing nonclinical-related tasks (Bohanske & Franczak, 2007).

Such favorable results led to an expansion of the pilot project. Two additional SBHS clinics—one urban and one rural—were chosen to participate. The administration was anxious to see the effects of the changes on staff productivity. Two additional sites, providing services as usual, were selected for comparison. At the outset, productivity rates were the same at all four sites, an abysmal 30% to 40% of expected therapeutic encounters. For the preceding 2 years, this rate had not fluctuated more than 10% in either direction. Many consider these rates typical for the population being served in public behavioral health agencies.

Within 4 months, productivity rates rose dramatically, in one clinic nearly doubling. It is important to note that the increase was achieved with no change in the population being served, the types of treatments offered, or the clinical staff providing services. What is more, a notable side effect was observed among prescribers not directly involved in either the training or use of the new approach. Within this group, productivity rates soared 33% at the same time no-shows dropped by more than 70%. All this was taking place in the context of improved client outcomes and shorter lengths of stay. With regard to the latter, the average time spent in in-home services declined by 150 days and 90 days in traditional outpatient care (Bohanske & Franczak, 2007).

With the full implementation of CDOI clinical services, comparisons were made between formalized feedback (CDOI) and traditional behavioral health services. A review of data over the first 18-month implementation period, involving over 1,500 clients, resulted in dramatic increases in client-reported successful completion of treatment, up over 20%. Concurrently, length of stay was reduced by 3 months while reducing clinician caseloads substantially. The conclusion was inescapable: The principles and practices were having an impact on the broader organizational culture.

During this time, other agencies reported similar positive results. For instance, Community Health and Counseling Services in Bangor, Maine experienced dramatic increases in the effectiveness and efficiency of services provided to clients traditionally characterized as "severely and persistently mentally ill." Over a 3-year period, no-show and cancellation rates were reduced by 30%, and the average length of stay decreased by 59% (see Table 10.1). At the same time, the need for long-term, ongoing support in the form of either residential treatment or case management dropped by 50% and 72%, respectively—all this while consumer satisfaction with services markedly improved (Bohanski, Plum, Albert, & Haynes, 2006).

Striking results, too, were achieved at the Center for Alcohol and Drug Treatment (CADT) in Duluth, Minnesota. In brief, this facility, the third largest of its kind in the state, provides services to more than 6,000 new clients per year in a variety of programs including medical detox, intensive outpatient, residential, inpatient, prison-based, and free-standing halfway houses. Akin to SBHS, the CADT was plagued by a high dropout rate (>50%), declining reimbursement rates, and ever-changing regulatory and documentation requirements. Between 2002 and 2006, the center significantly improved retention and success rates, streamlined service delivery, reduced paperwork, and increased revenue and cash flow. When compared with similar agencies in Minnesota, program completion rates were on average 15% higher at CADT, and lengths of stay for inpatient and intensive outpatient were 20% and 43% lower. With the significant reduction in lengths of stay, costs concomitantly decreased for both by 36% (see Table 10.2). Meanwhile, outcomes have steadily improved, currently matching the level seen in carefully controlled randomized clinical trials.

Today, approximately 5 years into the transformation process, all services provided by SBHS and the MC are guided by CDOI. The systemwide change required continuous dedication from both administration and staff. Beyond the demands inherent in learning and implementing any new approach, constant vigilance was required to resist returning to the dominant deficit-based paradigm. If that were not enough, it proved necessary to take steps to preserve the dynamism central to the success of this way of working. Circumventing mere compliance, given the diverse settings, services, and providers involved was no small task. Organizations, by their very nature, must have structure to survive. However, such structures routinely morph

TABLE 10.1
Average Length of Stay, in Years, for Treatment Programs
at Community Health and Counseling Services

| Program | Pretransformation | Posttransformation | Length of stay reduction (%) |
|---|---|---|---|
| Case management | 2.50 | 0.7 | 72 |
| Outpatient therapy | 1.45 | .6 | 59 |
| Residential treatment | 1.90 | 1.0 | 47 |

TABLE 10.2

Comparison of Average Length of Stay (LOS), in Days, at Center for Alcohol and Drug Treatment (CADT) and the State of Minnesota in 2006

| Program | CADT | State of Minnesota | LOS difference (%) | Cost savings |
|---|---|---|---|---|
| Inpatient | 20 | 25 | 20 | $3,094 |
| Outpatient therapy | 28 | 16 | 43 | $896 |

into the most expedient methods to meet contractual obligations. Finally, the changes at SBHS did not take place in a vacuum. While the revolution in service delivery was in motion, the organization was forced to simultaneously attend to new policies, procedures, and program requirements imposed by stakeholders. Competition for staff time and energy was keen. In the end, considerable effort was expended keeping the eye on the prize.

## Critical Steps

Looking back, it is possible to identify a series of steps critical to success experienced at SBHS and MC. Although it is far from a paint-by-numbers prescription for organizational change, they do distill our experience born out of a series of right moves, false starts, and lucky breaks. The same basic template, proposed by Miller, Mee-Lee, Plum, and Hubble (2005) and Duncan and Sparks (2007), is being used in numerous sites around the globe. In order, the steps include the following.

### Secure the Cooperation and Commitment of Agency Administrators

Staff members at PBH agencies are accustomed to constant changes in policy and procedure. Over time, many learn to cope by hunkering down and waiting out the latest edict dictated by management. Circumventing the self-protective skepticism of the staff is critical. They must be convinced that the call for transformation is sincere and will actually take place. To borrow an analogy from sports, agency administrators must be more than team owners; they must leave their glass booth at the top of the stadium and get down on the field. They have to then listen to the players and coach play by play. Mixing metaphors, organizational change is best viewed as a marathon, not a sprint. And no agency to date has achieved the organizational changes described in this chapter in less than 3 years. In the case of SBHS and MC, what tipped the balance for administration were the favorable results from other agencies and our own pilot projects.

## Start Small

Think evolution not revolution. PBH agencies are among the most regulated and controlled entities in health care. They are beholden to numerous stakeholders and regulatory bodies. Wholesale changes in programs, policies, and procedures are, consequently, likely to provoke resistance from top to bottom. With that in mind, would-be change agents are advised to think small and go slow. For example, start by piloting the approach in one setting. Then, use the findings to secure ongoing commitment from administration and address the inevitable conflicts between the approach and existing policy and procedure.

## Create a Transition Oversight Group

It is not uncommon for conflict to arise between administration and line staff whenever change is contemplated and undertaken. Each holds the other responsible for ensuring successful implementation. The result is often a stalemate. Staff, feeling that they are already doing all they can, look to administration for relief. The administration, responding to the whims of payers and regulators, wants staff to comply. Preventing such standoffs and facilitating continued forward movements is the purpose of the transition oversight group (TOG).

Briefly, the TOG is a small group made up of several line staff, at least one administrator, supervisors from programs outside the pilot, and anyone else with an investment or shared interest in the outcome of the transformation project (e.g., payers, regulators, local politicians). This body has two principle duties. First, ensure the success of the pilot. Second, use ongoing results to plan for future implementation across the entire organization.

One way to ensure the success of the pilot is to maintain a constant flow of information between clinicians and the TOG. It is at this stage that conflicts between the new approach and existing treatment philosophy and practice should be identified and resolved. To illustrate, considerable time and forethought at SBHS went into streamlining the intake process and associated paperwork, a constant stress for clinicians and a barrier to consumer-directed services. The existing progress note was replaced with one focused on the client's experience of his or her improvement as well as his or her view of the clinical relationship, goals, and methods. In addition, intake forms were radically revised, changing from an emphasis on deficit and diagnosis to strength and recovery. The successful resolution of this and other issues encountered in the pilot project facilitated the introduction of the approach across the organization.

## Provide Ongoing Training, Consultation, and Supervision

The clinical staffs' initial exposure to the CDOI approach was through the typical training seminar format. This was followed and reinforced quickly by attendance at the Heart and Soul of Change Conference. At the conference, SBHS staff received the *Heroic Agencies* book, which provided a nuts and bolts workbook approach that speaks to all levels of behavioral health care staff within an organization.

Notwithstanding, as anyone who has attended a workshop knows, enthusiasm quickly dissipates and readily lapses into frustration if continued instruction and support are unavailable. For this reason, it is incumbent on the TOG to create a formal system of training to ensure success. Whereas at SBHS such a system allowed for occasional attendance at formal workshops or presentations, most energy and effort was directed toward making training a routine part of daily clinical activities. For instance, staff was helped in both supervision and case conferences to present information about clients consistent with the CDOI framework. Supervision is key. Supervision became outcome focused as supervisees were required to bring client graphs to supervision. As already discussed, paperwork was changed to reflect the client input regarding progress and treatment relationship. Finally, on the basis of the information gathered from the multiple pilot projects, the TOG prepared a series of training manuals and videos as a resource for existing staff as well as new hires.

*Systematize a Continuum of Care*

No one therapist, treatment program, or agency can be all things to all people. All too often, the fickle finger of responsibility points in one of two directions when the treatment offered fails. Traditionally, the client is blamed; they are unmotivated, resistant, or simply too sick. Of late, it has become fashionable to hold therapists responsible; they lack the training and skills necessary to be effective.

With regard to treatment failure, it bears mentioning that rates in randomized clinical trials approach 57% to 67% (Hansen, Lambert, and Foreman, 2002). That so many fall short in these kinds of studies is all the more compelling given the many advantages afforded to experimenters. In point of fact, randomized clinical trials are frequently stacked for success. Clinicians in PBH settings do not have the luxury, for example, of handpicking the people they will see. They must, by contrast, take all comers, many whose complicated lives and histories would be an immediate cause for exclusion in research settings.

Fixing blame on therapists or clients merely perpetuates more of the same. Clients deemed resistant continued with the same clinician or program despite a lack of progress. On the other hand, clinicians are sent to one continuing education event after another, though not a scintilla of evidence exists that such training improves outcome. Put bluntly, failure needs to be recognized for what it is: a common and normal part of service delivery. Knowing this in advance means that systems must have an organized and formal method in place for moving people within a system of care, whether to another therapist, treatment program, or even service outside of PBH (e.g., housing, medical, legal, spiritual). PBH must learn to fail successfully (Duncan, Miller, & Sparks, 2004).

At SBHS and MC, the traditional continuum of care has been replaced by a system of care expanded greatly by the use of peer supports. Instead of acting as junior counselors, this resourceful group works as partners to clients, using their own experience to help families and individuals stay on course and reach their goals. By using peers as change partners in the recovery process, as suggested by Duncan (2005), the authors of this chapter have been able to demonstrate both the effectiveness of peer support and the importance of individualized client direction on the recovery journey. To date, involvement of these recovery support specialists has resulted in attendance and improvement rates rivaling those of professional staff (Franczak & Bohanske, 2006).

*Prepare for Fallout*

The psychologist Sheldon Kopp (1972) once observed, "All solutions breed new problems" (p. 223). The CDOI transformation of PBH is no exception. Although it is impossible to anticipate all complications, the difficulties encountered at SBHS fell into three general categories: (a) maintaining momentum, (b) molding new relationships with stakeholders, and (c) managing ineffective clinicians and treatment programs.

Over time and facing relentless, competing demands, staff enthusiasm for any new approach naturally wanes. The vigilance required to sustain anything new naturally dwindles. It is at this point, approximately 1 year into the transformation, that many agencies lose their way. Then, the approach is in danger of being jettisoned or simply becoming another chore. The solution to this problem is leadership, generally one person who by force of personality and their tireless commitment inspires continued participation and sustained effort to eliminate barriers to implementation. Across implementations, no service setting has succeeded without such a leader. This was certainly the case at SBHS and MC, as it was for CFS, Community Health and Counseling Services, and CADT.

No doubt, organizing services around client preferences and progress will challenge conventional wisdom about how to provide treatment and disrupt business as usual. As a result, involving stakeholders in the transformation project is critical, as established relationships will need to be modified. Referrers, for example, accustomed to fixed lengths of stay, pathology-based assessments and characterizations, and circumscribed client roles, often take exception to programmatic changes. As to the latter, some mightily struggled with the practice of involving clients as full partners in all aspects of clinical decision making.

For the long term, considerable thought needs to be directed toward developing clear and consistent policies and procedures for managing ineffective programs and providers. The good news is that data gathered from other treatment settings show that feedback improves the outcome of most clinicians. To illustrate, at Resources for Living®, an international behavioral wellness organization, the percentage of counselors with below average outcomes dropped 80% in the 18 months that feedback was provided. At the same time, differences in outcome between clinicians decreased as overall effectiveness increased (see Figure 10.1). CFS experienced a similar effect on therapist performance. Unfortunately, feedback alone does not improve the outcome of all therapists or programs. In such instances, it is important to use the core principles of CDOI work. First, provide ongoing feedback regarding the therapist's or program's performance. Second, engage the clinician or program staff in problem solving when performance lags behind agency averages. Third, follow up. Where improvement is not forthcoming, be prepared to end the program or move staff to other settings or positions. In most cases, poorly performing clinicians have sought input on how or what to change, requested reassignment, or quit on their own.

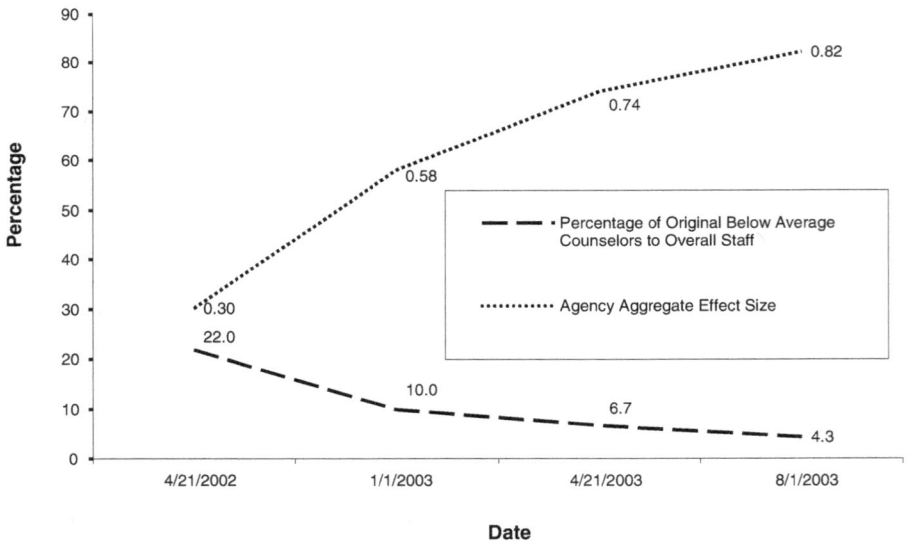

*Figure 10.1.* Effects of feedback on outcome of below average counselors.

# CONCLUSIONS

This chapter demonstrates the power of CDOI practices to transform PBH, to address the problems of mental and health and substance abuse service delivery, and to embrace the recommendations of the PNFCMH. However, there is of course no panacea. PBH remains PBH. Even though CDOI has been designated a best practice in the State of Arizona, the very nature of state government, with its constant change in personnel and political whims, threatens its continuation. At a recent meeting of the Best Practice Committee, for example, financial support for continuing transformation of the PBH system was slashed. Knowing the very real differences that this way of working makes in the lives of people empowered us to argue convincingly for reaffirming the state's commitment to CDOI and to seek alternative sources of funding. In short, this small setback resulted in renewed energy and direction. Such is the fabric of PBH.

Some of the implications of CDOI are as follows:

- CDOI principles and practices answer the call of the PNFCMH and align with the Substance Abuse and Mental Health Services Administration's fundamental components of recovery. In addition, establishing a system of formalized feedback meets the American Psychological Association Task Force on Evidence-Based Practice (2006) recommendations for monitoring client response to treatment.
- Transformation of behavioral health service delivery requires much more than attendance at a conference or training program. It is not a one shot in the arm process. It is a long-term commitment to change the environmental values of practice. Agencies must undergo a cultural shift to support transformation. Organizational change requires consistent leadership. Clinical change requires clinical leadership, vision, and commitment.
- Such a change must involve all aspects of service delivery from policy and procedure through administrative, support, and clinical staff commitment. New staff orientation, consumer referral and intake process, documentation, treatment planning, and case staffing must all value consumer voice and choice.
- Empowering the value of formalized feedback has the effect of making clinical documents (progress notes and treatment plans) living records rather than required paperwork used only for audits and accountability. A continued focus on feedback keeps the consumer central.

- Use of feedback increases in value when extended past the clinical session. Case staffing, case presentation, peer review, and clinical supervision are all enriched, and the feedback environment is reinforced when such activities and meetings are driven by the consumer's view of his or her progress.
- For systemic change (transformation) to take root, it must be nourished. Outcome data can be used to demonstrate program and clinician effectiveness and efficiency. Although process measures can and in many settings will still be required, increases in clinician productivity (through decreased no-show rates), decreases in the length of episodes of care, and increased consumer satisfaction lead to increased staff morale. The data also establish the proof of value of PBH services.

## QUESTIONS FROM THE EDITORS

1. *When the data in favor of CDOI are so compelling, what accounts for the continued fascination with empirically supported treatments?*

In short, it is the rush to answer complex questions with simple solutions. The longer answer lies in the need of our behavioral health system to model itself after the developments in the medical community. Evidence-based medicine has established a clear set of interventions for diagnostic conditions and established a standard of care we have come to expect from our health care providers. In behavioral health, the diagnostic schema we have adopted is much less clear and significantly less reliable, yet many have attempted to hold to the medical model. As such, evidence-based practice, like many worthy concepts, has been either misunderstood or corrupted by many state, federal, and managed care organizations, placing too much emphasis on the standardized practices side of the equation instead of the evidence or outcome side. It has become accepted that adherence to a model (fidelity) is a better measure (process) than the actual client outcome that should be based on the ongoing feedback from the client receiving treatment. Using the person's response to treatment as measured by such tools as the Outcome Rating Scale provides a valid and reliable measure of effectiveness and has the effect of enhancing the effects of any empirically supported treatments. Simply measuring adherence to evidence-based practices continues the long tradition of PBH systems misdirecting their attention to measuring processes rather than outcomes.

2. *Staff turnover is notoriously high in public behavioral health settings. What effects, if any, have been observed in turnover rates at SBHS and MC following transformation?*

The PBH system has traditionally experienced a high turnover in clinical staff. Reasons cited are high case loads, paperwork overload, and low compensation. The various state professional credentialing boards also require supervised experience in an agency setting (in many jurisdictions), resulting in early career clinicians. In Arizona, the agencies often experience a 20% to 40% annual turnover in clinical staff. Additionally, both SBHS and MC are partners in the Training Institute, a multilevel, multidisciplinary professional training program for pre- and postdoctoral psychology students, social workers, and professional counselors.

In the 2 years since CDOI was implemented at the MC, there has been no turnover in the outpatient clinic staff. The past year at SBHS saw a marked reduction in turnover in outpatient clinical staff from an unusual high of 60% to a current rate of 20%. Although the transformation of our services to an outcome-informed approach does little for the high paperwork demands and low compensation rates, there has been a marked decrease in case load. Clients involved in the project had shorter lengths of stay by an average of over 100 days in outpatient programs at SBHS. Clinicians report higher levels of satisfaction when noting client improvement and an increased sense of accomplishment. Prior to implementation, few cases were discharged in a mutual agreed on fashion. Following implementation there are few unilateral discharges. It is interesting that of those young clinicians who move on, most continue outcome-informed practices.

3. *Many PBH organizations serve a large number of people diagnosed as "seriously and persistently mentally ill." Has the client-directed approach improved the outcome of this population at SBHS and MC?*

The transformation of the PBH system into a more inclusive and recovery-oriented paradigm has resulted in an increased emphasis on consumer voice and choice in service planning and delivery. As there has been less focus on the medical (deficit) model (symptoms and function) and a greater focus on how consumers live, work, play, and dream, consumers' input and direction has increased in importance. At both SBHS and MC, clients both with and without serious mental illness (SMI) are served using the same approach. In many ways this is a distinction without a difference. A number of individuals without SMI are served who have poorer current functioning than clients with SMI. There has been no difference in the results obtained. Length of stay in various levels of support continues to decrease, and objectives are easier to define and more related to consumer hope and expectations.

4. *If a person picked up this chapter, was inspired by the results, and wanted to implement the program, what would they do?*

Each organization or agency has its own unique strengths and challenges. The variations in stakeholders, funding, and services provided (child or adolescent, substance abuse, family, couples) as well as the distance the agency has traveled in becoming recovery oriented all play a part. In brief, we recommend planning for a 2- to 3-year transition period. Change can be slow, and the adoption of a clinical culture change requires a good deal of commitment at every level of the organization. The early adopters in the clinical staff can and will demonstrate the advantages of formalized feedback with decreases in no-show rates as well as decreases in length of stay. Yet giving consumers a directive voice and choice in their own care can be a threatening idea. The organizations' administration must be willing to support the change in culture and allow the adaptation of policies and procedures that allow for supervision and peer review as well as quality assurance programs to use the new approach. Support staff should be oriented to value consumer feedback and choices in every contact from initial call to scheduling or referral. Service (treatment) plans and progress notes can be modified to a consumer-directed format. Perhaps most important, all agency staff must be willing to allow the feedback to inform the operation of the services provided. Allowing the consumers goals to trump the programs goals can be a struggle for some. For a more complete explanation and supportive resource, we recommend the book *Heroic Clients, Heroic Agencies: Partners for Change* (Duncan & Sparks, 2002). A revised edition is available on the Heart & Soul of Change Project Web site (http://www.heartandsoulofchange.com).

## REFERENCES

American Psychological Association Presidential Task Force on Evidence-Based Practice. (2006). Evidence-based practice in psychology. *American Psychologist, 61*, 271–285.

The Annapolis Coalition on the Behavioral Health Workforce. (2007). *An action plan on behavioral health workforce development*. Retrieved May 13, 2008, from http://www.annapoliscoalition.org/files/Strategic_Planning/WorkforceAction Plan.pdf

Arizona Department of Health, Division of Behavioral Health Services. (2007, June). *Best Practice Committee meeting minutes*. Phoenix, AZ.

Baekeland, F., & Lundwall, L. (1975). Dropping out of treatment: A critical review. *Psychological Bulletin, 82*, 738–783.

Barber, J. P., Connolly M. B., Crits-Christoph, P., Gladis, L., & Siqueland, L. (2000). Alliance predicts patients' outcome beyond in-treatment changes in symptoms. *Journal of Consulting and Clinical Psychology, 68*, 1027–1032.

Barzun, J. (1959). *The house of intellect*. New York: Harper & Row.

Bohanske, R. T., Plum, W., Albert, P. & Haynes, M. (2006, June). *Changing the face of mental health and substance abuse services*. Panel presentation at the Heart and Soul of Change 3 International Conference, Bar Harbor, ME.

Bohanske, R. T., & Franczak M. (2007, June). *Improving engagement and achieving better outcomes using the client directed outcome informed clinical approach*. Paper presented at the United States Psychiatric Rehabilitation Association Annual Training Conference, Orlando, FL.

The Campaign for Mental Health Reform. (2005). *Emergency response: A roadmap for federal action on America's mental health crisis.* Retrieved May 14, 2008, from http://www.mhreform.org/Portals/0/1.3_EmergencyResponseExecutive Summary.pdf

Claud, D., Duncan, B., Kinchen, K., Miller, S., Sparks, J., & Walt, J. (2004, June). Giving clients the voice they deserve: The heroic agency/ISTC movement. Panel presentation at the Heart and Soul of Change 2 International Conference, Austin, TX.

Duncan, B. (2005). *What's right with you: Debunking dysfunction and changing your life.* Deerfield Beach, FL: Health Communications.

Duncan, B., Miller, S., & Sparks, J. (2004). *The heroic client: A revolutionary way to improve effectiveness via client directed outcome informed therapy.* San Francisco: Jossey Bass.

Duncan, B. & Sparks, J. (2002). *Heroic clients, heroic agencies: Partners for change.* Fort Lauderdale, FL: Author.

Duncan, B. & Sparks, J. (2007). *Heroic clients, heroic agencies: Partners for change* [Electronic version]. Fort Lauderdale, FL: Author. Available at http://www. heartandsoulofchange.com

Franczak, M., & Bohanske, R.T. (2006, March). *An analysis of retention and treatment outcomes from peer support services using a client-directed outcome-informed treatment approach.* Paper presented at the National State of the Knowledge Conference on Psychiatric Disabilities, University of Pennsylvania Medical School, Philadelphia, PA.

Hansen, N. B., Lambert, M. J., & Forman, E. V. (2002). The psychotherapy dose–response effect and its implications for treatment delivery services. *Clinical Psychology: Science and Practice, 9,* 329–343.

Issakidis, C., & Andrews G. (2004) Pretreatment attrition and dropout in an outpatient clinic for anxiety disorders. *Acta Psychiatrica Scandinavica, 109,* 426–433.

Johnson, A. B. (1990). *Out of bedlam: The truth about deinstitutionalization.* New York: Basic Books.

Kopp, S. (1972). *If you meet the Buddha on the road, kill him!* Palo Alto, CA: Science & Behavior Books.

Layard, R. (2006). *Mental health: Britain's biggest social problem: The case for psychological treatment centres* (RL447; 2nd ed.). Retrieved March 24, 2008, from http://cep. lse.ac.uk/textonly/research/mentalhealth/RL447_version2.pdf

Miller, S. D., Mee-Lee, D., Plum, B., & Hubble, M. (2005). Making treatment count: Client-directed, outcome-informed clinical work with problem drinkers. In J. Lebow (Ed.), *Handbook of clinical family therapy* (pp. 281–308). New York: Wiley.

Mark, T. L., Coffey, R. M., McKusick, D. R., Harwood, H., King, E., Bouchery, E., et al. (2005). *National estimates of expenditures for mental health services and substance abuse* treatment, *1991–2001* (SAMHSA Publication No. SMA 05-3999). Rockville, MD: U.S. Government Printing Office.

National Consensus Conference on Mental Health Recovery and Mental Health Systems Transformation. (2004a). *National consensus statement on mental health recovery.* Retrieved September 22, 2007, from http://mentalhealth.samhsa.gov/publications/allpubs/sma05-4129/

National Consensus Conference on Mental Health Recovery and Mental Health Systems Transformation. (2004b). *The ten fundamental components.* Retrieved September 22, 2007, from http://mentalhealth.samhsa.gov/publications/allpubs/sma05-4129/

President's New Freedom Commission on Mental Health. (2002). *Interim report* (DHHS Pub. No. SMA-03-3932). Retrieved September 21, 2007, from http://www.mentalhealthcommission.gov/reports/interim_toc.htm

President's New Freedom Commission on Mental Health. (2003). *Achieving the promise: Transforming mental health care in America. Final report* (DHHS Pub. No. SMA-03-3832). Retrieved September 21, 2007, from http://www.mental healthcommission.gov/reports/FinalReport/toc.html

Osterberg, L., & Blaschke, T. (2005) Adherence to medication. *New England Journal of Medicine, 353,* 487–497.

Pekarik, G. (1985). Coping with dropouts. *Professional Psychology Research and Practice, 16*(1), 114–123.

Southwest Behavioral Health Services. (2007). *Who we are.* Retrieved July 2, 2009, from http://www.sbhservices.org/index.php?page=who_we_are

Whitaker, R. (2005). Anatomy of an epidemic: Psychiatric drugs and the astonishing rise of mental illness in America. *Ethical Human Psychology and Psychiatry, 7*(1), 12–34.

Wierzbicki, M., & Pekarik, G. (1993). A meta-analysis of psychotherapy dropout. *Professional Psychology Research and Practice, 24*(2), 190–195.

# III

# SPECIAL POPULATIONS

# 11

# EVIDENCE-BASED TREATMENTS AND COMMON FACTORS IN YOUTH PSYCHOTHERAPY

SUSAN DOUGLAS KELLEY, LEONARD BICKMAN,
AND EARTA NORWOOD

Improving personal and organizational performance without constant feedback is like trying to pin the tail on the donkey when we're blindfolded. Only through knowing where we are, can we change where we are going.
—Jim Clemmer, *Don't Wait to See the Blood*

*Evidence-based treatment* (EBT) is not just a fashionable phrase to describe empirically supported approaches for specific childhood disorders; it is fast becoming a practice mandate by market forces and a centerpiece of policy recommendations (Bickman, 2005; Kazdin & Whitley, 2006). At the same time, EBT has spurred some of the most spirited debates in the history of mental health (Norcross, Beutler, & Levant, 2006). For example, EBT proponents argue "for compelling evidence that some techniques are clearly the treatment of choice for the various problems that children and adolescents bring to treatment" (Kazdin, 2004, p. 580). Contrast that with Miller, Wampold, and Varhely's (2008) conclusion that "current attempts aimed at identifying and codifying a list of 'best practices' for the treatment of children and adolescents can at best viewed as premature and at worst misleading" (p. 12). It is no wonder that many mental health professionals are seeking guidance on whether and how to incorporate EBTs into practice.

The preparation of this article was partially supported by National Institute of Mental Health Grant MH068589-01 and the Lowenstein Foundation. Susan Douglas Kelley and Leonard Bickman report that they and Vanderbilt University have a financial interest in the computerized version of Contextualized Feedback Intervention and Training (CFIT).

In 2006, the American Psychological Association (APA) Presidential Task Force on Evidence-Based Practice (APA Task Force, 2006) proposed a different way of viewing the evidence, more comprehensive than the narrower EBT or empirically supported treatment (EST) approach. Calling this approach *evidence-based practice in psychology* (EBPP), the APA Task Force stated,

> ESTs start with a treatment and ask whether it works for a certain disorder or problem under specified circumstances. EBPP starts with the patient and asks what research evidence . . . will assist the psychologist in achieving the best outcome. (APA Task Force, 2006, p. 273)

The policy statement on EBPP clearly called for the integration of research, clinical expertise, and context, including practice setting and client characteristics as they influence care (APA Task Force, 2006). It acknowledged the importance of diverse research designs, including but not limited to randomized clinical trials. Further, the APA Task Force called for research exploring specific and common factors as mechanisms of change as well as the effects of feedback on treatment outcomes.

The EBPP policy has great promise to transform youth psychotherapy research by including evidence that is not solely based on specific treatments. This is timely, given that we cannot state with great confidence that most treatments considered to be evidence based are better than care as usual. This chapter seeks to make sense of the EBT debate and to clarify the role of both specific and common factors in youth psychotherapy, and in so doing, address whether the dodo verdict rings true for children and adolescents, as is claimed for adults with mental health (see chap. 2, this volume) and substance abuse problems (see chap. 13) as well as in couple and family therapy (see chap. 12). In addition, this chapter embraces the APA Task Force recommendation for outcome monitoring and argues that the systematic collection of feedback is an evidence-based approach (see chap. 8) that both improves clinical services and furthers an understanding of the factors accounting for change. We are not seeking to exclude any rational approach to improving the quality of treatment but to broaden what types of research and treatment should be supported.


YOUTH PSYCHOTHERAPY: DOES IT WORK AND WHY?

Simply stated, treatment is better than no treatment, and youth psychotherapy appears similarly effective to adult psychotherapy (Kazdin, 2004). But why it works and under what conditions is not quite so straightforward. By and large, research in child and adolescent mental health has adopted a *specific effects assumption*, or the belief that treatment models have unique aspects that can be demonstrated as more helpful than others for particular problems or diagnoses. Consequently, the bulk of the evidence has focused on the efficacy of a particular therapeutic approach for a given disorder (e.g., cognitive–behavioral therapy [CBT] for depression, reinforced practice and participant modeling for phobias). Given that there are more than 550 child psychotherapies in use (Kazdin, 2000), it seems logical that looking for specific effects in randomized clinical trials would first narrow the field by identifying what works and then ultimately lead to transporting these findings via manuals and other training approaches to real-world practice.

Despite this compelling rationale and the popularity of the specific effects assumption, recent reviews and meta-analyses have exposed significant limitations in this knowledge base, leading to the suggestion that EBTs "may be clearing a very low threshold" (Jensen, Weersing, Hoagwood, & Goldman, 2005, p. 71). Meta-analyses synthesize effect sizes (ESs) across multiple studies, providing a more comprehensive picture of the field as a whole (Schmidt, 1992). Cohen's (1988) benchmarks (small ES = 0.20, medium ES = 0.50, large ES = 0.80) are widely used to evaluate meta-analytic findings.

To make sense of the evidence for youth treatment efficacy, first consider a meta-analysis of 35 EBT studies for youth depression (Weisz, McCarty, & Valeri, 2006). When compared with non-EBT controls (wait list, treatment as usual [TAU], or attention controls), the overall ES (0.34) was much lower than in published meta-analyses of adult psychotherapy (e.g., ES = 0.80; Wampold, 2001). Further, this investigation noted that the ES decreased at follow-up, with no lasting effect for EBTs at 1 year or longer after treatment ended. Aside from having a larger pool of studies available, Weisz, McCarty, and Valeri (2006) attributed the difference to the inclusion of the following: nonpublished studies, thereby reducing publication bias (chap. 6); additional information from study authors needed for calculations; only randomized control trials; and all outcome measures reported to calculate ESs. A further methodological improvement was the use of random effects analyses versus fixed effects analyses for computing ES, deemed a more appropriate estimation technique for youth depression psychotherapy studies that also increases generalizability of findings (Weisz, McCarty, & Valeri, 2006).

But do improved meta-analytic methods account for the less than exemplary performance of the EBTs? A fundamental weakness is the type of control group used in the individual studies. Consider that the majority of youth psychotherapy efficacy studies compare EBTs with passive control groups, such as waitlist or no-treatment controls (Weisz, 2004). It is known that comparison of an EBT with an active versus passive control results in lower ESs (Baskin, Tierney, Minami, & Wampold, 2003; Kazdin, Bass, Ayers, & Rodgers, 1990). Comparisons with active treatments, such as TAU, also known as *usual care* (UC), or attention-only groups has been promoted as a method of exploring whether an EBT is "*specifically* effective, over and above simple compassion, friendliness, attention, and belief" (Jensen et al., 2005, p. 54). Weisz, McCarty, and Valeri (2006) identified a subset of 14 studies that compared an EBT with an active control group in the youth depression psychotherapy meta-analysis mentioned above. The ES was smaller (0.24) than for the remainder of studies that used passive control groups (ES = 0.41). In other words, when EBTs were compared with TAU, the ES decreased considerably. The small ES of 0.24 is similar to the ES of comparisons between different bona fide treatment approaches in youth psychotherapy, described later.

In a separate meta-analysis of 32 studies comparing EBT with UC, Weisz, Jensen-Doss, and Hawley (2006) found a small to moderate ES of 0.30. The authors then conducted a series of comparisons to address several limitations of EBT research, focusing on subsamples of studies to identify the influence of study characteristics of the treatment and therapist (e.g., treatment dose, homework assignment, therapist training, supervision), client (e.g., minority status, severity, comorbidity), and design (e.g., therapists from the same pool, different treatment settings, purity of EBT and UC comparison, involvement of EBT developer). In almost all cases, the ESs decreased considerably. In other words, when the EBT and UC were similar in intensity, therapist training, setting, and other characteristics, the superiority of the EBT on client outcomes disappeared (Minami & Wampold, 2008).

A second confound that challenges comparisons of EBT and UC is the *allegiance effect*, the researcher's belief or commitment to a particular treatment. Allegiance bias is a threat known to influence outcomes in psychotherapy trials (see Luborsky et al., 1999; Wampold, 2001). In Weisz, Jensen-Doss, and Hawley's (2006) meta-analysis, the ES produced by studies not conducted by EBT developers was very small and nonsignificant (ES = 0.09). The allegiance effect may reflect research design artifacts that favor EBT therapists, such as extensive training and supervision, therapist selection on the basis of skill, and fewer clients. It is also possible that UC therapists, aware that they are delivering the control treatment, may have a decreased belief in the efficacy of the treatment (Baskin et al., 2003), an important common factor discussed in the next section.

Therefore, it is surprising that Weisz, Jensen-Doss, and Hawley (2006) concluded that their findings "support the view that EBTs have generally outperformed UC in direct, randomized comparisons" (p. 684), although the authors indicated several limitations of the meta-analyses. Particularly notable, they reported, is the striking lack of detail typically reported for the control condition is a significant problem in relying on comparisons of EBT with UC. The finding of a small to medium ES overall further led the authors to recommend several improvements to EBT development and efficacy research. They advised practitioners that "those who are selecting treatments for youths in clinical care cannot safely assume that any EBT they choose will improve on any form of

UC" (Weisz, Jensen-Doss, & Hawley, 2006, p. 685). Indeed, Weisz and Gray (2008) called for a greater emphasis on documenting and studying UC as a potentially promising intervention.

Direct comparison of two or more bona fide treatments is a far more appropriate design to demonstrate differential effects of specific treatments (Wampold, Mondin, et al., 1997). Wampold, Mondin, et al. (1997) provided criteria to classify treatments as bona fide, including the following: therapist characteristics (e.g., therapy-specific training, relevant degree and level of education), treatment format (e.g., face-to-face meetings, individualized treatment), and validity of treatment (e.g., use of treatment guidelines or a manual, referencing an established therapeutic approach or process, identification of active treatment ingredients with citations).

Two recent meta-analyses used these criteria to conduct direct comparisons of bona fide treatments for youth mental health disorders (Miller et al., 2008; Spielmans, Pasek, & McFall, 2007). Given the lack of specificity in the literature, the comparison of two or more bona fide treatments is still largely unexplored territory. It is noteworthy that although there are countless outcome studies in youth treatment—more than 1,500 by some estimates—only 16 identified by Spielmans et al. (2007) and 23 by Miller et al. (2008) examined differential efficacy of two or more bona fide treatments. It is not surprising that Spielmans et al. found that bona fide CBTs were more efficacious than non–bona fide treatments for youth anxiety and depression. The authors also suggested that CBT was no more efficacious than other bona fide treatments; however, this conclusion was based on only one identified study that directly compared CBT with interpersonal therapy for depression, with no studies in the anxiety literature identified.

In a meta-analysis that included efficacy studies of child and adolescent therapies for depression, anxiety, conduct disorder, and attention-deficit/hyperactivity disorder, Miller et al. (2008) found that ESs were not homogeneously distributed around zero, thereby suggesting the possibility of differential effects of the various treatments. However, the difference between treatments had an ES of only 0.22 at the upper bound, which is consistent with the small effect size reported for adult treatments (cf. Wampold, Mondin, et al., 1997). Furthermore, when results were adjusted for researcher allegiance, there was no difference found among bona fide therapies, with an ES around zero. In other words, the allegiance effect could be used to explain all the observed differences among treatments.

Finally, one other study that examined differential efficacy is worthy of note: the Cannabis Youth Treatment Study (Dennis et al., 2004). This sophisticated randomized clinical trial of 600 adolescents with a substance abuse disorder compared five short-term outpatient interventions, including CBT (Dennis et al., 2004). All five treatments were similarly effective in pre–post improvement in youth outcomes, with small ESs. The only predictor of ultimate treatment outcome was the alliance as rated by the client (see chap. 12, this volume, for details).

Is there sufficient support to uphold the dodo bird verdict? On the one hand, the modest ESs associated with comparisons of EBTs and UCs and the lack of findings when direct comparisons of bona fide treatments are made suggest that different youth psychotherapies are similarly effective. On the other hand, varying ESs across individual studies suggest that some treatments may be more efficacious than others (Jensen et al., 2005; Weisz, Jensen-Doss, and Hawley, 2006). To put it more accurately, some treatments, whether EBT or UC, may work better for some youth in some settings. Yet reviews of recent efficacy studies in child and adolescent psychotherapy have indicated that almost none identify or test the mechanisms of change in the treatment process (Jensen et al., 2005; Weersing & Weisz, 2002; Weisz, McCarty, & Valeri, 2006). As noted earlier, researchers do not have a clear understanding of the moderators and mediators of treatment outcomes (Kazdin, 2004; Kazdin & Whitley, 2006; Jensen et al., 2005; Weisz, 2004; Westen, Novotny, & Thompson-Brenner, 2004). The existing research is simply not sophisticated enough to answer questions related to the impact of client and clinician characteristics, relationship factors, and other ingredients of the therapeutic process that are common to any psychotherapy, regardless of treatment modality or model. These factors, as well as characteristics of the intervention and service setting, should inform future research on EBTs (Hoagwood, Burns, Kiser, Ringeisen, & Schoenwald, 2001).

Taken as a whole, greater caution is warranted in the promotion of the evidence base as it currently stands. Those in the field of clinical child and adolescent psychotherapy need to better understand the contributions of both specific effects and common factors on treatment outcomes (Bickman, 2005; Ollendick & Davis, 2004). Rather than a seemingly endless quest to simply prove the superiority of EBTs or common factors, a more nuanced approach is needed to provide understanding of the components of treatment that actively work to improve youth outcomes.

Our stance, described in the next section, is that the importance of common factors has been established and does not depend on demonstrating that specific factors are unimportant. Rather, there is a need for further research on the relative importance of each common factor, the interrelationships among them, and the contribution of common factors to enhancing the impact of specific therapeutic techniques for individual clients. Most important, we need to move beyond descriptive correlational studies and test common factors interventions in real-world settings.

We are not aware of any published study that has evaluated the effectiveness of a common factors intervention despite the central importance of this construct in psychotherapy. The absence of such research is mystifying. Perhaps it is due to a lack of clarity regarding what a common factors intervention might be. Because common factors are indeed common to any treatment, they could not be directly experimentally manipulated (e.g., therapists randomly assigned to form or not form a relationship). Although it is not possible to remove the common factors processes from typical treatment, it is certainly possible to vary client exposure to common factors. For example, stand-alone bibliotherapy could be compared with therapist-directed treatment. Bibliotherapy does not have three of the four common factors that Jerome Frank (1961) identified for effective therapies (helping confidential relationship, a healing setting, the active participation of client and clinician), although it does have a conceptual theme (which may also serve as the basis for its bona fide status). Another example is to experimentally vary training in common factors (e.g., therapeutic alliance) to establish if such training improves alliance and subsequent client improvement. We are indeed testing such a common factors training intervention as part of a larger study funded by the National Institute of Mental Health. As Jensen et al. (2005) pointed out, if a common factors approach is found effective, it may be less expensive and more acceptable to focus on training therapists to maximize these nonspecific aspects of therapy as opposed to continuing the current emphasis on manual-based treatments.

## COMMON FACTORS IN CHILD AND ADOLESCENT TREATMENT

Clinical care for children and adolescents is characterized not only by high levels of symptom severity and comorbidity (Angold, Costello, & Erkanli, 1999) but also by parent and family stressors (Hammen, Rudolph, Weisz, Burge, & Rao, 1999). Access to and maintenance of treatment for youth is typically initiated by caregivers or other adults (Yeh & Weisz, 2001), necessitating the formation of an ongoing therapeutic relationship with both the youth and the parents. Treatment dropout rates range from 28% to 85% (Garcia & Weisz, 2002). As such, it is not surprising that some researchers have shifted their attention toward the study of common factors that may influence treatment access, engagement, and outcomes for youth and their families.

An exhaustive review of the common factors literature (Karver, Handelsman, Fields, & Bickman, 2005, 2006) organized common factors in child and adolescent psychotherapy into a dozen separate yet interrelated constructs. For example, therapist reactions, perceptions, and feelings were posited as important mediating links between therapist and client pretreatment characteristics and therapist behaviors. The current volume (see chap. 1 and 2) describes the common factors in five broad categories: client factors, therapist effects, therapeutic alliance or relationship, and both general and specific model or technique effects. Client factors include both demographic variables (e.g., age or developmental status, race or ethnicity, socioeconomic status, gender) and characteristics directly related to therapy (e.g., resilience, severity, presenting problems, interpersonal functioning, motivation). Similarly, therapist qualities include demographic variables and characteristics directly related to therapy (e.g., theoretical orientation, years of experience, interpersonal skills, training). More recently, therapist effectiveness has come to the attention of researchers although this trend has yet to reach the youth psychotherapy literature. The therapeutic relationship, the most researched factor, is a broad category that includes the alliance, engagement, and transference. Similar to the adult literature, the alliance in youth psychotherapy is the most investigated of the common factors. Specific model or technique factors represent defined theories or strategies that influence treatment outcomes, whereas the more general aspects of model or technique refer to the provision of a treatment structure as well as the hope and expectancy engendered in clients via a credible rationale for the youth problem and the rituals to address it.

Common factors are generally supported in the literature as important factors in treatment outcomes, potentially more powerful than the specific ingredients of different therapies (e.g., Lambert & Barley, 2002; Wampold, 2001). In addition, the finding that a substantial amount of client improvement occurs very early in treatment may be interpreted as support for the common factors perspective, indicating that specific treatment effects had not had sufficient time to be effective (Cromley & Lavigne, 2008; Dennis et al., 2004; Snyder, Michael, & Cheavens, 1999). Although this finding is quite promising, it is not clear which common factors may be contributing to early gains, although client or other extratherapeutic factors have been posited (Duncan, Miller, & Sparks, 2004).

There are several difficulties in extrapolating this evidence on common factors to practice with children and adolescents. Much of the research to date has been conducted with adult populations, although the literature base for common factors in working with youth is growing. There has not been a systematic approach to the study of common factors, with most studies using a wide variety of measures and lacking a cohesive theory base to drive hypotheses (Shirk & Karver, 2003). Although common factors have been acknowledged as important mediators of treatment outcome (Lambert & Ogles, 2004), a current weakness is that almost all of the research is correlational (e.g., Kazdin & Whitley, 2006).

In this section, we focus on those common factors in child and adolescent psychotherapy for which instrumentation and theory have been proposed (see Bickman et al., 2007) and links to client outcomes studied. These include the therapeutic relationship and client characteristics such as parent and family functioning, motivation for treatment, expectancies about treatment, and hope (also considered a change process). We also discuss change processes and treatment structure in terms of general and specific treatment techniques. The following discussion relies heavily on the Karver et al. (2006) meta-analysis of 49 studies of common factors in youth treatment. Although Karver et al.'s investigation addressed the relationships among process variables as well, here the focus is largely on the relationships found between a given variable and treatment outcome.

## Client Factors

As one might suspect, the characteristics that youths and their parents bring to treatment have a prominent impact on how therapy proceeds and on the ultimate outcome of treatment. Wampold (see chap. 2, this volume) has assigned little of the variance in therapy outcomes to specific therapeutic interventions. Throughout this discussion, it is worthwhile to consider how the various common factors interact with one another. As noted in chapter 1 of this volume, the factors are not discrete or separate, but rather they dynamically interact and overlap with one another. Therapist behaviors, for example, are contingent on the pretreatment characteristics that clients (youth, parents, family members) bring to therapy (Karver et al., 2005). Karver, Lambert, and Bickman (2003) found that therapists were most likely to point out strengths in those youths who entered therapy with the most pretreatment strengths. It is unfortunate that research addressing client factors in youth treatment is sparse, largely retrospective, hardly robust, and has focused on the traditional client characteristics identified in the adult literature, which have found little replicated relationship to outcome. For example, although there is a growing body of research about youth resilience (e.g., Bonanno & Mancini, 2008), the relationship of this pretreatment characteristic to treatment outcomes is largely unknown. Here, we focus on parent and family functioning as well as youth motivation for and participation in treatment.

### Caregiver and Family Functioning

Caregivers and family, obviously, have an important role in child and adolescent psychotherapy. Parent and family members' interpersonal functioning, mental health, intelligence, family environment, and expectancies about treatment have all been identified as factors impacting youth participation in treatment and outcomes (Fields, Handelsman, Karver, & Bickman, 2004; Hutchings, Appleton, Smith, Lane, & Nash, 2002; Kazdin & Wassell, 2000). Caregiver strain, a related but distinct construct from parental psychological distress (Brannan & Heflinger, 2001), is an important outcome of treatment and may also influence participation in treatment. The demands of caring for a troubled child have been tied to increased use of youth mental health services (Angold et al., 1998; Brannan & Heflinger, 2005; Brannan, Heflinger, & Foster, 2003; Farmer, Burns, Angold, & Costello, 1997) as well as parental involvement in youth treatment (Yatchmenoff et al., 1998). Parent empowerment in dealing with mental health services has been studied experimentally. Although empowerment can be enhanced through training, it has not been shown to have any effect on clinical outcomes (Bickman, Heflinger, Northrup, Sonnichsen, & Schilling, 1998; Heflinger, Bickman, Northrup, & Sonnichsen, 1997).

## Motivation and Participation

Motivation has been identified as a predictor of seeking and staying in services (Simpson, 2001) as well as of better treatment outcomes in the field of adolescent substance abuse (Breda & Heflinger, 2004), with equal promise in the field of child and adolescent mental health. Conceptualizations of youth and parental motivation often identify two broad components: extrinsic and intrinsic motivation. External sources of motivation can come from parents or legal authorities who exert pressure on the individual to seek or stay in treatment. Intrinsic motivation reflects the respondent's own problem recognition, desire for help, and treatment readiness, dimensions that have been found to be important for treatment involvement and outcome (Simpson, 2001).

The Karver et al. (2006) meta-analyses focused on youth and parent willingness to participate in treatment (acceptability and commitment) and participation in treatment (effort and engagement). Although moderately correlated with outcomes, few studies were identified that linked youth (one) or parent (two) willingness to participate to youth outcomes. The association between participation in treatment and youth outcomes was also in the moderate range for youth and parent participation in treatment, although there was wide variation across the studies identified. It is important to note that although these correlations should not be interpreted as treatment effects or group differences, these findings do indicate that client and parent motivation for and participation in treatment all have an important influence on youth outcomes. In addition, equal consideration should be given to the therapist and treatment context. Motivation, willingness to participate, and actual participation in treatment are not solely found in the youth or parents themselves but rather in the interplay among the participants (including the therapist) and the match of the services with the goals of the consumers.

## Therapist Effects

As with client characteristics, there has been minimal study of the impact of therapist characteristics on ultimate treatment outcome. There is no consistent support for the notion that the academic degree of the therapist or the number of years of experience affects treatment outcomes (Beutler et al., 2004; Lambert & Ogles, 1997; Sapyta, Riemer, & Bickman, 2005; Wampold & Brown, 2005). However, an analysis of 60 clinicians in UC found that some therapists are consistently more effective than others in treating adults (Wampold & Brown, 2005). Karver et al. (2006) found a moderate average association in several studies that linked counselor interpersonal skills (e.g., empathy) to youth outcomes, although as with client participation there was a great deal of variability in the individual studies. Recent studies using more sophisticated analytic techniques have confirmed the existence of a therapist effect (Dinger, Strack, Leichsenring, Wilmers, & Schauenburg, 2008; Lutz, Leon, Martinovich, Lyons, & Stiles, 2007). However, methodological issues still trouble this area of research (Crits-Christoph & Mintz, 1991; Wampold & Bolt, 2007).

Considering the prominent role of therapists in delivering therapy to their clients, the paucity of studies is quite amazing. In the mental health literature in general, and specifically in the youth treatment literature, research is needed to explore therapist qualities that are linked to positive client outcomes. More important, such research should focus on how the field may act to support and train therapists in improving their effectiveness. This critical point is addressed later in the chapter.

**Therapeutic Alliance**

The *therapeutic alliance* (TA) between clinician and client has been cited as one of the most important elements of effective therapy (Karver et al., 2006). TA is commonly defined as consisting of three components: (a) the bond or rapport between the client and the therapist and their agreement on (b) therapeutic goals and (c) tasks (i.e., specific activities that occur in therapy) (Bordin, 1979, 1994). The bond component consists of a general perception of the working relationship, including communication, trust, and therapist helpfulness and competence.

Meta-analyses of child and caregiver alliance studies (Karver et al., 2006; Shirk & Karver, 2003) have provided support for the importance of TA in youth psychotherapy, although the effects were small. Both child and parent TA have been found to be associated with youth outcomes even after accounting for type of disorder (Green, 2006; McLeod & Weisz, 2005); treatment characteristics, including the use of EBTs and other client characteristics, such as severity (Kazdin, Whitley, & Marciano, 2006; McLeod & Weisz, 2005); and type of treatment setting, including outpatient, inpatient, and community clinics (e.g., Garcia & Weisz, 2002; Green, 2006; Kazdin, Marciano, & Whitley, 2005). TA is particularly important in light of a recent finding that perceived barriers associated with treatment participation resulted in less therapeutic change among youth receiving EBT for externalizing disorders (Kazdin & Whitley, 2006). Given that TA has been noted as a major factor in treatment dropouts (e.g., Garcia & Weisz, 2002), it is possible that a stronger alliance may increase treatment participation.

Strong TA may be an even more critical issue for youth psychotherapy than adult therapy, given that child and adolescent clients are typically not self-referred and caregivers or extended family usually play a vital role in treatment (Shirk & Karver, 2003). It follows that developing a strong therapeutic relationship with young clients and their family members may facilitate engagement by providing a stable, accepting, and supportive context in which therapy may take place. It should be noted that child and parent TA may exhibit different mechanisms of change. They have been found to be independent (Green, 2006), and it has been suggested that although youth TA is more predictive of symptom improvement, parent TA is associated with greater participation in treatment (Hawley & Weisz, 2005; Karver et al., 2006).

The TA may influence outcomes of youth treatment in several different ways: as a necessary relational change mechanism, as a catalyst for other treatment processes that lead to positive outcomes, or as a moderator of therapist-offered interventions (Bickman et al., 2004; Shirk & Karver, 2003). The therapeutic relationship with the parent may also impact outcomes of treatment in several ways: The treatment may be focused on directly changing parent behavior that will impact child behavior, and thus, engaging the parent will be critical, or the treatment may be focused on the child, so engaging the parent will be important because parents schedule and keep appointments, provide information about the child to the therapist, encourage the child's treatment adherence, and promote generalization of treatment gains outside of therapy sessions (Fields et al., 2004). A parent who has a strong TA with the therapist is likely to convey hope and other positive attitudes about treatment that may generally encourage the child's participation in treatment, which then in turn may influence youth outcomes. These are all reasonable expectations of the benefits of a positive TA; however, rigorous empirical research has yet to be accomplished that could provide evidence of such effects.

## Specific and General Aspects of Model and Technique

Currently, research is only suggestive of the potential effect of different change processes and treatment structures on youth psychotherapy outcomes, given the rarity of mediator analyses in existing efficacy studies (e.g., Jensen et al., 2005; Weersing & Weisz, 2002; Weisz, McCarty, & Valeri, 2006). However, there is some evidence that general techniques, not specific to any particular therapy—such as provision of a treatment rationale, collaborative treatment planning, and goal clarification—may be associated with improved youth outcomes. Karver et al. (2006) found that "therapist direct influence skills" (p. 53), including the clear presentation of information and provision of an understandable treatment rationale, was a strong predictor of youth treatment outcome. Hawley and Weisz (2003) found that collaborative goal setting, a component of goal clarification and a central feature of the TA, was associated with positive youth outcomes.

Client expectations and hope about treatment, considered pretreatment client factors, play fundamental roles in the delivery of any techniques or models of therapy. Historically, the literature has focused on expectancies about role (both of the client and the therapist) and outcome (that therapy will lead to change; Arnkoff, Glass, & Shapiro, 2002). More recent research has focused on process expectations, that is, the activities involved in and feelings elicited by treatment (Dew & Bickman, 2005). It has been suggested that client expectations and hope about outcome will accompany any treatment model that provides both a rationale for the client's problem and a ritual for its solution (Frank, 1973).

In a recent review of the literature, Dew and Bickman (2005) found that outcome expectations were significantly related to youth treatment outcomes in 10 of 13 studies reviewed. Client expectations are likely related to the treatment process as well, although far fewer studies have been conducted in this area. For example, TA has been linked with positive outcome expectations, but little research has focused on TA's association with role expectations. It would make sense that client expectations would be related to premature termination from treatment, but the research base in this area is considered weak and difficult to interpret (e.g., dropout is not consistently correlated with either high or low expectations across studies). Although this research is promising, more research is needed to understand how expectations about treatment may affect both treatment process and outcomes. It would be interesting to assess how child and adolescent expectations are influenced by unique aspects of youth psychotherapy, such as whether the typical lack of self-referral has a negative impact on youth expectations. Another question is whether and how concordance or discordance in youth and caregiver expectations influences TA.

Youth hopefulness is related to but distinct from expectations about treatment and can be conceptualized as both a moderator (i.e., level of hope pretreatment) and a mediator (i.e., increased hopefulness over time) of treatment outcomes. Although there is some controversy in the literature as to whether hope is predominantly a cognitive or emotional construct, most authors agree that both cognitions and emotions are involved in the experience of hope (Hinds et al., 1999; Snyder, 2002; Snyder et al., 1997; Valle, Huebner, & Suldo,

2004). In broad terms, *hope* is a way of thinking about goals: a wish or desire for something accompanied by the expectation of obtaining it. Snyder et al. (1999) defined hope as the perceived ability to produce pathways to attain goals (pathway thinking) and move on the path toward those goals (agency thinking). Dew and Bickman (2005) suggested that client expectations and hope may influence each other over the course of treatment: Positive outcome expectations may increase client hope of improvement, which in turn may augment further expectations about treatment.

Efforts to tease out the elements of a therapy that are specifically effective are typically found in component studies, in which a full treatment group is compared with one or more groups with varying levels of intensity or dose of the same treatment. Meta-analytic results for youth psychotherapy for anxiety and depression found no difference in full CBT approaches (e.g., CBT plus parent training) over their components (e.g., CBT only; Spielmans et al., 2007). Meta-analyses comparing cognitive treatments with noncognitive approaches (e.g., behavioral) for youth depression have also found no difference in treatment outcomes (Spielmans et al., 2007; Weisz, McCarty, and Valeri, 2006), raising the possibility that specific alteration of cognitions may not contribute to better outcomes. A systematic review of recently published efficacy studies in youth psychotherapy (regardless of disorder) found less than half of those comparing treatments of differing intensity had significant findings (Jensen et al., 2005). It should be noted that a significant limitation of all these findings is the use of the therapy as the unit of analysis, making it difficult to identify the differential effectiveness of specific techniques found within a larger intervention. Chorpita, Daleiden, and Weisz (2005) have proposed an innovative methodology for identifying specific therapeutic techniques extracted from manuals and intervention studies. This "tool kit" would then be matched to client characteristics and contextual variables to maximize effectiveness. Such an approach would be an elegant solution to the development of an evidence base more in keeping with the eclectic approach to treatment espoused by many therapists in the real world.

## What Next?

Our review of the common factors literature in youth psychotherapy reveals similar findings to investigations of the common factors in adult psychotherapy, although on the basis of far fewer studies. A look at client factors reveals a growing emphasis on positive pretreatment characteristics as well as the phenomena of early change and its relationship to ultimate treatment outcome. The importance of therapists to treatment outcome is just beginning to take hold in the research literature, and future studies will likely focus on what differentiates more successful from less successful therapists, and more important, how therapists can improve. Therapeutic alliance and its connection to youth outcomes appears to transcend treatment type and client population. Finally, hope, expectations, specific therapeutic techniques, and the more general functions of providing treatment also mirror findings in the adult psychotherapy literature. But the question remains: How does one apply this research? How does knowing about the aggregate data about the common factors help youth clinicians with the troubled child and worried family in the office now?

## LEARN FROM EVERY CHILD: PRACTICE-BASED EVIDENCE USING A MEASUREMENT FEEDBACK SYSTEM

Given the limitations of the specific effects assumption and the need for a more pragmatic and individualized application of common factors research, the field of child and adolescent mental health requires a change in direction. More precisely, it needs a complete reversal of direction. Instead of the medical model research paradigm, proceeding from laboratory to field, a development flow from field to laboratory may yield far more practical results. This practice-based evidence (PBE) approach promotes the systematic and frequent measurement of youth treatment progress and process in clinical service settings within a continuous quality improvement (CQI) framework (Duncan et al., 2004; Howard, Moras, Brill, Martinovich, & Lutz, 1996; Lambert, 2005; Margison et al., 2000). We have labeled this a *measurement feedback system* (MFS; Bickman, 2008; Kelley & Bickman, 2009).

By using available computer technology, an MFS could provide a relatively inexpensive infrastructure to improve research through the mining of large data sets, contributing to randomized trials and correlational analyses to better identify the relationship between (and among) youth outcomes and specific therapies and common factors across treatments. Moreover, practice improvements could include feedback to clinicians and clients on individual client progress and process, thereby allowing the application of research findings in ways never dreamed possible in laboratory settings. Clinical service sites could become learning organizations by aggregating data for their own clinical trials. It is important to note that an MFS engages the clinical community and consumers as full partners in building the knowledge base in terms of identifying effective strategies, improving outcomes, and providing data from the field instead of the lab. This emphasis on engaging practitioners in research efforts using data from community and clinical settings is consistent with practice research networks (Bradley, Sexton, & Smith, 2005; Smith, Sexton, & Bradley, 2005), a promising approach that incorporates many of the features of MFSs.

## The Evidence for Feedback in Mental Health Care

Although the ultimate goal is to improve outcomes, the importance of the clinician in the adoption of any new approach is often overlooked. Changing clinician practice behavior is not an easy endeavor. Dissemination of guidelines may increase clinician access to information but do not create lasting behavior change without the addition of enabling or reinforcing strategies, such as feedback (Davis et al., 1999). To learn effectively from experience, clinicians need reliable knowledge about the success or failure of performance (Kluger & DeNisi, 1996). However, the environmental cues of success available to mental health clinicians are often vague and unsystematic (Bickman, 1999). Feedback interventions overcome this barrier by providing systematic knowledge of results, a potentially powerful tool to change clinician behavior.

Research strongly suggests that systematic feedback to clinicians about the outcome of clinical services improves outcomes in adult mental health (see chap. 8, this volume; Hawkins et al., 2004; Lambert, 2007; Lambert et al., 2001). Providing feedback to therapists seems to be of particular benefit for adult clients who were either not improving or deteriorating. If designed appropriately, feedback interventions provide practitioners with knowledge about the outcomes of their performance and enhance intrinsic motivation to change their behavior. The success, however, of any feedback system depends primarily on its adoption and use by clinicians and in service settings. Any system must be seen as both feasible and clinically relevant by therapists for widespread utilization to occur.

For example, the Mental Health Outcomes and Assessment Tools is a set of standardized clinical instruments for use in youth mental health treatment settings, intended to be administered at intake, every 13 weeks during treatment, and on discharge (NSW Department of Health, 2004). Although mandated by the government, a review found that the measures were generally not being completed or used (Patterson, Matthey, & Baker, 2006). The authors identified several barriers that contributed to the lack of adherence, including concerns about the relevance of resulting feedback to client care and issues related to a "passive resistance," namely, concerns about reduced clinical autonomy and perceived lack of value added to existing mechanisms for review of client progress (e.g., case review and supervision). In addition, organizational factors such as climate and culture can influence clinician behavior (e.g., Glisson & Hemmelgarn, 1998; Hemmelgarn, Glisson, & James, 2006). It is important to note that although outcomes monitoring has been promoted as a method for increasing program accountability (e.g., Hernandez, Hodges, & Cascardi, 1998), feedback is fundamentally different in that the focus is on individual client progress and change over time. This is a critical point and separates accountability as a management oversight device from feedback as a way to enhance outcomes.

The provision of an MFS within a larger CQI framework may enhance clinician and organizational acceptance through consultation, ongoing training, and built-in flexibility within the feedback system to meet local needs. Hodges and Wotring (2004) described such an approach in an ongoing state-based initiative to promote continuous outcome monitoring for public sector youth mental health providers. Providers complete the Child and Adolescent Functional Assessment Scale (Hodges, 2000) for youth with serious emotional disturbances at intake, every 3 months during treatment, and at discharge. In addition to state- and agency-aggregated data reports, clinicians are provided with monthly assessment reports on individual clients to be used in treatment planning. Building from the active use of outcome monitoring by individual providers and agencies, the initiative has promoted a variety of CQI activities, from the identification of champion users available for consultation to the introduction of state-based training in EBTs (Hodges & Wotring, 2004). The impact on treatment outcome, however, is unknown.

Feedback factors, such as the timing, source, content, format, and sign (positive or negative) are also likely to impact the perceived utility of feedback (Riemer & Bickman, in press; Riemer, Rosof-Williams, & Bickman, 2005; Sapyta et al., 2005). It is worthwhile to note here that retrospective feedback, as exemplified by the Child and Adolescent Functional Assessment Scale, is quite different than real-time feedback, as illustrated by the Youth Outcome Questionnaire (YOQ; Burlingame, Wells, & Lambert, 1996). The YOQ is a parent-report questionnaire on youth symptoms and functioning (an adolescent-report version is also available). Weekly feedback based on the YOQ was found to be clinically useful in determining the dose–response relationship for the number of sessions needed for clinically significant change (Asay, Lambert, Gregersen, & Goates, 2002). This study is notable in that the feedback system was successfully implemented and found to be valuable for tracking individual clients and improving the therapeutic process for a clinician in private practice.

Caregivers or other adults typically initiate or maintain mental health services for youth (Yeh & Weisz, 2001). To enhance client engagement in services, Duncan, Sparks, Miller, Bohanske, and Claud (2006) emphasized the importance of giving youths and their caregivers a voice about both the outcome and fit of provided services in their Partners for Change Outcome Management System (PCOMS). PCOMS utilizes the Child Outcome Rating Scale (Duncan, Miller, & Sparks, 2003) for children 6 to 12 years of age (the first self-report outcome measure for children under 13 years) and the Outcome Rating Scale (Miller & Duncan, 2000) for youths 13 years and older. Both scales consist of only four items and are completed by the client and caregiver on a session-by-session basis. The Child Outcome Rating Scale and the Outcome Rating Scale provide brief measures of global subjective distress and, consequently, a feasible way to track benefits and enable real-time feedback in each session. PCOMS also includes the routine monitoring of the alliance from both caretaker and youth perspectives. These measures exhibit good reliability, moderate validity, and sensitivity to change (Duncan et al., 2006; measures available for free download at http://www.talkingcure.com). It is important that PCOMS provides a large clinical database for normative comparisons, an example of how PBE can be put to practical use. PCOMS has demonstrated the positive effects of feedback with adults (see chap. 8, this volume) and couples (see chap. 12).

The Ohio Youth Problems, Functioning, and Satisfaction Scales (Ohio Scales, Short Form; Ogles, Melendez, Davis, & Lunnen, 1999) were developed for use in treatment planning and outcomes monitoring for youths 5 to 18 years of age, with caregiver, adolescent, and clinician versions. In addition to youth problem severity and functioning, the Ohio Scales include questions on hopefulness and satisfaction with services. A recent study of monthly feedback in wraparound services for youth and families (Ogles et al., 2006) found that provision of feedback (a maximum of four times), using the Ohio Scales, did not contribute to improved youth outcomes or family functioning in comparison with a no-feedback control group. However, parents who received feedback perceived more positive outcomes than caregivers who did not receive feedback. A significant limitation of this study is the small sample size, which reduces the possibility of finding the most powerful effects of feedback, namely for clients who are either not improving or deteriorating.

## Contextualized Feedback Intervention and Training

On the basis of our brief review of EBTs, common factors, and feedback in child and adolescent therapy, we recommend that feedback include an added focus on the common factors (e.g., therapeutic alliance, expectancy, client characteristics). Our model, which we have termed *contextual feedback intervention and training* (CFIT), synthesizes the valuable knowledge provided by basic and applied researchers into one coherent model of clinician behavior change (Bickman, Riemer, Breda, & Kelley, 2006; Riemer & Bickman, in press; Riemer et al., 2005; Sapyta et al., 2005).

Motivation to change and commitment to the target goal are necessary but not sufficient for therapist change to occur. The clinician must also believe that the goal is yet to be accomplished. In this model, client-level feedback provides the information needed for a clinician to make that judgment. CFIT provides valid and reliable feedback about a client's current status through the use of the Peabody Treatment Progress Battery, a set of brief psychometrically sound instruments targeting client progress and the treatment process (Bickman et al., 2007; measures are available for free use at http://peabody.vanderbilt.edu/ptpb). Once entered into the CFIT web-based system, these questionnaires—administered on a weekly basis to clients, caregivers, and clinicians—can provide immediate feedback on client current scores, change since last administration, and trends over time using computerized algorithms. The feedback is hierarchical in nature, offering more detailed views at the press of a button. Attention to and acceptance of the feedback depend largely on the perceived credibility of the feedback source, the value of the information contained within, and the form of the feedback. The Peabody Treatment Progress Battery contains instruments related to both treatment progress (e.g., symptom reduction) and the treatment process (e.g., TA). Further, at least 3 informants (youth, caregiver, and clinician) provide multiple perspectives as an approach to increasing perceived value of the information.

Clinicians may still reject the feedback message if it is too inconsistent with their own perceptions. The clinician is likely to experience cognitive dissonance with unexpected feedback (e.g., client or caregiver responses not consistent with clinical experience) or negative feedback (e.g., client symptoms and functioning are worsening over the course of treatment). CFIT identifies this dissonance as a leverage point for targeting motivation for behavior change. For clinicians to be motivated to change, it is vital to provide them with the tools, training, and supervision that could support their feelings of self-efficacy and responsibility for providing more effective services.

Consistent with the construct of a learning organization (Marsick & Watkins, 2003), CFIT addresses the need for individual learning through provision of online training in common therapeutic factors, and collective learning and organizational support by directly involving supervisors in the intervention. CFIT has promising implications for guiding both supervision and training for clinicians by providing an evidence-directed approach. It has been suggested that client-level feedback brings the voice of the client and caregivers directly into the supervisory session, a valuable addition to the clinician's perceptions in the discussion of individual clients (Duncan & Miller, 2000; Worthen & Lambert, 2007). Supervisors can assist clinicians in targeting areas for growth, as well as agency-wide training needs, by reflecting on patterns of strengths and weaknesses across multiple clients on the basis of case characteristics and treatment process data. The online learning modules on common factors include not only information but specific tools that can be used in supervision and clinical sessions. Finally, an innovative aspect of CFIT's design is the inclusion of implementation feedback to supervisors, intended to ease attendance to administrative matters.

By targeting clinicians as the agents of change, CFIT may help us get inside the black box of treatment and the service setting to see if change in clinician behavior and the task environment of the setting can generate positive outcomes at both the client and organizational levels.

## CONCLUSIONS AND IMPLICATIONS

We started this chapter by describing the evidence-based treatment debate and then examining the most recent meta-analytic studies to make sense of the confusing array of contradictory opinions. We have noted that the supporting data for the putative effectiveness of EBTs are not as strong as some would think. Thus, is it justifiable to base treatments in the community on approaches developed in the laboratory that have limited empirical support? Instead, we have argued for a different approach to improving outcomes that emphasizes common factors (but does not ignore EBTs) and the evidence developed not in the lab but in the community: PBE. Specifically, we believe that clinical service settings should be responsible for using an MFS to collect, process, and analyze data collected concurrent with treatment. Such a focus would significantly broaden our understanding of the factors that contribute to success, improve outcomes via consumer feedback to clinicians, and provide performance-enhancing training in the common factors to clinicians.

On the basis of our review of the literature, we offer the following implications for practice:

- The new APA definition of EBPP should be widely disseminated. Policymakers and third-party payers should recognize that rigorously collected and analyzed PBE is indeed an evidence-based practice. Given the apparent lack of demonstrated differential efficacy of approaches to child and adolescent problems, the field should no longer only promote specific approaches for specific disorders as examples of best practice nor tolerate unsupported claims of model superiority. Specific treatments for specific disorders are worthy of consideration but do not yet merit practice mandates by agencies, policy makers, or payers. Reliable and valid measurement of client response to treatment should be the guiding metric of best practice.
- The apparent low return on investment yielded by EBT over UC or TAU and the initial evidence for feedback suggests that available resources may be better used to support therapists in practice through such means as providing them with outcome feedback and supervision that promotes an outcome orientation to performance.

- As Lambert concludes in chapter 8 of this volume, it is indeed time for all youth practitioners to routinely measure child and adolescent outcomes and use PBE to make adjustments to tailor services to individual clients. It is time for all youth mental health agencies to partner with consumers to measure outcomes while simultaneously collecting and analyzing data to improve effectiveness and efficiency of services.
- High-quality community-based research in real clinical settings should become a priority to those who deliver mental heath services to children and adolescents. This PBE can further understanding of both specific treatments and common factors, improve outcomes, and directly evaluate different forms of training on outcome. It could further serve to facilitate meaningful engagement between the research and practice communities. This is a vital step to increasing both the use of research findings by practitioners and the clinical utility of youth mental health services research.
- MFSs are not a panacea nor are they simple and inexpensive to implement with high fidelity. MFSs will not work unless sufficient resources are provided for the required software, training, and supervision. Moreover, the culture of the setting has to become more receptive to the use of data-based decision making and ultimately more accountable for the services provided. Greater support from funders and policymakers are also necessary ingredients for success.

## QUESTIONS FROM THE EDITORS

1. *Given the state of research evidence on children and adolescents, where do you think research should be focused that would be most likely to produce results vital to improving mental health services to this population?*

The core issue to improving mental health services to children and adolescents is gaining greater understanding of clinical practice and how to change those practices. The field is only in the early stages of exploring the processes of practice, such as therapeutic alliance. Not knowing what clinicians do in UC settings has contributed to an approach to EBT that has discounted the process of therapy, as if what clinicians were doing prior to following a treatment manual does not matter. We believe that this is related to the larger problem of understanding how to integrate EBTs (such as a feedback system) into clinical practice. It is vital that the field promotes research that is conducted in real-world settings and acknowledges the complex interactions among client, clinician, and organizational factors as they influence implementation.

2. *Clearly, some child and adolescent therapists are more effective than others. You have indicated that clinical feedback is critical to improving the benefits of therapy. But this leaves open the question, "What are the characteristics and actions of the more effective therapists?"*

Although there is research that shows some therapists are more effective than others (e.g., Kim, Wampold, & Bolt, 2006; Wampold & Brown, 2005), the evidence is limited in its practical application. The number of clients and client sessions needed to conduct research on individual therapist differences is a significant obstacle. For example, if the individual clinician contributes only 3% of the variance, one would need more than 100 clients to determine the effectiveness of that clinician at 80% reliability. A systematic feedback system that includes weekly or biweekly measurement of therapeutic processes and client outcomes could make research on individual differences in therapist effectiveness more feasible.

Just the provision of feedback is necessary for improvement, but it is not sufficient. So our response to the question about clinician characteristics is the all too common and worn-out request for more research. We are equally ignorant about what actions clinicians should take. We can provide a specific example from our experience in learning from the clinicians and supervisors involved in our ongoing evaluation of CFIT. The therapeutic alliance is one of those processes that is considered central to all treatments, yet we could not find an experiment that tested whether alliance can be improved. Can it be taught or are you born with it? Once you have it, do you have it ever after? It is interesting that initial perceptions of our CFIT client-level feedback focused more on the value of feedback for new clinicians as opposed to those with more experience. Yet, clinicians and supervisors do not hesitate to support the need for supervision as a mechanism for learning, no matter how many years of practice one has had. In part, we believe this contradictory stance stems simply from the fact that supervision is standard practice, yet feedback to therapists on clients is new, and innovation can feel threatening. However, perhaps an attitude of openness and growth is an important characteristic of the effective clinician.

3. *You have described a feedback system that appears grounded in the research on psychotherapy as well as an understanding of how feedback is used generally. What is the role of supervisors and managers in feedback systems, and why is this human element missing in most systems? Just as clients often need the relationship with a therapist to change, perhaps therapists need the relationship with a supervisor to change.*

In our ongoing evaluation of CFIT, we have identified supervision as a key mechanism for supporting clinician's integration of feedback into clinical practice. We have provided resources for ongoing coaching with supervisors across the country to empower them to better support clinicians in their use of CFIT. Clinical supervision typically encompasses three realms through a consultative process between the supervisor and the clinician: monitoring individual client welfare and progress, enhancing the clinician's professional growth, and attending to administrative issues, such as completion of required paperwork (e.g., Bernard & Goodyear, 2004; Falender & Shafranske, 2004). CFIT directly supports all three of these supervisory functions. Supervisors have full access to client-level feedback to review on their own and together with the clinician during supervision. The addition of the client's voice to supervision could support exploration of the clinician's perceptions of treatment processes or specific therapeutic events. CFIT is an excellent tool for supervisors and managers to identify learning opportunities by aggregating data across multiple clients. With regard to support for administrative issues, supervisors are provided with their own feedback reports on implementation. This includes real-time information on rates of questionnaire completion and feedback viewing by clinicians. However, supervision also appears to be one of those areas in which there is a huge amount of material written about it but little empirical research to support that material. As a final note, we also discovered that in many sites supervisor training was not sufficient for good implementation. We now include counselor training in CFIT.

## REFERENCES

American Psychological Association Presidential Task Force on Evidence-Based Practice. (2006). Evidence-based practice in psychology. *American Psychologist, 61,* 271–285.

Angold, A., Costello, J. E., & Erkanli, A. (1999). Comorbidity. *Journal of Child Psychology and Psychiatry, 40,* 57–87.

Angold, A., Messer, S. C., Stangl, D., Farmer, E. M., Costello, E. J., & Burns B. J. (1998). Perceived parental burden and service use for child and adolescent psychiatric disorders. *American Journal of Public Health, 88,* 75–80.

Arnkoff, D. B., Glass, C. L., & Shapiro, S. J. (2002). Expectations and preferences. In Norcross, J. C. (Ed.), *Psychotherapy relationships that work: Therapist contributions and responsiveness to patients* (pp. 335–356). New York: Oxford University Press.

Asay, T. P., Lambert, M. J., Gregersen, A. T., & Goates, M. K. (2002). Using patient-refocused research in evaluating treatment outcome in private practice. *Journal of Clinical Psychology, 58,* 1213–1225.

Baskin, T. W., Tierney, S. C., Minami, T., & Wampold, B. E. (2003). Establishing specificity in psychotherapy: A meta-analysis of structural equivalence of placebo controls. *Journal of Consulting and Clinical Psychology, 71,* 973–979.

Bernard, J. M., & Goodyear, R. K. (2004). *Fundamentals of clinical supervision* (3rd ed.). Needham Heights, MA: Allyn & Bacon.

Beutler, L. E., Malik, M., Alimohamed, S., Harwood, T. M., Talebi, H., & Noble, S. (2004). Therapist variables. In M. J. Lambert (Ed.), *Bergin and Garfield's handbook of psychotherapy and behavior change* (5th ed., pp. 227–306). New York: Wiley.

Bickman, L. (1999). Practice makes perfect and other myths about mental health services. *American Psychologist, 54,* 958–973.

Bickman, L. (Ed.). (2005). A common factors approach to improving mental health services [Special issue]. *Mental Health Services Research, 7*(1).

Bickman, L. (2008). A measurement feedback system (MFS) is necessary to improve mental health outcomes. *Journal of the American Academy of Child and Adolescent Psychiatry, 47,* 1114–1119. doi:10.1097/chi.0b013e3181825af8

Bickman, L., Heflinger, C. A., Northrup, D., Sonnichsen, S., & Schilling, S. (1998). Long-term outcomes of family caregiver empowerment. *Journal of Child and Family Studies, 7,* 269–282.

Bickman, L., Riemer, M., Breda, C., & Kelley, S. D. (2006). CFIT: A system to provide a continuous quality improvement infrastructure through organizational responsiveness, measurement, training, and feedback. *Report on Emotional and Behavioral Disorders in Youth, 6*(4), 86–87, 93–94.

Bickman, L., Riemer, M., Lambert, E. W., Kelley, S. D., Breda, C., Dew, S. E., et al. (Eds.). (2007). *Manual of the Peabody Treatment Progress Battery* [Electronic version]. Nashville, TN: Vanderbilt University.

Bickman, L., Vides de Andrade, A. R., Lambert, E. W., Doucette, A., Sapyta, J., Boyd, A. S., et al. (2004). Youth therapeutic alliance in intensive treatment settings. *Journal of Behavioral Health Services & Research, 31*(2), 134–148.

Bonanno, G. A., & Mancini, A. D. (2008). The human capacity to thrive in the face of potential trauma. *Pediatrics, 121,* 369–375.

Bordin, E. S. (1979). The generalizability of the psychoanalytic of the working alliance. *Psychotherapy: Theory, Research, and Practice, 16,* 252–260.

Bordin, E. S. (1994). Theory and research on the therapeutic working alliance: New directions. In A. O. Horvath, & L. S. Greenberg (Eds.), *The working alliance: Theory, research, and practice* (pp. 13–37). Oxford, England: Wiley.

Bradley, L. J., Sexton, T. H., & Smith, H. B. (2005). The American Counseling Association Practice Research Network (ACA-PRN): A new research tool. *Journal of Counseling & Development, 83,* 488–491.

Brannan, A. M., & Heflinger, C.A. (2001). Distinguishing caregiver strain from psychological distress: Modeling the relationships among child, family, and caregiver variables. *Journal of Child and Family Studies, 10,* 405–418.

Brannan, A. M., & Heflinger, C.A. (2005). Child behavioral health service use and caregiver strain: Comparison of managed care and fee-for-service Medicaid systems. *Mental Health Services Research, 7,* 197–211.

Brannan, A. M., Heflinger, C. A. & Foster, E. M. (2003). The role of caregiver strain and other family variables in determining children's use of mental health services. *Journal of Emotional and Behavioral Disorders, 11,* 78–92.

Breda, C., & Heflinger, C. A. (2004). Predicting incentives to change among adolescents with substance abuse disorder. *American Journal of Drug and Alcohol Abuse*, *30*, 251–267.

Burlingame, G. M., Wells, M. G., & Lambert, M. J. (1996). *The Youth Outcome Questionnaire*. Stevenson, MD: American Professional Credentialing and Services.

Chorpita, B. F., Daleiden, E. L., & Weisz, J. R. (2005). Identifying and selecting the common elements of evidence based interventions: A distillation and matching model. *Mental Health Services Research*, *7*, 5–20.

Cohen, J. (1988). *Statistical power analysis for the behavioral sciences* (2nd ed.). Hillsdale, NJ: Erlbaum.

Crits-Christoph, P. & Mintz, J. (1991). Implications of therapist effects for the design and analysis of comparative studies of psychotherapies. *Journal of Consulting and Clinical Psychology*, *59*, 20–26.

Cromley, T., & Lavigne, J. V. (2008). Predictors and consequences of early gains in child psychotherapy. *Psychotherapy*, *45*, 42–60.

Davis, D. A., Thomson, M. A., Freemantle, N., Wolf, F. M., Mazmanian, P., & Taylor-Vaisey, A. (1999). The impact of formal continuing medical education: Do conferences, workshops, rounds, and other traditional continuing activities change physician behavior or health care outcomes? *Journal of the American Medical Association*, *282*, 867–874.

Dennis, M., Godley, S. H., Diamond, G., Tims, F. M., Babor, T., Donaldson, J., et al. (2004). The Cannabis Youth Treatment (CYT) Study: Main findings from two randomized trials. *Journal of Substance Abuse Treatment*, *27*, 197–213.

Dew, S. E., & Bickman, L. (2005). Client expectancies about therapy. *Mental Health Services Research*, *7*, 21–33.

Dinger, U., Strack, M., Leichsenring, F., Wilmers, F., & Schauenburg, H. (2008). Therapist effects on outcome and alliance in inpatient psychotherapy. *Journal of Clinical Psychology*, *64*(3), 344–354.

Duncan, B. L., & Miller, S. D. (2000). *The heroic client: Doing client-directed, outcome-informed therapy*. San Francisco: Jossey-Bass

Duncan, B. L., Miller, S. D., & Sparks, J. A. (2003). *The Child Outcome Rating Scale*. Ft. Lauderdale, FL: Authors.

Duncan, B. L., Miller, S., & Sparks, J. (2004). *The heroic client: A revolutionary way to improve effectiveness through client-directed, outcome-informed therapy*. San Francisco: Jossey-Bass.

Duncan, B. L., Sparks, J., Miller, S., Bohanske, R., & Claud, D. (2006). Giving youth a voice: A preliminary study of the reliability and validity of a brief outcome measure for children, adolescents, and caretakers. *Journal of Brief Therapy*, *5*, 5–22.

Falender, C. A., & Shafranske, E. P. (2004). *Clinical supervision: A competency based approach*. Washington, DC: American Psychological Association.

Farmer, E. M., Burns, B. J., Angold, A., & Costello, E. J. (1997). Impact of children's mental health problems on families: Relationships with service use. *Journal of Emotional and Behavioral Disorders, 5*, 230–238.

Fields, S., Handelsman, J., Karver, M. S., & Bickman, L. (2004). *Parental and child factors that affect the therapeutic alliance.* Paper presented at the 17th Annual Meeting of the Florida Mental Health Institute's A System of Care for Children's Mental Health: Expanding the Research Base, Tampa, FL.

Frank, J. (1961). *Persuasion and healing.* Baltimore, MD: Johns Hopkins University Press.

Frank, J. (1973). *Persuasion and healing: A comparative study of psychotherapy* (2nd ed.). Baltimore, MD: Johns Hopkins University Press.

Garcia, J. A., & Weisz, J. R. (2002). When youth mental health care stops: Therapeutic relationship problems and other reasons for ending youth outpatient treatment. *Journal of Consulting and Clinical Psychology, 70*, 439–443.

Glisson, C., & Hemmelgarn, A. (1998). The effects of organizational climate and interorganizational coordination on the quality and outcomes of children's service systems. *Child Abuse and Neglect, 22*, 401–421.

Green, J. (2006). Annotation: The therapeutic alliance—A significant but neglected variable in child mental health treatment studies. *Journal of Child Psychology and Psychiatry, 47*, 425–435.

Hammen, C., Rudolph, K., Weisz, J. R., Burge, D., & Rao, U. (1999). The context of depression in clinic referred youth: Neglected areas in treatment. *Journal of the American Academy of Child & Adolescent Psychiatry, 38*, 64–71.

Hawkins, E. J., Lambert, M. J., Vermeersch, D. A., Slade, K., & Tuttle, K. (2004). The therapeutic effects of providing client progress information to patients and therapists. *Psychotherapy Research, 10*, 308–327.

Hawley, K. M., & Weisz, J. R. (2003). Child, parent and therapist (dis)agreement on target problems in outpatient therapy: The therapist's dilemma and its implications. *Journal of Consulting and Clinical Psychology, 71*, 62–70.

Hawley, K. M., & Weisz, J. R. (2005). Youth versus parent working alliance in usual clinical care: Distinctive associations with retention, satisfaction, and treatment outcome. *Journal of Clinical Child and Adolescent Psychology, 34*, 117–128.

Heflinger, C. A., Bickman, L., Northrup, D., & Sonnichsen, S. (1997). A theory-driven intervention and evaluation to explore family caregiver empowerment. *Journal of Emotional and Behavioral Disorders, 5*, 184–191.

Hemmelgarn, A. L., Glisson, C., & James, L. R. (2006). Organizational culture and climate: Implications for services and interventions research. *Clinical Psychology: Science and Practice, 13*, 73–89.

Hernandez, M., Hodges, S., & Cascardi, M. (1998). The ecology of outcomes: System accountability on children's mental health. *The Journal of Behavioral Health Services & Research, 25*, 136–150.

Hinds, P. S., Quargnenti, A., Fairclough, D., Bush, A. J., Betcher, D., Rissmiller, G., et al. (1999). Hopefulness and its characteristics in adolescents with cancer. *Western Journal of Nursing Research, 21,* 600–620.

Hoagwood, K., Burns, B., Kiser, L., Ringeisen, H., & Schoenwald, S. K. (2001). Evidence-based practice in child and adolescent mental health services. *Psychiatric Services, 52,* 1179–1189.

Hodges, K. (2000). *Child and adolescent functional assessment scale* (2nd ed.). Ypsilanti: Eastern Michigan University.

Hodges, K. & Wotring, J. (2004). The role of monitoring outcomes in initiating implementation of evidence-based treatments at the state level. *Psychiatric Services, 55,* 396–400.

Howard, K. I., Moras, K., Brill, P. L., Martinovich, Z., & Lutz, W. (1996). Evaluation of psychotherapy: Efficacy, effectiveness, and patient progress. *American Psychologist, 51,* 1059–1064.

Hutchings, J., Appleton, P., Smith, M., Lane, E., & Nash, S. (2002). Evaluation of two treatments for children with severe behavior problems: Child behavior and maternal mental health outcomes. *Behavior and Cognitive Psychology, 30,* 279–295.

Jensen, P. S., Weersing, R., Hoagwood, K. E., & Goldman, E. (2005). What is the evidence for evidence based treatments? A hard look at our soft underbelly. *Mental Health Services Research, 7,* 53–74.

Karver, M. S., Handelsman, J. B., Fields, S., & Bickman, L. (2005). A theoretical model of common process factors in youth and family therapy. *Mental Health Services Research, 7,* 35–51.

Karver, M. S., Handelsman, J., Fields, S., & Bickman, L. (2006). Meta-analysis of therapeutic relationship variables in youth and family therapy: The evidence for different relationship variables in the child and adolescent treatment outcome literature. *Clinical Psychology Review, 26,* 50–65

Karver, M. S., Lambert, W., & Bickman, L. (2003, March). *Strength based assessment: The Vanderbilt Positive Functioning Index—Revised.* Paper presented at the 16th Annual Meeting of the Florida Mental Health Institute's A System of Care for Children's Mental Health: Expanding the Research Base, Tampa, FL.

Kazdin, A. E. (2000). *Psychotherapy for children and adolescents: Directions for research and practice.* New York: Oxford University Press.

Kazdin, A. E. (2004). Psychotherapy for children and adolescents. In M. J. Lambert (Ed.), *Bergin and Garfield's handbook of psychotherapy and behavior change* (5th ed., pp. 543–589). New York: Wiley.

Kazdin, A. E., Bass, D., Ayers, W. A., & Rodgers, A. (1990). Empirical and clinical focus of child and adolescent psychotherapy research. *Journal of Consulting and Clinical Psychology, 58,* 729–740.

Kazdin, A. E., Marciano, P. L., & Whitley, M. K. (2005). The therapeutic alliance in cognitive–behavioral treatment for children referred for oppositional, aggressive, and antisocial behavior. *Journal of Consulting and Clinical Psychology, 73,* 726–730.

Kazdin, A. E., & Wassell, G. (2000). Predictors of barriers to treatment and thera-peutic change in outpatient therapy for antisocial children and their families. *Mental Health Services Research, 2*, 27–40.

Kazdin, A. E., & Whitley, M. K. (2006). Comorbidity, case complexity, and effects of evidence-based treatment for children referred for disruptive behavior. *Journal of Consulting and Clinical Psychology, 74*, 455–467.

Kazdin, A. E., Whitley, M., & Marciano, P. L. (2006). Child–therapist and parent–therapist alliance and therapeutic change in the treatment of children referred for oppositional, aggressive and antisocial behavior. *Journal of Child Psychology and Psychiatry, 47*, 436–445.

Kelley, S. D., & Bickman, L. (2009). Beyond outcomes monitoring: Measurement feedback systems in child and adolescent clinical practice. *Current Opinion in Psychiatry, 22*, 363–368.

Kim, D. M., Wampold, B. E., & Bolt, D. M. (2006). Therapist effects in psycho-therapy: A random-effects modeling of the National Institute of Mental Health Treatment of Depression Collaborative Research Program data. *Psychotherapy Research, 16*, 161–172.

Kluger, A. N., & DeNisi, A. (1996). Effects of feedback intervention on performance: A historical review, a meta-analysis, and a preliminary feedback intervention theory. *Psychological Bulletin, 119*, 254–284.

Lambert, M. J. (Ed.). (2005). Enhancing psychotherapy outcome through feedback [Special issue]. *Journal of Clinical Psychology, 61*(2).

Lambert, M. J. (2007). Presidential address: What we have learned from a decade of research aimed at improving psychotherapy outcome in routine care. *Psycho-therapy Research, 17*(1), 1–14.

Lambert, M. J., & Barley, D. E. (2002). Research summary on the therapeutic rela-tionship and psychotherapy outcome. In J. C. Norcross (Ed.), *Psychotherapy rela-tionships that work: Therapist contributions and responsiveness to patients* (pp. 17–32). Oxford, England: Oxford University Press.

Lambert, M. J., & Ogles, B. M. (1997). The effectiveness of psychotherapy supervision. In E. C. Watkins Jr. (Ed.), *Handbook of psychotherapy supervision* (pp. 421–446). Hoboken, NJ: Wiley.

Lambert, M. J., & Ogles, B. M. (2004). The efficacy and effectiveness of psycho-therapy. In M. J. Lambert (Ed.), *Bergin and Garfield's handbook of psychotherapy and behavior change* (5th ed., pp. 139–193). New York: Wiley.

Lambert, M. J., Whipple, J. L., Smart, D. W., Vermeersch, D. A., Nielsen, S. L., & Hawkins, E. J. (2001). The effects of providing therapists with feedback on patient progress during psychotherapy: Are outcomes enhanced? *Psychotherapy Research, 11*, 49–68.

Luborsky, L., Diguer, L., Seligman, D. A., Rosenthal, R., Krause, E. D., Johnson, S., et al. (1999). The researcher's own therapy alliances: A "wild card" in compar-isons of treatment efficacy. *Clinical Psychology: Science and Practice, 6*, 95–106.

Lutz, W., Leon, S. C., Martinovich, Z., Lyons, J. S., & Stiles, W. B. (2007). Therapist effects in outpatient psychotherapy: A three-level growth curve approach. *Journal of Counseling Psychology, 54*(1), 32–39.

Margison, F. R., Barkham, M., Evans, C., McGrath, G., Clark, J. M., Audin, K., & Connel, J. (2000). Measurement and psychotherapy: Evidence-based practice and practice-based evidence. *British Journal of Psychiatry, 177*, 123–130.

Marsick, V. J., & Watkins, K. E. (2003). Demonstrating the value of an organization's learning culture: The dimensions of the Learning Organization Questionnaire. *Advances in Developing Human Resources, 5*, 132–151.

McLeod, B. D., & Weisz, J. R. (2005). The Therapy Process Observational Coding System-Alliance Scale: Measure characteristics and prediction of outcome in usual clinical practice. *Journal of Consulting and Clinical Psychology, 73*, 323–333.

Miller, S. D., & Duncan, B. L. (2000). *The Outcome Rating Scale*. Chicago: Authors.

Miller, S. D., Wampold, B., & Varhely (2008). Direct comparisons of treatments for youth disorders: A meta-analysis. *Psychotherapy Research, 18*, 5–14.

Minami, T., & Wampold, B. E. (2008). Adult psychotherapy in the real world. In B. W. Walsh (Ed.), *Biennial review of counseling psychology* (pp. 27–45). New York: Routledge/Taylor & Francis Group.

Norcross, J. C., Beutler, L. E., & Levant, R. F. (2006). *Evidence-based practices in mental health: Debate and dialogue on the fundamental questions*. Washington, DC: American Psychological Association.

NSW Department of Health. (2004). *Your guide to MH-OAT. Clinician's reference guide to NSW mental health outcomes and assessment tools*. Sydney, Australia: Author.

Ogles, B. M., Carlston, D., Hatfield, D., Melendez, G., Dowell, K., & Fields, S. A. (2006). The role of fidelity and feedback in the wraparound approach. *Journal of Child and Family Studies, 15*, 115–129.

Ogles, B. M., Melendez, G., Davis, D. C., & Lunnen, K. M. (1999). *The Ohio Youth Problems, Functioning, and Satisfaction Scales (Short Form): User's manual*. Athens: Ohio University.

Ollendick, T. H., & Davis, T. E. (2004). Empirically supported treatments for children and adolescents: Where to from here? *Clinical Psychology: Science and Practice, 11*, 289–294.

Patterson, P., Matthey, S., & Baker, M. (2006). Using mental health outcome measures in everyday clinical practice. *Australasian Psychiatry, 14*, 133–136.

Riemer, M., & Bickman, L. (in press). Using program theory to link social psychology and program evaluation. In M. M. Mark, S. I. Donaldson & B. Campbell (Eds.), *Social psychology and program/policy evaluation*. New York: Guilford Press.

Riemer, M., Rosof-Williams, J., & Bickman, L. (2005). Theories related to changing clinician practice. *Child and Adolescent Psychiatric Clinics of North America, 14*, 241–254.

Sapyta, J., Riemer, M., & Bickman, L. (2005). Feedback to clinicians: Theory, research, and practice. *Journal of Clinical Psychology, 6,* 145–153.

Schmidt, F. L. (1992). What do data really mean? Research findings, meta-analysis, and cumulative knowledge in psychology. *American Psychologist, 47,* 1173–1181.

Shirk, S. R., & Karver, M. (2003). Prediction of treatment outcome from relationship variables in child and adolescent therapy: A meta-analytic review. *Journal of Consulting and Clinical Psychology, 71,* 452-464.

Simpson, D. D. (2001). *Evidence for the TCU treatment process model.* Retrieved July 14, 2009, from http://www.ibr.tcu.edu/presentations/PDF/tpm-evidence.PDF

Smith, H. B., Sexton, T. H., & Bradley, L. J. (2005). The practice research network: Research into practice, practice into research. *Counselling & Psychotherapy Research, 5,* 285–290.

Snyder, C. R. (2002). Hope theory: Rainbows in the mind. *Psychological Inquiry, 13,* 249–275.

Snyder, C. R., Hoza, B., Pelham, W. E., Rapoff, M., Ware, L., Danovsky, M., et al. (1997). The development and validation of the Children's Hope Scale. *Journal of Pediatric Psychology, 22,* 399–421.

Snyder, C. R., Michael, S. T., & Cheavens, J. S. (1999). Hope as a psychotherapeutic foundation of common factors, placebos, and expectancies. In M. A. Hubble, B. L. Duncan, & S. D. Miller (Eds.), *The heart and soul of change: What works in therapy* (pp. 179–200). Washington, DC: American Psychological Association.

Spielmans, G. I., Pasek, L. F., & McFall, J. P. (2007). What are the active ingredients in cognitive and behavioral psychotherapy for anxious and depressed children? A meta-analytic review. *Clinical Psychology Review, 27,* 642–654.

Valle, M. F., Huebner, E. S., & Suldo, S. M. (2004). Further evaluation of the Children's Hope Scale. *Journal of Psychoeducational Assessment, 22,* 320–337.

Wampold, B. E. (2001). *The great psychotherapy debate: Models, methods, and findings.* Mahwah, NJ: Erlbaum.

Wampold, B. E., & Bolt, D. M. (2007). The consequences of "anchoring" in longitudinal multilevel models: Bias in the estimation of patient variability and therapist effects. *Psychotherapy Research, 17,* 509–514.

Wampold, B. E., & Brown, G. S. (2005). Estimating variability in outcomes attributable to therapists: A naturalistic study of outcomes in managed care. *Journal of Consulting and Clinical Psychology, 73,* 914–923.

Wampold, B. E., Mondin, G. W., Moody, M., Stich, F., Benson, K., & Ahn, H. (1997). A meta-analysis of outcome studies comparing bona fide psychotherapies: Empirically, "all must have prizes." *Psychological Bulletin, 122,* 203–215.

Weersing, V. R., & Weisz, J. R. (2002). Mechanisms of action of youth psychotherapy. *Journal of Child Psychology & Psychiatry and Allied Disciplines, 43,* 3–29.

Weisz, J. R. (2004). *Psychotherapy for children and adolescents: Evidence-based treatments and case examples.* Cambridge, England: Cambridge University Press.

Weisz, J. R., & Gray, J. S. (2008). Evidence-based psychotherapy for children and adolescents: Data from the present and a model for the future. *Child and Adolescent Mental Health, 13*(2), 54–65.

Weisz, J. R., Jensen-Doss, A., & Hawley, K. M. (2006). Evidence-based youth psychotherapies versus usual clinical care: A meta-analysis of direct comparisons. *American Psychologist, 61*, 671–689.

Weisz, J. R., McCarty, C. A., & Valeri, S. M. (2006). Effects of psychotherapy for depression in children and adolescents: A meta-analysis. *Psychological Bulletin, 132*, 132–149.

Westen, D., Novotny, C. M., & Thompson-Brenner, H. (2004). The empirical status of empirically supported psychotherapies: Assumptions, findings, and reporting in clinical trials. *Psychological Bulletin, 130*, 631–663.

Worthen, V. E., & Lambert, M. J. (2007). Outcome oriented supervision: Advantages of adding systematic client tracking to supportive consultations. *Counseling and Psychotherapy Research, 7*, 48–53.

Yatchmenoff, D. K., Koren, P. E., Friesen, B. J., Gordon, L. J, & Kinney, R. F. (1998). Enrichment and stress in families caring for a child with a serious emotional disorder. *Journal of Child and Family Studies, 7*, 129–145.

Yeh, M., & Weisz, J. R. (2001). Why are we here at the clinic? Parent–child (dis)agreement on referral problems at outpatient treatment entry. *Journal of Consulting and Clinical Psychology, 69*, 1018–1025.

# 12

## COMMON FACTORS IN COUPLE AND FAMILY THERAPY: MUST ALL HAVE PRIZES?

JACQUELINE A. SPARKS AND BARRY L. DUNCAN

Great doubt: great awakening. Little doubt: little awakening. No doubt: no awakening.

—Zen mantra

Marriage and family therapy (MFT),[1] though fashionably late, has taken a seat at the empirically validated table. Many argue that determining what is and who defines *empirically validated* entails significant implications for the field's future and its very identity (Duncan, Miller, & Sparks, 2004; Sexton, Ridley, & Kleiner, 2004; Sprenkle, Blow, & Dickey, 1999). What would seem to be common sense—use of evidence-based practice—is intertwined with politics and power. As Norcross, Beutler, and Levant (2006) put it, "defining evidence, deciding what qualifies as evidence, and applying what is privileged as evidence are complicated matters with deep philosophical and huge practical consequences" (p. 7).

This chapter furthers this discussion, exploring the question, "Does the dodo verdict—uniform not differential efficacy—hold true for systemic therapy?" For couple and family approaches, have all won and must all have prizes? A review of the evidence for absolute and relative efficacy for MFT is followed by a critical analysis of major comparative trials. Next, the role of

---

[1]This chapter uses *marriage and family therapy* and *couple and family therapy* interchangeably, recognizing that although MFT is a common identifier, marriage does not represent all couples.

common factors in the MFT empirical literature is examined. The chapter concludes with implications for practice, training, and research.[2]

## EFFICACY OF COUPLE AND FAMILY THERAPY

*Absolute efficacy*, the effects of treatment compared with no treatment, addresses the question "Does it work?" (Wampold, 2001; see chap. 2, this volume). Historical and current data indicate the answer to be an unequivocal "yes." Shadish and Baldwin (2002) meta-analyzed 20 published and unpublished meta-analytic studies of family, couple, and couple enrichment intervention. They found an average effect size (ES) of 0.58 for 12 meta-analyses comparing MFT with no-therapy controls. These findings approximate the 0.51 ES for the 70 trials comparing MFT with controls in Shadish et al. (1993). In answer to the question of clinical significance (Jacobson & Truax, 1991), Shadish and Baldwin (2002) indicated that MFT clients moved from distressed to non-distressed ranges 40% to 50% of the time. Confirming this estimate, in a large study of 134 couples, Christensen et al. (2004) reported that 48% of couples reached recovered status.

Controlled outcome studies for drug abuse, conduct disorders, delinquency, alcoholism, relationship enhancement, marital difficulties, schizophrenia, and other problems show robust efficacy for family and couple interventions (Sprenkle, 2003). Carr (2000a, 2000b) examined reviews and controlled trials for family intervention through the 1990s and found effects superior to no treatment. Cottrell and Boston (2002) also reported favorable results for family therapy over no treatment for conduct disorders,[3] substance misuse, and eating disorders. Finally, in a review of home-based family treatment, Diamond and Josephson (2005) found superiority of family intervention over no treatment both as a stand-alone and augmentation modality for youth depression, anxiety, conduct and attention-deficit disorders, and drug abuse.

Noteworthy is the finding that marital therapy ESs are somewhat larger than those for family therapy. In Shadish and Baldwin (2002), the average ES for marital therapy was 0.84 compared with 0.58 for family therapy. Regarding specific approaches, Shadish and Baldwin (2005) meta-analytically examined randomized trials of behavioral marital therapy (BMT) and found it significantly more effective than no treatment ($d = 0.59$). Gollan and Jacobson (2002) identified five couple treatments

---

[2]This chapter does not exhaustively or historically review all the studies concerning covered topics but rather chooses more contemporary studies that are representative of the issues at hand.
[3]The word *disorder* is used only to report the research findings and in no way endorses the science or ethics of diagnosis.

in addition to BMT with proven efficacy over no treatment: emotionally focused therapy (EFT; Greenberg & Johnson, 1988); integrative couple therapy (Jacobson & Christensen, 1996), cognitive–behavioral marital therapy (CBMT; Baucom & Epstein, 1990), strategic therapy (Goldman & Greenberg, 1992); and insight-oriented marital therapy (IOMT; Snyder & Wills, 1989). Finally, Christensen et al. (2004) found an ES of 0.86 for traditional behavioral couple therapy (TBCT) and integrative behavioral couple therapy (IBCT).

In sum, it can be justifiably concluded that family and couple therapy, in comparison with no treatment, is efficacious in alleviating a range of symptomatic complaints. Although posttest treatment gains tend to diminish somewhat at follow-up and as many as half of clients do not progress to nonclinical functioning, when compared with no treatment, MFT offers a viable opportunity for positive change. The only qualification to these conclusions concerns the dearth of data collected in real-world practice settings (Addison, Sandberg, Corby, Robila, & Platt, 2002; Shadish & Baldwin, 2002) and whether current research encompasses the diversity of a growing segment of family and couple clientele (Northey, 2002).

*Relative efficacy*, the effects produced by comparing two treatments, addresses the question, "Does one work better than another?" (Wampold, 2001). Unlike the response to the question of absolute efficacy, the answer here is controversial. Is the dodo bird correct or mistaken in declaring that all are winners and all must have prizes? If models contain unique ingredients that are responsible for outcome effects, then variations in efficacy will be found in comparative trials (differential efficacy). If common factors are responsible for outcome, then outcomes will generally be homogenous in head-to-head model comparisons (uniform efficacy).

On one hand, some have reported differential effects of one approach over another. For example, summarizing the findings of all examined trials at the time, Pinsof and Wynne (1995) concluded that there was convincing evidence for MFT superiority over individual approaches for certain problems and populations. They particularly noted studies that revealed superior outcomes for persons diagnosed with schizophrenia who received psychoeducational family therapy compared with treatment as usual (TAU; Goldstein & Miklowitz, 1995). Similarly, Stanton and Shadish's (1997) meta-analysis of 15 drug abuse outcome studies found superior effects for family–couple interventions over individual and group therapies. Some see these findings as just scratching the surface. For example, Sexton, Ridley, and Kleiner (2004) expressed the belief that future meta-analyses that examine approaches adhering to treatment-specific protocols will confirm the relative efficacy of models and the critical relationship between technique and outcome.

On the other hand, meta-analyses over the past 17 years and recent comparative investigations have not found evidence for differential efficacy nor the predicted advantage of models adhering to specific protocols. The Shadish et al. (1993) meta-analysis of 163 randomized trials did not find significant differential effects of couple and family therapy over individual therapy or differences between various MFT orientations. In a later review of 20 meta-analyses of MFT interventions, Shadish and Baldwin (2002) similarly found few significant differences among various models. When comparing MFT approaches with alternative treatments, any differences were small and tended to get smaller over time. Confirming this conclusion, a recent meta-analysis of differential efficacy in the treatment of youth disorders, including family therapy, found some differences in efficacy among treatments, but the upper bound of the difference was small (Miller, Wampold, & Varhely, 2008

Couple therapy follows suit. In Dunn and Schwebel's (1995) meta-analysis of BMT, CBMT, IOMT, and EFT, weighted mean ESs were not significantly different at either posttreatment or follow-up on marital behavior, including target complaint. IOMT was significantly better on relationship ratings at posttreatment, but not at follow-up. Christensen and Heavey's (1999) review of couple therapy noted that the few studies showing the superiority of one treatment over another favored the investigator's treatment and had not been replicated. They concluded, "In short, there is no convincing evidence at this point that any one couple therapy is better than another" (p. 173). Confirming that conclusion in a comparison of TBCT and IBCT, Christensen et al. (2004) reported, "For the most part, TBCT and IBCT performed similarly across measures, despite being demonstrably different treatments" (p. 188).

In the Cannabis Youth Treatment (CYT) Study (Dennis et al., 2004), considered by many to be the largest and most methodologically sound investigation of adolescents to date, 600 adolescents were assigned either to treatment with motivational enhancement therapy plus cognitive–behavioral therapy (5 or 12 sessions), family education and therapy, adolescent community reinforcement approach, or multidimensional family therapy (MDFT). Comparisons between conditions found roughly equivalent significant pre–post treatment effects that were stable in terms of days of abstinence and percent in recovery by the end of the study. The similarities in outcome in the CYT, the authors noted, are consistent with studies with adults comparing multiple interventions for substance abuse.[4]

---

[4]Cost-effectiveness comparisons did indicate moderate to large differences between treatment conditions, with motivational enhancement therapy, cognitive–behavioral therapy, and adolescent community reinforcement the most cost effective, and family education and therapy and MDFT the least.

## MUST ALL HAVE PRIZES?

Although the preponderance of the evidence suggests the dodo verdict to be true to form in MFT, the view that some approaches are better than others persists. To resolve this apparent conundrum, one must take a closer look at what constitutes claims of superiority in those studies that report differential efficacy. Two factors must always be kept in mind when a report of differential efficacy is advanced: allegiance factors and unfair comparisons.

### Allegiance

As noted in chapter 2 and throughout this volume, *allegiance* refers to researchers' belief in and commitment to a particular approach. Allegiance can exert a large influence on outcome in comparative studies. For example, Luborsky et al. (1999) used three types of allegiance measures (reprint method, ratings by colleagues, and researcher self-ratings) and found that allegiance explained 69% of the variance in outcomes. In Miller et al.'s (2008) analysis of differential treatment of youth disorders, researcher allegiance was found to be strongly associated with the difference in ESs; when allegiance was controlled, the differences among treatments vanished. Often, allegiance-bound therapists are compared with colleagues without similar ties to models. As a point of comparison, in the CYT mentioned above, the principal investigators had no particular allegiance to the models compared, and the therapists believed their approach to be superior and were equally committed to their models. As a result, no differences were found.

One step further, when therapists in trials are trained and supervised by the model advocate, at a site where the model is taught, and in a study designed by a model proponent, they most likely will have allegiance to the researcher or trainer's model (Wampold, 2001). Consider the role of allegiance in findings for the efficacy of EFT. Johnson (2003) referred to a meta-analysis of four EFT studies (Johnson, Hunsley, Greenberg, & Schindler, 1999), indicating an ES of 1.3. This estimate significantly outstrips the 0.84 reported by Shadish and Baldwin (2002) for couple therapy. Calling the dodo bird verdict the "dodo cliché," Johnson (2003) explained, "Some researchers . . . believe that, like the Dodo bird, the idea of some models of intervention being more effective than others is extinct" (p. 367). Setting aside this erroneous interpretation of the dodo bird verdict, an examination of allegiance in the meta-analyzed studies addresses the assertion that "EFT appears to demonstrate the best outcomes at present" (Johnson, 2003, p. 365).

First, two trials of the four compared EFT with a wait-list control group and predictably found superior outcomes; demonstrations of efficacy over placebo or no treatment are not comparisons with other approaches and therefore have no bearing on the dodo verdict. Two studies investigated differential effects. In Johnson and Greenberg (1985), EFT was superior to problem-solving treatment on 6 of 13 outcome indices at termination and 2 of the 5 reported at 8-week follow-up. Both EFT and problem-solving treatment achieved significant differences over the waitlist and clinically significant change (recovery into a nondistressed range), with equivalent maintenance of that change. This article acknowledged that the first author had served as a therapist in the study and that the authors developed EFT, raising concerns about therapist allegiance to the contrasted approach conducted in an EFT hotbed. In the second trial addressing differential efficacy, Goldman and Greenberg (1992), researchers had comparable allegiance to the treatments delivered—EFT and integrated systemic therapy—and no significant differences were found.

Researcher allegiance may lead to distortions (Wampold, 2001). For example, Johnson (2003) described the EFT meta-analysis as follows: "This analysis found that EFT was associated with a 70% to 73% recovery rate for relationship distress" (p. 367). However, in the meta-analysis, Johnson et al. (1999) stated that "in most studies, over half of the EFT treated couples met criteria for recovery (i.e., no longer maritally distressed)" (pp. 71–72). Recovery rates for the four meta-analyzed trials averaged 57.5%, a figure comparable with other estimates for couple intervention. The quoted rates of 70% to 73% are, in fact, rates of improvement, not recovery.[5] Christensen and Heavey (1999) have suggested that measurement of durability is essential in determining an intervention's true effect. However, follow-up data from the four analyzed studies was selective in Johnson et al., with the omission of the striking posttreatment regression for EFT clients in Goldman and Greenberg (1992). EFT couples failed to maintain gains on the Dyadic Adjustment Scale (DAS), Target Complaints (TC), and Goal Attainment Scale (GAS) at 4 months posttreatment, whereas the comparison approach (integrated systemic therapy) held onto posttest levels.

In all four EFT studies cited by Johnson et al. (1999), authors are model developers or developers' students or trainees, and study sites are locations where model creators trained, facts acknowledged by the authors. It is worthy to note that in the only direct comparison of EFT with another couple approach in which the comparative model was delivered by therapists with equal allegiance, no differences in outcomes were reported. Magnitudes of ESs and claims of superiority in the EFT meta-analysis clearly must be interpreted with allegiance as a point of reference. The robust impact of allegiance factors

---

[5]These percentages were reported by Johnson et al. (1999) in only two of the original studies. Only one original study indicated attrition rates, making it difficult to determine if recovery and improvement rates were derived from the intent-to-treat sample or completers only.

illustrated in these instances suggests that the portion of outcome variance attributable to allegiance factors in the MFT literature in general warrants close scrutiny in evaluating claims of differential efficacy.

## Unequal Comparisons

Inequality in important attributes between treatments constitutes a significant confound in evaluating comparative trial findings (Duncan et al., 2004; Wampold, 2001). Looking for unfair comparisons speaks to the old but relevant question, "Compared with what?" Unequal comparisons significantly inflate the meanings often attributed to results. For example, on average, any systematically applied treatment is 4 times more effective than no treatment (Lambert & Ogles, 2004). So when a study of functional family therapy (FFT) reported a 41% recidivism rate in the no-treatment group whereas FFT achieved a 9% rate (Gordon, Arbuthnot, Gustafson, & McGreen, 1988), the findings are laudable but nothing more than would be expected. Moreover, comparisons with no treatment have no relevance to differential efficacy.

The meta-analysis claiming differential efficacy conducted by Stanton and Shadish (1997) further illustrates unequal comparisons. Synthesizing drug abuse outcomes for 13 studies, this investigation compared MFT with non-MFT modalities. Five studies (one study report could not be located) found a difference between MFT and non-MFT intervention. First, in McLellan, Arndt, Metzger, Woody, and O'Brien (1993), methadone plus minimal counseling and methadone plus individual counseling were compared with an enhanced package of methadone, individual counseling, medical or psychiatric service, employment, and family therapy. The sheer amount of time given to the enhanced group would increase the chances that participants would fare better than those in other groups. This study cannot say, however, whether the key ingredient responsible for better outcomes is family therapy, only that the entire array of intervention proved superior. Next, in Stanton, Todd, and Associates (1982), outcome results (days abstinent from opiates), from most to least effective intervention, were paid family therapy, unpaid family therapy, paid family movie, TAU. Here, TAU is compared with the carefully coordinated efforts of family treatment teams who contacted families, elicited engagement, and provided a well-defined treatment modality supervised by approach advocates. The study reported that TAU therapists were skeptical that clients would respond positively to treatment, whereas clinicians in the family conditions believed that significant change was possible. This study teaches much about the value of an intensive and hopeful response to addiction. Whether it constitutes a head-to-head comparison and definitive evidence for superiority of family intervention is questionable.

Two trials involving multisystemic therapy (MST) in Stanton and Shadish's (1997) analysis found differences between family and nonfamily approaches (see chap. 6, this volume, for further critique of MST). MST therapists meet in the home and engage the targeted clients' significant social and community networks. The first study, Henggeler, Melton, and Smith (1992), compared MST with probation monitoring and therefore was not a fair contest but rather a control or no-treatment comparison. The second study (Borduin et al., 1995) described MST conducted in the home, involving parents and other interacting systems, by therapists with limited caseloads (students of principal investigator) who were regularly supervised (2.5 hr per week by a founder of the approach). MST was compared with therapy of the adolescent only, conducted in a clinic by therapists with no special supervision or allegiance and with full caseloads. These therapists, supposedly to remain true to an individual orientation, involved only the adolescent in services more than 90% of the time. Regardless of orientation, it is a questionable practice to ignore relevant individuals and systems (parents, schools, courts) in the treatment of adolescents (especially parents). This comparison goes beyond just a TAU contrast and enters the realm of a sham treatment comparison, one that is unlikely to be delivered in actual practice.

In Joanning, Thomas, Quinn, and Mullen (1992), family drug education (FDE) and adolescent group therapy had outcomes inferior to family therapy. FDE provided educational material to families, whereas "discussion of problems or concerns unique to a particular family was discouraged" (p. 349); it is obvious that this was not a bona fide treatment designed to be therapeutic. The other comparison, adolescent group therapy, was delivered by two students in a family therapy doctoral program in which one or more study researchers presumably taught and supervised. As the authors noted, "A possible confounding factor in the study was the fact that all therapists and one of the two FDE leaders were doctoral students in a family therapy program" (p. 348). The final study favoring family therapy is unpublished, though Stanton and Shadish (1997) described the comparison condition as "teacher sponsor," clearly not an intervention and not on a par with family therapy. Stanton and Shadish's meta-analysis stated the obvious: When more time is spent, more systems are involved, and with approaches intended to be therapeutic, outcomes improve.

Psychoeducation (Goldstein & Miklowitz, 1995) has been cited as superior to other forms of intervention for the treatment of schizophrenia (e.g., see McFarlane, Dixon, Lukens, & Lucksted, 2003; Pinsof and Wynne, 1995), though inclusion of it in evidence-based practice lists for serious mental illness, including bipolar diagnoses, primarily focuses on its efficacy relative to standard individual approaches (Dixon et al., 2001). An inspection of unequal comparisons challenges differential efficacy. Psychoeducation as a model involves multiple components in addition to psychoeducation, including early engagement of the family in a no-fault atmosphere' recommendations for coping, communication, and problem-solving training; and crisis intervention. Goldstein and Miklowitz (1995) acknowledged that without empirically comparing varying aspects of treatment strategies, evidence that psychoeducation (or some other ingredient) produces reduction in relapse cannot be determined (Goldstein & Miklowitz, 1995). Moreover, Goldstein and Miklowitz reported a narrowing of differences between the experimental and comparison conditions in their 1995 review.

A later review (McFarlane et al., 2003) suggested that core elements of family psychoeducation are even more extensive: minimum 6 months intervention, social network expansion, behavioral skills, employment training, and cultural and contextual adaptations (p. 231). Sprenkle (2003) noted that "subsequent research has demonstrated that, when these core ingredients are present, disparate methods work about equally well" (p. 93). In sum, psychoeducation is a multifaceted, time- and resource-intensive modality, obviously not comparable to, and more likely to succeed than, the most frequent comparison condition: individual, office- or institution-based therapy.

A critical review of the differential efficacy data demonstrates few exceptions to the dodo verdict when allegiance is considered, comparisons are fair, and bona fide treatments are contrasted, eroding claims of differential efficacy and giving credence to the claim that all have won prizes. Indeed, Sexton, Alexander, and Mease (2004), in their comprehensive review of family therapy efficacy, appeared to concur, "The results of these treatments [evidence based] appear to be maintained in relation to treatment-as-usual control groups but have not been found to be superior to other alternative treatments" (p. 633).[6]

## MFT AND THE COMMON FACTORS: EXTRATHERAPEUTIC (CLIENT) FACTORS AND TREATMENT EFFECTS

The lack of meaningful differences among MFT approaches, as suggested by Rosenzweig (see Prologue, this volume) so long ago, points to aspects found across all couple and family interventions that account for outcome. To understand these common factors, it is first necessary to separate the variance due to

---

[6]This conclusion begs the question of financial pragmatics. Costs of implementation of evidence-based treatments are not insignificant. For example, FFT costs for training only one working group has been cited at $47,500, excluding expenses (National Center for Mental Health Promotion and Youth Violence Prevention, n.d.). Considering this cost in the context of the usual high therapist turnover rate in agencies challenges the practicality of implementing evidence-based treatments in a continually changing environment.

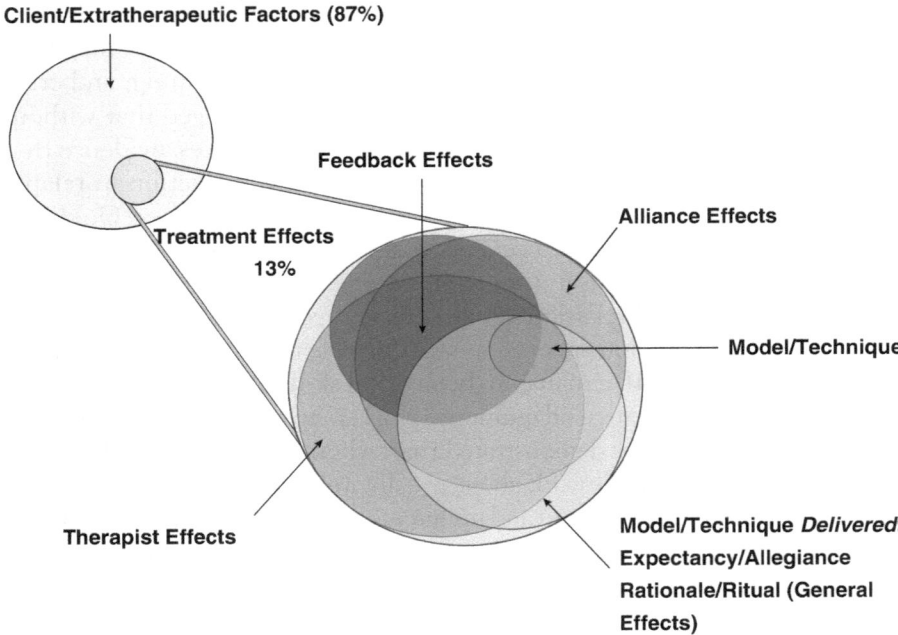

**Client/Extratherapeutic Factors (87%)**

**Feedback Effects**

**Alliance Effects**

Treatment Effects
13%

**Model/Technique**

**Therapist Effects**

**Model/Technique** *Delivered*:
Expectancy/Allegiance
Rationale/Ritual (General
Effects)

*Figure 12.1.* The common factors with a proposed feedback factor.

therapy from that attributed to extratherapeutic factors: those variables incidental to the treatment model, idiosyncratic to the specific client, and part of the client's life circumstances that aid in recovery despite participation in therapy (Asay & Lambert, 1999). These variables consist of the client's strengths, struggles, motivations, distress, supportive elements in the environment, and even chance events. Client factors, including unexplained and error variance, account for 87% of the variance of change, leaving 13% accounted for by treatment (Wampold, 2001). An inspection of Figure 12.1 reveals that the proportion of outcome attributable to extratherapeutic factors and treatment is represented by the circle on the left. The variance accounted for by treatment is depicted by the small circle nested within client factors (at the lower right side of the figure). For the sake of perspective, consider that model and technique differences have an ES of 0.2 at best, equating to only about 1% of the overall variance of outcome. Consequently, the impact of extratherapeutic factors on outcome flies in the face of the oft-told story: The heroic therapist galloping in on the white stallion of theoretical purity brandishing a sword of empirically supported treatments to rescue the helplessly disordered patient or dysfunctional family terrorized by the psychic dragon of mental illness. On the basis of the data, Duncan et al. (2004) called for a recasting of the therapeutic drama to assign clients their rightful "heroic" roles in change.

Perhaps the quintessential representation of client preexisting resources is found in pretreatment change (PTC). Weiner-Davis, de Shazer, and Gingerich (1987) published the original family therapy study about PTC and found that 66% of their clients reported positive, treatment-related gains prior to the formal initiation of therapy when asked about such change at the beginning of their first session. Other research has established a link between PTC and outcome. For example, solution-focused researchers Beyebach, Morejon, Palenzuela, and Rodriguez-Arias (1996) found that clients who reported PTC were 4 times more likely to finish treatment with a successful outcome. In Allgood, Parham, Salts, and Smith (1995), PTC predicted whether therapy termination was planned or unplanned; when clients reported no PTC, the therapy was likely to end prematurely. These findings suggest that clients harness pretherapy personal, interpersonal, or social resources to begin reaching their own particular change objectives.

That clients far outweigh specific technique in relative contribution to outcome is supported by the empirical literature (see chap. 3, this volume). Despite this, systemic research about the client's contribution to change is sparse. Client demographic characteristics (age, gender, race, ethnicity, education) have not shown consistent influence on outcome (Hampson & Beavers, 1996; Snyder, Mangrum, & Wills, 1993). Johnson & Talitman (1997) found that only one demographic factor, male age, was related to outcome in their study of EFT. Older men were more likely to be maritally satisfied 3 months after therapy than their younger counterparts, though the authors acknowledged that this may reflect more a match between the client and the approach than the ability of younger men to benefit.

One review of dropout in the MFT literature found that client socioeconomic status (SES) was associated with premature termination of therapy; clients of lower SES had higher rates of dropout than those with higher incomes (Bischoff & Sprenkle, 1993). However, in another study of 88 couples, SES did not predict marital outcome variance (Waldron, Turner, Barton, Alexander, & Cline, 1997). Bischoff and Sprenkle (1993) found that dropout rates were higher when the ethnic backgrounds of the therapist and client diverged. Although there is some empirical evidence that ethnic and racial matching may enhance outcome, ethnicity and race are likely only two among many characteristics that influence a good client–therapist fit (Zane, Hall, Sue, Young, & Nunez, 2004). One study found that although different client–therapist matching on race and gender impacted couples' perceptions of early sessions, this effect decreased over time, indicating that these variables were not static (Gregory & Leslie, 1996).

Client characteristics that are responsive to therapy appear to play larger roles in systemic therapy outcomes. These include pretherapy relational patterns and degree of system distress as well as those attributes specific to the therapy (e.g., motivation and engagement). Jacobson and Christensen (1996) found that BMT was best suited for clients who were highly committed to each other, had similar goals, and high emotional engagement. In a study of 55 couples receiving either BMT or IOMT, high levels of relationship distress predicted poorer outcomes at termination and at a 4-year follow-up, though the predictive value of this variable was greater for shorter term outcomes (Snyder et al., 1993). In contrast, Johnson and Talitman (1997) found that initial levels of marital satisfaction only modestly predicted outcome. This study found that couples with men who were unlikely to seek out their partners for comfort and support, and men who were rated as inexpressive by their partners, made the most gains. The alliance was found to be the largest predictor of outcome in this study, suggesting that the degree to which couple or individual client characteristics influenced outcome can be viewed as nested within this variable.

In a study of 434 families, families scoring high on measures of family competence fared better than those scoring low prior to therapy (Hampson & Beavers, 1996). There is some evidence that the level of expressed emotion (rejection, protectiveness, fusion) in families is predictive of whether family therapy is beneficial for persons experiencing psychotic-type symptoms (Askey, Gamble, & Gray, 2007). A recent study, however, found that expressed emotion levels varied according to the severity of the family member's symptoms rather than existing prior to, or precipitating, psychotic-type experiences (McFarlane & Cook, 2007).

Although the research appears to be a hodgepodge of findings, investigating client factors is hampered by largely ex post facto analysis and the complexity of the topic (see chap. 3, this volume). Clarkin and Levy (2004) suggested that disentangling client, therapist, and alliance variables is difficult at best and that "pretreatment variables have a plausible impact on the therapy, but as soon as therapy begins, the client variables are in a dynamic and ever changing context of therapist variables and behavior" (p. 215). The findings also suggest that the largest source of variance is not easily generalized because these factors differ with each client. These unpredictable differences can only emerge one client, one therapist, and one alliance at a time.

### Therapist Factors

Figure 12.1 also illustrates the second step in understanding the common factors. It depicts the overlapping elements that comprise the 13% of variance attributable to treatment (the second circle in the center of the figure). Visually, the relationship among the common factors, as opposed to a static pie-chart depicting discreet elements adding to a total of 100%, is more accurately represented with a Venn diagram, using overlapping circles and shading to demonstrate mutual and interdependent action. The factors, in effect, act in concert and cannot be separated into disembodied parts (Duncan, Solovey, & Rusk, 1992).

First, consider *therapist factors*, defined as the amount of variance attributable not to the model wielded but rather to who the therapist is. Variability among therapists is the rule rather that the exception (Beutler et al., 2004). In the individual literature, therapist factors have emerged as potent and predictive aspects of therapeutic services, capturing more of the variance of outcome than any treatment provided and accounting for 6% to 9% of the variance (Wampold & Brown, 2005), or in other words, about 6 to 9 times more than model differences. Although a growing area of research, the only couple or family therapy investigation to parcel out therapist effects has been the Norway Couple Feedback Project (Anker, Duncan, & Sparks, 2009; Anker, Owen, Duncan, & Sparks, 2009; Anker, Sparks, Duncan, & Stapnes, 2009; Owen, Anker, Duncan, & Sparks, 2009). Limited to only 10 therapists, Anker et al. (2009) reported somewhat smaller therapist effects than reported in the individual literature, about 4% of the variance. However, Owen et al. (2009), with a larger pool of therapists (20) reported that 8% of the variance was attributed to therapist effects.

Little has been known about what differentiates practitioners, but interesting findings are beginning to emerge after a period of a dearth of results. Traditionally, systemic researchers have explored therapist characteristics associated with outcome. Bischoff and Sprenkle (1993) could not find evidence that therapist static traits impacted retention in marriage and family therapy. In a study of 434 families receiving family therapy, therapist income level, ethnicity, and gender did not discriminate between families that improved and those that did not (Hampson & Beavers, 1996). Research on the impact of matching client preferences for ethnically or racially similar therapists is inconsistent. Beutler et al. (2004) concluded, "Whatever small advantages might be attributable to ethnic similarity are not consistent across ethnic groups and are thereby a very weak basis for definitive conclusions" (p. 234). However, research on the importance of therapist qualities of warmth, empathy, and the ability to structure is more conclusive and has been found to be related to positive outcomes (Green & Herget, 1991). Counselor use of interpersonal skills (empathy, warmth, etc.) and direct influence skills predicted positive treatment outcomes in a meta-analysis of relationship variables in child and family therapy (Karver, Handelsman, Fields, & Bickman, 2006). Qualitative reviews of client perceptions have added to the evidence that clients feel connected to therapists whom they view as empathic, accepting, caring, supportive, and personable (Bischoff & McBride, 1996). Moreover, Owen et al. (2009), in a study of 20 couple therapists and 250 couples, found that increases in alliance ratings accounted for approximately 40% of the variability between therapists. Therapist ability to manage the alliance appears to be an important contributor to therapist differences in couple therapy. Although more research is needed, this finding follows recent trends in the individual literature (e.g., Baldwin, Wampold, & Imel, 2007).

Several investigations of systemic treatments have focused on the therapist's adherence to the model and treatment outcome (Sexton, Alexander, & Mease, 2004). For example, Huey, Henggeler, Brondino, and Pickrel (2000) found that youth, caregiver, and therapist ratings of therapist adherence to MST protocol, as assessed on the MST Adherence Measure, were significantly associated with improved family relations and decreased delinquent behavior. Huey et al. (2000) stated, however, that treatment adherence is not a unitary concept; MST guidelines are "flexible and intended to fit the individual needs and strengths of the family" (p. 464). The conflation of alliance and model variables and the fact that therapist behaviors may vary considerably yet still qualify as adhering to protocol suggest that these studies may represent evidence for common factors rather than for any unique aspect of MST. What observers saw conformed with what studies across many modalities have indicated: the importance of the alliance and therapist ability to establish relationships, even in the midst of conflict and with multiple family members.

The direction of the link between therapist experience and outcome is equivocal. On one hand, Raytek, McCrady, Epstein, and Hirsch (1999) found a significantly positive association between therapist experience and observer ratings of the alliance and completion of treatment for a spouse's substance use, though not for overall outcome. Owen et al. (2009) found that therapist experience in couple therapy accounted for more than 50% of the variability in outcomes among therapists, suggesting that experience may matter more in couple work. On the other hand, others have found the evidence for the value of experience weak and even have reported that paraprofessionals may do as well as professionals (Beutler et al., 2004; Christensen & Jacobson, 1994). The lack of a consistent association between therapist experience and outcome can be viewed as an indication of the role of nonspecific variables in psychotherapy and systemic therapy. It appears that the person of the therapist, his or her own style of engaging with others and appreciating clients, and general attributes of warmth and communicated caring are strong contributors to success, as is the therapist's ability to form strong alliances.

## Alliance Factors

Researchers repeatedly have found that a positive alliance is one of the best predictors of outcome in psychotherapy (see chap. 4, this volume). Depending on which meta-analysis is cited, the amount of variance attributed to the alliance ranges from 5% (Martin, Garske, & Davis, 2000) to 7% (Horvath & Symonds, 1991), 5 to 7 times the impact of model and technique.

Karver et al.'s (2006) meta-analysis of relationship variables in youth and family therapy examined 49 studies and found that counselor interpersonal and direct influence skills as well as youth and parent willingness to participate and actual participation in treatment were the best predictors of outcome. In the CYT, client self-report of the alliance early in treatment predicted substance-related problems at 3- and 6-month follow-up (Tetzlaff et al., 2005). Shelef, Diamond, Diamond, and Liddle (2005) examined adolescent–therapist and parent–therapist alliances, dropout, and outcome in the MDFT condition of the CYT. Positive parent–counselor alliance scores predicted retention, and adolescent alliance predicted fewer substance abuse symptoms, accounting for 7% of the variance; the Adolescent × Parent alliance interaction accounted for an additional 6% of the variance. In addition, early adolescent alliance predicted days of drug use during the 90 days immediately following treatment, accounting for 14% of the variance. Shirk and Karver's (2003) meta-analytic review of relationship factors in child and adolescent therapy confirmed the robust effect of this variable. The authors concluded that "in this respect, it appears that the therapeutic relationship represents a hardy nonspecific factor in therapy" (p. 461).

In couple therapy, the therapeutic relationship, with variations based on gender in heterosexual couples, has predicted outcome. The alliance explained as much as 22% of outcome variance in a study of EFT (Johnson & Talitman, 1997). Keep in mind that treatment accounts for, on average, 13% of the variance. The alliance in this study accounted for more of the variance by itself, illustrating how the percentages are not fixed and depend on the particular context of client, therapist, alliance, and treatment model.

Quinn, Dotson, and Jordan (1997) found that couples' views of the alliance at the third session predicted outcome. In a study of 80 people treated with marital therapy, the alliance did not predict progress at the individual level but accounted for 5% to 22% of the variance of improvement in marital distress (Knobloch-Fedders, Pinsof, & Mann, 2007). Women's midtreatment alliance was a better predictor of improvement in marital distress than early treatment alliance, but couples who had strong first-session alliances were more likely to remain through Session 8. Additionally, treatment response was uniquely correlated with women's perceptions of the couples' alliance to treatment. The authors speculated that these findings indicate that alliances in couple therapy form early, are relatively stable, and account for treatment participation.

Of interest to systemic therapy researchers are assessments of these variables from multiple sources in the expanded treatment system (Sprenkle et al., 1999). Systemic instruments (e.g., Pinsof & Catherall's, 1986, integrative alliance scales) measure the alliance not only on the dimensions defined by individual therapy (Bordin, 1979) but also the clients' perceptions of the therapist's relationship with other family subsystems and the family as a whole. Family alliance research considers systems conflict, coalitions, hierarchy (Karver et al., 2006; Sprenkle et al., 1999), and the impact of differences in alliance scores within subsystems (Pinsof & Catherall, 1986). Robbins, Alexander, Turner and Perez (2003) looked at the relationship between alliance and retention in family therapy for adolescents with behavior problems. For the 34 families studied, discrepancies between adolescent–therapist and parent–therapist alliances (unbalanced alliances) predicted dropout. In a study of 40 families, the majority of families that dropped out had a moderately or severely split alliance in at least one session (De La Peña, Freidlander, & Escudero, 2009). Symonds and Horvath (2004) found that mutual agreement between marital partners regarding the strength of the alliance and alliance increases for both partners between Sessions 1 and 3 were robust predictors of outcome. In Knobloch-Fedders et al.'s (2007) study, when men scored the alliance higher at Session 8 than did their partners, couples showed greater overall improvement. Nonetheless, outcomes for couples with a *split alliance* (difference of 1 standard deviation or more on one subscale alliance measure) did not significantly differ from those with an *intact alliance*, though this finding is limited by the study's small sample size. Anker, Owen, et al. (2009), in contrast, in a study of 250 couples, found that split alliances (mild, moderate, and severe) at the first session had no impact on outcome whereas those alliances that were moderately or severely split at the last session had diminished outcomes. Further, they reported that first session alliances were not predictive of outcome whereas last session alliance scores were and that men's alliance scores at the last session predicted both their own and their partners' outcomes better than women's alliance scores at the last session. In a small study, Quinn et al. (1997) found evidence for differential impacts on outcome when wives disagreed with their husbands on the tasks dimensions of the alliance and in perceptions of their husbands' relationship to the therapist. In a 6-month follow-up qualitative analysis of 742 client responses about their experiences of couple therapy, Anker, Sparks, et al. (2009) confirmed the importance of the relational dimension of the alliance to both genders but also found the most complaints to be associated with an aspect of the alliance that is not often studied: the nuts and bolts aspects of the task dimension, such as scheduling, cancellation, and between-session contacts.

The plethora of views, often at odds with one another, encountered with more people in the room compounds the complexity of alliance influences and negotiations. Findings from the current couple and family therapy literature, however, suggest that the alliance is a potent predictor of treatment success and accounts for a measurable portion of variance.

## Model and Technique Delivered: Expectancy, Allegiance, and General Effects

Consider that the delivery of any model or technique has both general and specific effects. Specific effects, or the amount of variance attributable to model differences, accounts for about 1% of the variance of change (ES of 0.2). In the CYT, model differences accounted for less than 1% with an ES of 0.1. The general effects of delivering a model of treatment include the client's expectation for recovery (placebo or expectancy) and the therapist's belief in the intervention administered or allegiance factors. Model and technique are considered here as acting in concert with allegiance, expectancy, and placebo factors, as the model and technique delivered.

Breaking down this constellation of variables, consider the general aspects of treatment models. Model and technique factors are the assumptions and procedures unique to specific treatments. Although differing in content, all include a rationale, an explanation for the client's difficulties, a ritual, and strategies to follow for resolving them (Frank & Frank, 1991). Whether instructing clients to talk to one another, alter their communication styles, or understand family dynamics, couple and family therapists are engaging in healing rituals. In both medicine and psychotherapy, when the placebo or technically inert condition is offered in a context that creates positive expectations, it reliably produces effects almost as large, or as large as the treatment itself (Wampold, Minami, Tierney, Basking, & Bhati, 2005).

Allegiance and expectancy are mirror images: the belief by both the therapist and the client in the restorative power of the therapy's rationale and related rituals. The degree to which the therapist delivering the treatment believes the chosen therapy to be efficacious, as noted earlier, weighs in as a strong determinant of outcome in clinical trials. Meta-analytic investigations of allegiance have generally found effects ranging up to an ES of 0.65 (Wampold, 2001). Therapist allegiance to an approach contributes to the client's coming to believe in a treatment as well. Placebo factors may also be fueled by a therapist's belief that change occurs naturally and almost universally; human beings, shaped by millennia of survival, tend to find a way out of their difficulties, even out of the heart of darkness (Sparks, Duncan, & Miller, 2007).

Allegiance and expectancy effects cannot occur independently of model and technique. The clinician must have a model in which to place his or her faith (one hopes many models), and a rationale and ritual is required to satisfy the client's expectation that he or she is being treated by a credible psychotherapist. Given this interdependence, the act of administering treatment becomes the vehicle that carries allegiance and placebo effects in addition to the specific effects of a given approach. Although findings regarding expectancy loom large in treatment effects in individual therapy (Baskin, Tierney, Minami,

& Wampold, 2003), research on expectancy variables in the MFT literature are scant but reinforcing (Sprenkle et al., 1999).

Regarding specific technique, Orlinsky Rønnestad, and Willutzki (2004) noted that some effective treatment interventions, although housed in contrasting "treatment packages," appear largely similar; this sheds light on the comparability of results from one model to another (p. 363). For example, providing a nonblaming rationale for the presenting problem (*reframing* or *reattribution*) has been found to be helpful across treatment contexts (Robbins, Alexander, Newell, & Turner, 1996) and in the reduction of family negativity (Sexton, Alexander, & Mease, 2004). Orlinsky et al. (2004) further asserted that experimental designs, largely used to test specific techniques, are not well-suited to answering many of the questions posed in process–outcome research. Friedlander and Tuason (2000) noted that process–outcome research largely consists of ex post facto observations of verbal behavior. Correlations between process and outcome do not provide information about important contextual variables, and caution regarding interpretation is warranted. For example, Hogue, Dauber, Somuolis, and Liddle (2006) connected process to outcome using observational ratings of therapist interventions to predict outcomes at 6 and 12 months for 63 families receiving MDFT. The study found that a high-dose mix of both family and adolescent techniques predicted reduction of adolescent externalization and family conflict at 6-month follow-up; greater use of family-focused techniques was related to decrease in adolescent internalizing symptoms at 6 months and family cohesion at 1 year. The description of MDFT techniques in this study encompassed broad domains of therapist–client process, including the engagement of the adolescent and parent and the facilitation of changes in interactional patterns, activities found in many family approaches. The authors noted that the focus on technical aspects of treatment in the study excluded nontechnical components that may be as much or more responsible for outcomes.

## Feedback

The measurement and management of change, from the client's perspective, has been catapulted to the forefront of research and practice, and for good reason: Monitoring client-based outcome, when combined with feedback to the clinician, significantly increases the effectiveness of services (see chap. 8, this volume). Although the individual literature has seen an expanding body of research on feedback, couple and family research has produced very little in this area. This may be due in part to the fact that feedback is a relatively new development but also because measuring outcome with couples and families can be inherently cumbersome. Most available outcome measures, although reliable and valid, are long and intended more for oversight or research purposes, thereby presenting an arduous task for both clinicians and clients. A small recent study of feedback in wraparound services for youth and families (Ogles et al., 2006) found that provision of feedback using the 48-item Ohio Scales (Ogles, Melendez, Davis, & Lunnen, 2001) did not contribute to improved youth outcomes or family functioning in comparison with a no-feedback group. Feedback, however, was restricted to just four times over the course of the treatment process.

Conversely, a strong feedback effect was found in a recent couples study. Anker et al. (2009) conducted the only randomized clinical trial to date that compared feedback with a nonfeedback condition with couples. In the largest randomized clinical trial ever conducted with couples, Anker et al. recruited 205 couples in a naturalistic setting to examine the effect of feedback in routine practice. The Outcome Rating Scale (ORS; Miller, Duncan, Brown, Sparks, & Claud, 2003), a reliable and valid four-item, self-report instrument, provided outcome feedback, and the Session Rating Scale (SRS), also a reliable, valid, four-item, self-report measure (Duncan et al., 2003), provided alliance feedback. The study shared several characteristics with Lambert's feedback trials: use of consecutive cases seen in routine care regardless of diagnosis; random assignment of client to feedback and nonfeedback conditions; provision of different models and techniques; variations in clinician experience and discipline; use of the same therapists in feedback and nonfeedback; and determination of the length of care by therapists and clients rather than by the research design. Noteworthy is the fact that this study attempted to control for allegiance effects in addition to therapists serving as their own controls; therapists were naive to formal feedback and held attitudes about feedback that ranged from neutral to positive.

Feedback substantially increased positive outcomes (ES = 0.50), accounting for approximately 10% of the variability in change while simultaneously reducing the number of at-risk clients. The proportion of clients responding to treatment in the TAU group was 41.7% (both in couple, 22.6%) and in the feedback group was 64.6% (both in couple, 50.5%). The strong effect of feedback seems particularly noteworthy given the relative simplicity of the intervention and in light of the fact that the comparison group was in an active treatment. Feedback couples reached nondistressed levels nearly four times more than nonfeedback couples. The feedback condition maintained its advantage at 6-month follow-up and achieved nearly a 50% less separation or divorce rate.

Speaking directly to the issue of therapist variability discussed above, the effect of feedback varied significantly across therapists. Anker et al. (2009) reported that the correlation between the variability in the effectiveness of a therapist with no feedback and variability in the effect of feedback was unusually high ($r = -.99$). Although the authors cautioned that the small number of therapists (10) significantly limits any conclusions that can be drawn, it does suggest that the less effective therapists (those who had the worst outcomes without feedback) benefited more from feedback than the most effective therapists. Feedback, therefore, seems to act as a leveler among therapists, raising the effectiveness of lower or average therapists to that of their more successful colleagues. In fact, a therapist among the lower effectiveness group without feedback became the therapist with the best results with feedback![7] Nine of 10 therapists benefited from the effects of feedback.

On the basis of their findings, Anker et al. (2009) suggested continued reflection about the transportability of specific couple therapy approaches to clinical settings. As noted, couple therapy research has robustly demonstrated superiority over no-treatment controls for several approaches but has failed to find reliable superiority of one over another or TAU, especially at follow-up. At the same time, the financial investment for agency-wide implementation of a particular couple therapy orientation is substantial. For example, certification in emotionally focused couple therapy (EFCT) requires a minimum of 42 hours training and 32 hours of supervision with a certified EFCT supervisor (see International Centre for Excellence in Emotionally Focused Therapy, 2007). Conversely, the feedback condition in Anker et al.'s (2009) study demonstrated superior results to TAU at posttreatment and follow-up. Feedback methods are generic in nature and not tied to a single therapy modality and therefore represent a lower commitment of staff and money to implement. Therapists received only 17 hours of training in Anker et al.'s study. The authors concluded, "Feedback, therefore, seems more easily transportable to community settings compared with specific treatment packages, and more likely to yield a return on investment" (p. 701).

Feedback studies with families are in their infancy, hampered by a lack of feasible instruments that reliably track change from a youth's perspective. Until recently, persons under the age of 13 years have not had an opportunity to provide formal feedback to helpers about their views. To fill this void, the Child Outcome Rating Scale (CORS; Duncan, Sparks, Miller, Bohanske, & Claud, 2006) was developed. The CORS is similar in format to the ORS but contains child-friendly language and graphics to aid the child's understanding. With such instruments, children and their families can benefit from client-informed

---

[7]This finding, although preliminary, challenges the practice of giving referrals to only the most effective therapists as suggested in chapter 9, this volume, or providing incentives in general for therapist performance. Such policies risk turning therapists against measuring outcomes and could perhaps encourage therapists to cheat the system to ensure referrals and to gain a competitive edge. Given that feedback seems to act as a leveler of therapist performance that enables nearly all therapists to achieve good outcomes, such practices seem unnecessary and perhaps counterproductive. See chapter 14 of this volume for more discussion of the downsides of institutional data collection and provider profiling.

practice, and researchers have a tool for examining the impact of services at individual, family, and systems-wide levels.

On the basis of a growing body of compelling empirical findings, feedback seems to improve outcomes across client populations and professional discipline, regardless of the model practiced; the feedback process is thus a vehicle to modify any delivered treatment for client benefit. Given its apparent broad applicability and lack of theoretical baggage, feedback can be argued to be a factor that demonstrably contributes to outcome regardless of the theoretical predilection of the clinician. It therefore could be considered a common factor of change.

### Feedback as a Common Factor: A Proposal

At first blush, feedback may seem like an odd addition to the list of common factors. The process of attaining formal client feedback and using that input to tailor services, however, seems a worthy addition for several reasons. First, the effects of feedback are independent of the measures used; a variety of outcome instruments have demonstrated a positive impact on outcome. Second, systematic feedback improves outcome regardless of the specific process used, whether in collaboration with clients or merely giving the feedback to therapists—over the phone or face to face, paper and pencil administrations or electronic format, it matters not. Third, feedback increases client benefit across professional discipline, clinical setting, client population, and level of experience of the therapist. And fourth, feedback improves outcome regardless of the model practiced: The feedback process does not dictate what technique is used but rather is a vehicle to modify any delivered treatment for client benefit.

Finally, the conceptualization of feedback as a common factor follows the tradition of other factors that were initially recognized as important and later evolved an empirical backing and more systematic application. Consider the therapeutic alliance. Although appreciated early on (see Prologue, this volume), the alliance was not understood as a ubiquitous factor with particular components that influenced and predicted outcome until the groundbreaking research conducted in the 1980s.[8] Attaining informal client feedback about the benefit and fit of services is a common phenomenon among psychotherapies. Any goal-directed, symptom-oriented approach that openly discusses the outcome of services is incorporating informal client feedback into the therapeutic mix. Feedback speaks to an interpersonal process of give and take between the clinician and client and, at least to some extent, can be argued to be characteristic of many therapeutic encounters. Many clinicians believe that

---

[8]For an excellent discussion of the development of the alliance concept, see Gaston (1990).

attaining client feedback about the benefit and fit of services is part and parcel to their normal everyday activities with clients. Indeed, 9 out of 10 therapists in Anker et al.'s (2009) study reported that they already informally asked clients about progress and the relationship.

And the empirical support, as reported in this volume, is increasingly showing that feedback has an impressive impact on outcome. As Lambert reports in chapter 8, ESs for the difference between feedback and TAU ranges from 0.34 to 0.92, unusually large considering that the estimates of the ES of the difference between empirically supported and comparison treatments are about 0.20. Anker et al.'s (2009) study achieved an ES of 0.50. Feedback, then, like the alliance, has been initially viewed as an important aspect of conducting effective psychotherapy and is garnering a growing evidence base that supports a more formal understanding and systematic inclusion. Clearly, feedback is not an individual phenomenon but a systemic one, uniting multiple players in a common therapeutic process.

Figure 12.1 shows how feedback overlaps with and affects all the factors— it is the tie that binds them together—allowing the other common factors to be delivered one client at a time. Soliciting systematic feedback is a living, ongoing process that engages clients in the collaborative monitoring of outcome, heightens hope for improvement, fits client preferences, maximizes therapist–client fit, and is itself a core feature of therapeutic change.

### Summary

Common factors research provides clues and general guidance for enhancing those elements shown to be most influential in positive outcomes. The specifics, however, can only be derived from the client's response to any treatment delivered: the client's feedback regarding progress in therapy and the quality of the alliance. Feedback enables a reliable and valid method of tailoring services to the individual; therapists need not know what approach should be used with each disorder, but rather whether the delivered approach is a good fit for and beneficial to the client in the moment. As such, feedback assumes a role alongside the more widely researched client, therapist, and alliance variables, emerging as a potential common factor.

## ARE SOME MORE EQUAL THAN OTHERS?

Can both sides have a piece of the evidence pie? "All are equal, but some are more equal than others" is reminiscent of a well-known fable of barnyard animals in a hypothesized future society (Orwell, 1945). The "both–and" in this tale disguises the actual workings of power, in fact, there are clear winners and losers. Until greater evidence is brought forward that disputes what has now become one of the most replicated findings in the research literature, having it both ways is untenable. With very few exceptions, all approaches in the systemic literature appear to work equally well when the conditions of the delivery of the treatment are roughly equivalent. A different both–and point of view, however, is possible. Particular change mechanisms appear to overlap in MFT models. This finding invites exploration of how these mechanisms operate in systemic practice, with the understanding that they are common factors, and one approach is not promoted at the expense of others. Mandating the provision of certain approaches at the exclusion of others limits the ability of diverse pairings of therapists and clients to flexibly devise effective treatments.

The preponderance of research suggests that specific ingredients likely to produce variations in outcome are not, in fact, meaningfully operational in the systemic literature; the dodo thrives beyond its origins in the individual psychotherapy literature. This conclusion implies that practice, training, and research centralize common factors. Although emphases on the common factors in accordance with the amount of variance each accounts for makes strong empirical sense, codifying common factors to apply across therapies transforms a transtheoretical paradigm into a level of abstraction consistent with specific models (Duncan et al., 2004; Wampold, 2001). The common factors literature suggests instead that each therapy encounter is unique: one cannot know a priori what will work best. Obtaining consistent information from clients as therapy unfolds helps ensure that common factors do not devolve into specified strategies to be applied universally. The relative importance of common factors, with attention to the role of feedback, recommends the following practice directions:

- Family clinicians in a variety of settings advocate for ways to formally give voice to clients, via client-based outcome measures as well as other methods to form partnerships with consumers of MFT services.
- Family clinicians tailor treatment on the basis of the formal collection of client feedback using measures and means consistent with the language, customs, and cultural preferences of diverse clientele.
- Therapists creatively develop ways to invite client resources and resilience into therapy.
- Therapists initiate and facilitate the transformation from mandated protocols to more flexible procedures that fit client preferences in accordance with the new American Psychological Association definition of evidence-based practice (see chap. 1, this volume).

- Therapists incorporate measures of client views of progress and the alliance at each session (including children's and adolescents' perspectives) to respond to divergent goals and enhance individual and subsystem alliances as treatment progresses.
- Therapists become skilled in several approaches that have personal resonance and enhance their sense of confidence to provide a hopeful environment for client change.
- Therapists use client feedback to recognize when a different approach is warranted and are able to make this shift midstream when required.
- Family clinicians advocate for lower caseloads, more supervision, reliable feedback about the outcome of services, and training in models that fit therapist preferences rather than more costly mandated evidence-based treatment protocols in typical family service environments.

Although teaching relational skills and helping trainees develop allegiance to several approaches is consistent with the empirical findings, manualizing these is at odds with the minor importance of specific techniques in overall outcome. Training in and use of client feedback has the potential to help student therapists adapt skills to each situation. This can enable trainees falling in average or below average ranges of efficacy to more consistently produce outcomes that are above average. The following are common factors–informed recommendations for MFT academic and training programs:

- Curricula include a focus on the empirical basis for common factors in the systemic literature and the expertise to critically evaluate outcome research.
- Clinical trainees learn how to obtain and use formal feedback via outcome tools throughout practicum and internship experiences.
- Supervisors use client feedback to assist trainees to improve outcomes, expand skills, and enhance relational flexibility.
- Training sites systematically collect client-generated data to inform improvements to overall client service and program learning initiatives.

The race to win prizes in the evidence-based treatment (EBT) contest has produced results distracting from the factors most associated with change and, in some cases, misinformation for therapists and funders. Recognizing the preeminence of common factors in outcome entails a redirection of the research agenda to include the following:

- Exploration into how clients, families, and their communities mobilize resources to achieve preferred goals.

- A shift from the search for the best model for a given targeted group, problem, or therapist trait, to how therapists can best engage clients in each unique encounter.
- Greater attention to the role of therapist effects in couple and family practice.
- Continued exploration of the dynamics of multiple, interacting variables and therapeutic alliance in systemic work.
- Research into the role of feedback conditions in improving retention, recovery, and treatment durability.
- Increased qualitative research that can develop rich descriptions and give voice to people speaking from nondominant social locations.
- The inclusion in research of diverse individuals, couples, and families that reflect the changing demographics of family therapy's clientele and practice communities.

Wampold (2002) noted that RCTs are designed to show efficacy of treatments and not factors, such as who delivers them, who receives them, and their relationship. He concluded that the inclusion of minority groups in trials is based on the erroneous assumption that specific ingredients need to be tested for their interaction with set categories (e.g., race), without a critical examination of the social construction of those categories and the complexity of variables (e.g., values, attitudes, SES, gender) within them. A critical research lens, whether qualitative or quantitative, can undermine traditional diagnostic categories and focus analysis on factors such as discrimination, poverty, and the differential operations of social and institutional power, areas of inquiry consistent with the field's ecosystemic paradigm.

Inviting clients' voices to be part of the literature regarding what works and what is needed can only enrich treatment strategies and improve outcomes. Engaging clients as the most potent common factor requires a "culture of feedback" (Duncan et al., 2004) grounded in knowledgeable and affirming practice (Brown, 2006) and an appreciation of context. It also entails asking for, listening to, and valuing each client's meanings, hopes, and preferred forms of help at each therapy encounter. Tailoring intervention to each person and family ensures that clients' unique worldviews and values are not only respected but central.

There are now decades of family and couple practice and a venerable history of clinicians, scholars, and researchers elaborating systemic principles. Clearly, the systemic lens provides a compelling basis for effective psychotherapy across a spectrum of problems. Proving its worth may no longer be a necessity. And yet, the current emphasis on EBT insists on more: proving superiority. What is created is a context of competition. The "all must have prizes" verdict is singularly out of step in this environment. It would be useful to establish a dialogue that considers the impact of this development on the field, with voices pro and con. The stance proposed here is that a focus on common factors is empirically informed, enhances the viability of systems therapy in the market, facilitates a framework for training and research, and is accountable to clients, respecting their unique diversity.

## QUESTIONS FROM THE EDITORS

1. *You have made a strong case for the dodo verdict in MFT. Aren't EBTs, however, superior to TAU, and therefore shouldn't they be implemented?*

EBTs, actually, have not shown their superiority over usual care (UC) or TAU. For example, in a meta-analysis of 32 studies comparing EBT with TAU for child problems, Weisz, Jensen-Doss, and Hawley (2006) reported an ES of 0.30 in favor of EBT (see chap. 11, this volume). This meager difference becomes even more so when considering the following: (a) When the EBT was not added to the UC, which is a fairer comparison than comparing the combination with UC, the effect was smaller; (b) if the dose of EBT was not greater than the dose of UC, the difference became nonsignificant; and (c) several of the comparisons were between EBT and a UC that was not a psychotherapy (e.g., case management or minimal contact). When the UC was a psychotherapy, the effect was not significantly different from zero. Further, many comparisons did not draw the therapists for EBT and UC from the same pool. Given that it is likely that the EBT therapists were selected for their skill and that therapists differ consistently in their outcomes, this would advantage the EBT. When therapists were drawn from the same pool, the superiority of EBT was nonsignificant.

A recent investigation of Parent Management Training, the Oregon Model (PMTO) further illustrates. After an uncritical account of reviews claiming PMTO efficacy (see chap. 6, this volume, for the problems with such reviews), Ogden and Hagan (2008) reported that PMTO was effective in reducing parent-reported child externalizing problems, improving teacher-reported social competence, and enhancing parental discipline over TAU. They concluded that "the findings thus indicate that PMTO is an effective treatment program . . . with children exhibiting serious behavioral problems and moreover that an EBT program can be transported successfully to a new participant group" (p. 617).

The initial analysis that compared PMTO with TAU included 16 outcome measures. Only 4 found a difference favoring PMTO. On 1 of the 4 measures reporting a significant effect for PMTO (the Child Behavior Check List Total), the difference between the means at the end of treatment of PMTO versus TAU was 1.92 points. On another (Child Behavior Check List Externalizing Total), the difference between posttreatment means was 1.53 points. The clinical significance of these differences is questionable at best. The secondary analysis looked at treatment differences by age of the child. Once again, they found a superior finding for PMTO on 4 of 16 measures for children 7 years of age and younger only. No differences between TAU and PMTO on 15 of 16 measures for children 8 years of age and older; 1 measure favored TAU over PMTO. In other words, for children over 7 years of age, there was only one significant finding and that was for TAU.

In addition to these underwhelming results, the PMTO therapists received 18 months of training and ongoing support and supervision during the study, whereas the TAU therapists received no additional training, support, or supervision. Finally, the dose of treatment favored PMTO (work with parents; 40 vs. 21 hours). The meager results, no findings on 12 of 16 measures, and no effects favoring PMTO for children 8 years of age and over, combined with the confounds of the differential training and support of the two therapist groups and unequal doses of treatment, cast significant doubt on this study's conclusions. The cost effectiveness of implementing an approach that requires 18 months of training while yielding minimal results is dubious.

*2. You have asserted that including the client's voice is an important issue in graduate training. What are you (Jacqueline A. Sparks) doing in your MFT program at the University of Rhode Island?*

The MFT Program at the University of Rhode Island recently instituted an outcome-informed protocol that emphasizes the importance of systematically monitoring client feedback throughout therapy. Trainees are taught to collect, score, and use brief, valid measures of progress and relationship (ORS, SRS, CORS; see http://www.heartandsoulofchange.com) at each session to enhance therapist flexibility, evaluate outcome, and improve overall effectiveness. Additionally, our program uses a software system that allows automated data entry from the ORS, SRS, and CORS and real-time warnings to therapists when client ratings of either the alliance or outcome fall significantly outside of established norms. The program uses algorithms based on large normative samples to help trainees and supervisors identify clients who are at risk for a negative outcome or dropout. It allows data to be stored and analyzed efficiently, providing an extensive base for faculty and student research. Most important, therapists and clients receive immediate feedback about therapy progress, enhancing student learning and client engagement. The Family Therapy Program at the University of Rhode Island is one of only a handful of clinical training programs that can claim to train not only competent but effective clinicians.

*3. You mention that feasibility is important to the feedback process. Are you saying that at the practice level, outcome measures have to be brief?*

Yes. Long measures are largely impractical in the real world, especially in work with families. Consider our experience in our validation study of the CORS (Duncan et al., 2006). The 30-item instrument used as a measure of concurrent validity made the completion of this study doubtful at times. In one school site, following a donation to the school, 500 youth–parent dyads volunteered for the study. At the first assessment, only 200 completed the measures. Of that 200, only 25 returned for a second assessment. In total, over 2,500 research packets were disseminated that finally resulted in a nonclinical sample of 199 dyads, illustrative of the feasibility issue.

On the practitioner side of things, many therapists see outcome measurement as an add-on separate from actual clinical work and relevant only to management and other overseers. In addition to wanting measures to be brief, to be easy to integrate, and to have face validity, therapists want measures that are clinically useful. Is the measure intended to improve the effectiveness of rendered services or merely monitor them? Most youth outcome measures were developed primarily as pre–post or periodic outcome measures. Such instruments provide an excellent way to measure program effectiveness but are not feasible to administer frequently and, therefore, do not provide real-time feedback for immediate treatment modification before clients drop out or suffer a negative outcome; in short, they are not clinical tools as much as they are oversight tools.

## REFERENCES

Addison, S. M., Sandberg, J. G., Corby, J., Robila, M., & Platt, J. J. (2002). Alternative methodologies in research literature review: Links between clinical work and MFT effectiveness. *American Journal of Family Therapy, 30*, 339–371.

Allgood, S. M., Parham, K. B., Salts, C. J., & Smith, T. A. (1995). The association between pretreatment change and unplanned termination in family therapy. *American Journal of Family Therapy, 23*, 195–202.

Anker, M., Duncan, B., & Sparks, J. (2009). Using client feedback to improve couples therapy outcomes: A randomized clinical trial in a naturalistic setting. *Journal of Consulting and Clinical Psychology, 77*, 693–704.

Anker, M., Owen, J., Duncan, B., & Sparks, J. (2009). *Split alliances, gender, and partner influences in couple therapy: A randomized sample in a naturalistic setting.* Manuscript submitted for publication.

Anker, M., Sparks, J., Duncan, B., & Stapnes, A. (2009). *Footprints of couple therapy: Client reflections at six-month follow up after routine care.* Manuscript submitted for publication.

Asay, T. P., & Lambert, M. J. (1999). The empirical case for the common factors in therapy: Quantitative findings. In M. A. Hubble, B. L. Duncan, & S. D. Miller (Eds.), *The heart and soul of change: What works in therapy* (pp. 33–56). Washington, DC: American Psychological Association.

Askey, R., Gamble, C., & Gray, R. (2007). Family work in first-onset psychosis: A literature review. *Journal of Psychiatric and Mental Health Nursing, 14,* 356–365.

Baucom, D., & Epstein, N. (1990). *Cognitive–behavioral marital therapy.* New York: Brunner/Mazel.

Baskin, T. W., Tierney, S. C., Minami, T., & Wampold, B. E. (2003). Establishing specificity in psychotherapy: A meta-analysis of structural equivalence of placebo controls. *Journal of Consulting and Clinical Psychology, 71,* 973–979.

Beutler, L. E., Malik, M., Alimohamed, S., Harwood, T. M., Talebi, H., Noble, S., et al. (2004). Therapist effects. In M. J. Lambert (Ed.), *Bergin and Garfield's handbook of psychotherapy and behavior change* (5th ed., pp. 227–306). New York: Wiley.

Beyebach, M., Morejon, A. R., Palenzuela, D. L., & Rodriguez-Arias, J. L. (1996). Research on the process of solution-focused brief therapy. In S. Miller, M. Hubble, & B. Duncan (Eds.), *Handbook of solution-focused brief therapy* (pp. 299–334). San Francisco: Jossey-Bass.

Bischoff, R. J., & McBride, A. (1996). Client perceptions of couple and family therapy. *American Journal of Family Therapy, 24,* 117–128.

Bischoff, R. J., & Sprenkle, D. H. (1993). Dropping out of marriage and family therapy: A critical review of research. *Family Process, 32,* 353–376.

Bordin, E. (1979). The generalizability of the psychoanalytic concept of the working alliance. *Psychotherapy, 16,* 252–260.

Borduin, C. M., Mann, B. J., Cone, L. T., Henggeler, S. W., Fucci, B. R., Blaske, D. M., & Williams, R. A. (1995). Multisystemic treatment of serious juvenile offenders: Long-term prevention of criminality and violence. *Journal of Consulting and Clinical Psychology, 63,* 569–578.

Brown, L. S. (2006). The neglect of lesbian, gay, bisexual, and transgendered clients. In J. C. Norcross, L. E. Beutler, & R. L. Levant (Eds.), *Evidence-based practices in mental health: Debate and dialogue on the Fundamental Questions* (pp. 346–352). Washington, DC: American Psychological Association.

Carr, A. (2000a). Evidence-based practice in family therapy and systemic consultation: I. Child-focused problems. *Journal of Family Therapy, 22,* 29–60.

Carr, A. (2000b). Evidence-based practice in family therapy and systemic consultation: II. Adult-focused problems. *Journal of Family Therapy, 22,* 273–295.

Christensen, A., Atkins, D. C., Berns, S., Wheeler, J., Baucom, D., & Simpson, L. E. (2004). Traditional versus integrative behavioral couple therapy for significantly and chronically distressed married couples. *Journal of Consulting and Clinical Psychology, 72,* 176–191.

Christensen, A., & Heavey, C. L. (1999). Interventions for couples. *Annual Review of Psychology, 50,* 165–190.

Christensen, A. & Jacobson, N. S. (1994). Who (or what) can do therapy: The status and challenge of non-professional therapies. *Psychological Science, 5,* 8–14.

Clarkin, J. F., & Levy, K. N. (2004). The influence of client variables on psychotherapy. In M. J. Lambert (Ed.), *Bergin and Garfield's handbook of psychotherapy and behavior change* (5th ed., pp. 194–226). New York: Wiley.

Cottrell, D., & Boston, P. (2002). Practitioner review: The effectiveness of systemic family therapy for children and adolescents. *Journal of Child Psychology and Psychiatry, 43,* 573–586.

De La Peña, C. M., Friedlander, M., & Escudero, V. (2009). Frequency, severity, and evolution of split family alliances: How observable are they? *Psychotherapy Research, 19,* 133–142.

Dennis, M., Godley, S. H., Diamond, G., Tims, F. M., Babor, T., Donaldson, J., et al. (2004). The Cannabis Youth Treatment (CYT) Study: Main findings from two randomized trials. *Journal of Substance Abuse Treatment, 27,* 197–213.

Diamond, G., & Josephson, A. (2005). Family-based treatment research: A 10-year update. *Journal of the American Academy of child and adolescent psychiatry, 44,* 872–887.

Dixon, L., McFarlane, W. R., Lefley, H., Lucksted, A., Cohen, M., Fallon, I., et al. (2001). Evidence-based practices for services to families of people with psychiatric disabilities. *Psychiatric Services, 52,* 903–910.

Duncan, B. L., Miller, S. D., & Sparks, J. A. (2004). *The heroic client: A revolutionary way to improve effectiveness through client-directed, outcome-informed therapy.* San Francisco: Jossey-Bass.

Duncan, B. L., Miller, S. D., Sparks, J. A., Claud, D. A., Reynolds, L. R., Brown, J., & Johnson, L. D. (2003). The Session Rating Scale: Preliminary psychometric properties of a "working" alliance measure. *Journal of Brief Therapy, 3,* 3–12.

Duncan, B. L., Solovey, A., & Rusk, G. (1992). *Changing the rules: A client-directed approach.* New York: Guilford Press.

Duncan, B. L., Sparks, J., Miller, S., Bohanske, R., & Claud, D. (2006). Giving youth a voice: A preliminary study of the reliability and validity of a brief outcome measure for children. *Journal of Brief Therapy, 5,* 5–22.

Dunn, R. L., & Schwebel, A. I. (1995). Meta-analytic review of marital therapy outcome research. *Journal of Family Psychology, 9,* 58–68.

Frank, J. D., & Frank, J. B. (1991). *Persuasion and healing* (3rd ed.) Baltimore: Johns Hopkins University Press.

Friedlander, M. L., & Tuason, M. T. (2000). Processes and outcomes in couples and family therapy. In S. D. Brown & R. W. Lent (Eds.), *Handbook of counseling psychology* (pp. 797–824). New York: Wiley.

Gaston, L. (1990). The concept of the alliance and its role in psychotherapy: Theoretical and empirical considerations. *Psychotherapy, 27,* 143–152.

Goldman, A., & Greenberg, L. (1992). Comparison of integrated systemic and emotionally focused approaches to couple therapy. *Journal of Consulting and Clinical Psychology, 61*, 6–15.

Goldstein, M. J., & Miklowitz, D. J. (1995). The effectiveness of psychoeducational family therapy in the treatment of schizophrenic disorders. *Journal of Marital and Family Therapy, 21*, 361–376.

Gollan, J. K., & Jacobson, N. S. (2002). Developments in couple therapy research. In H. A. Liddle, D. A. Santisteban, R. F. Levant, & J. H. Bray (Eds.), *Family psychology: Science-based interventions* (pp. 105–122). Washington, DC: American Psychological Association.

Gordon, D. A., Arbuthnot, J., Gustafson, K., & McGreen, P. (1988). Home-based behavioral systems family therapy with disadvantaged juvenile delinquents. *American Journal of Family Therapy, 16*, 243–255.

Green, R. J., & Herget, M. (1991). Outcomes of systemic/strategic team consultation: II. The importance of therapist warmth and active structuring. *Family Process, 30*, 321–336.

Greenberg, L. S., & Johnson, S. M. (1988). *Emotionally focused couples therapy*. New York: Guilford Press.

Gregory, M. A., Leslie, L. A. (1996). Different lenses: Variations in clients' perception of family therapy by race and gender. *Journal of Marital and Family Therapy, 22*, 239–251.

Hampson, R. B., & Beavers, W. R. (1996). Measuring family therapy outcome in a clinical setting: Families that do better or do worse in therapy. *Family Process, 35*, 347–361.

Henggeler, S. W., Melton, G. B., & Smith, L. A. (1992). Family preservation using multisystemic therapy: An effective alternative to incarcerating serious juvenile offenders. *Journal of Consulting and Clinical Psychology, 60*, 953–961.

Hogue, A., Dauber, S., Samuolis, J., & Liddle, H. A. (2006). Treatment techniques and outcomes in multidimensional family therapy for adolescent behavior problems. *Journal of Family Psychology, 20*, 535–543.

Horvath, A. O., & Symonds, B. D. (1991). Relation between working alliance and outcome in psychotherapy: A meta-analysis. *Journal of Counseling Psychology, 38*, 139–149.

Huey, S. J., Henggeler, S. W., Brondino, M. J., & Pickrel, S. G. (2000). Mechanisms of change in multisystemic therapy: Reducing delinquent behavior through therapist adherence and improved family and peer functioning. *Journal of Consulting and Clinical Psychology, 68*, 451–467.

International Centre for Excellence in Emotionally Focused Therapy. (2007). *Certification*. Retrieved July 6, 2009, from http://www.iceeft.com/training2.htm

Jacobson, N. S., & Christensen, A. (1996). *Integrative couple therapy: Promoting acceptance and change*. New York: Norton.

Jacobson, N. S., & Truax, P. (1991). Clinical significance: A statistical approach to defining meaningful change in psychotherapy research. *Journal of Consulting and Clinical Psychology, 59*, 12–19.

Joanning, H., Thomas, F., Quinn, W., & Mullen, R. (1992). Treating adolescent drug abuse: A comparison of family systems therapy, group therapy, and family drug education. *Journal of Marital and Family Therapy, 18*, 345–356.

Johnson, S. M. (2003). The revolution in couple therapy: A practitioner–scientist perspective. *Journal of Marital and Family Therapy, 29*, 365–384.

Johnson, S. M., & Greenberg, L. S. (1985). Differential effects of experiential and problem-solving interventions in resolving marital conflict. *Journal of Consulting and Clinical Psychology, 53*, 175–184.

Johnson, S. M., Hunsley, J., Greenberg, L., & Schindler, D. (1999). Emotionally focused couples therapy: Status and challenges. *Clinical Psychology: Science and Practice, 6*, 67–79.

Johnson, S. M., & Talitman, E. (1997). Predictors of success in emotionally focused marital therapy. *Journal of Marital and Family Therapy, 23*(2), 135–152.

Karver, M. S., Handelsman, J. B., Fields, S., & Bickman, L. (2006). Meta-analysis of relationship variables in youth and family therapy: The evidence for different relationship variables in the child and adolescent treatment outcome literature. *Clinical Psychology Review, 26*, 50–65.

Knobloch-Fedders, L. M., Pinsof, W. M., & Mann, B. J. (2007). Therapeutic alliance and treatment progress in couple psychotherapy. *Journal of Marital and Family Therapy, 33*, 245–257.

Lambert, M., & Ogles, B. (2004). The efficacy and effectiveness of psychotherapy. In M. J. Lambert (Ed.), *Bergin and Garfield's handbook of psychotherapy and behavior change* (5th ed., pp. 139–193). New York: Wiley.

Luborsky, L., Diguer, L., Seligman, D. A., Rosenthal, R., Krause, E. D., Johnson, S., et al. (1999). The researcher's own therapy allegiances: A "wild card" in comparisons of treatment efficacy. *Clinical Psychology: Science and Practice, 6*, 95–106.

Martin, D. J., Garske, J. P., & Davis, M. K. (2000). Relation of the therapeutic alliance with outcome and other variables: A meta-analytic review. *Journal of Consulting and Clinical Psychology, 68*, 438–450.

McFarlane, W. R., Dixon, L., Lukens, E., & Lucksted, A. (2003). Family psychoeducation and schizophrenia: A review of the literature. *Journal of Marital and Family Therapy, 29*, 223–245.

McFarlane, W. R., & Cook, W. L. (2007). Family expressed emotion prior to onset of psychosis. *Family Process, 46*(2), 18–197.

McLellan, A., Arndt, I., Metzer, D., Woody, G., & O'Brien, C. (1993). The effects of psychosocial services in substance abuse treatment. *JAMA, 269*, 1953–1959.

Miller, S. D., Duncan, B. L., Brown, J., Sparks, J., & Claud, D. (2003). The Outcome Rating Scale: A preliminary study of the reliability, validity, and feasibility of a brief visual analog measure. *Journal of Brief Therapy, 2*, 91–100.

Miller, S. D., Wampold, B., & Varhely, K. (2008). Direct comparisons of treatment modalities for youth disorders: A meta-analysis. *Psychotherapy Research, 18,* 5–14.

National Center for Mental Health Promotion and Youth Violence Prevention. (n.d.). *Fact sheet: Functional family therapy.* Retrieved July 6, 2009, from http://www.promoteprevent.org/Publications/EBI-factsheets/FFT.pdf

Norcross, J. C., Beutler, L. E., & Levant, R. F. (2006). Prologue. In J. C. Norcross, L. E. Beutler, & R. L. Levant (Eds.), *Evidence-based practices in mental health: Debate and dialogue on the fundamental questions* (pp. 3–12). Washington, DC: American Psychological Association.

Northey, W. F. (2002). Characteristics and clinical practices of marriage and family therapists: A national survey. *Journal of Marital and Family Therapy, 28,* 487–494.

Ogden, T., & Hagen, K.A. (2008). Treatment effectiveness of Parent Management Training in Norway: A randomized controlled trial of children with conduct problems. *Journal of Consulting and Clinical Psychology, 76,* 607–621.

Ogles, B. M., Carlston, D., Hatfield, D., Melendez, G., Dowell, K., & Fields, S. A. (2006). The role of fidelity and feedback in the wraparound approach. *Journal of Child and Family Studies, 15,* 115–129.

Ogles B. M., Melendez, G., Davis, D.C., & Lunnen, K. M. (2001). The Ohio scales: Practical outcome assessment. *Journal of Child and Family Studies, 10,* 199–212.

Orlinsky, D. E., & Rønnestad, M. H. (2005). *How psychotherapists develop: A study of therapeutic work and professional growth.* Washington, DC: American Psychological Association.

Orlinsky, D. E., Rønnestad, M. H., & Willutzki, U. (2004). Fifty years of psychotherapy process–outcome research: Continuity and change. In M. J. Lambert (Ed.), *Bergin and Garfield's handbook of psychotherapy and behavior change* (5th ed., pp. 307–390). New York: Wiley.

Orwell, G. (1945). *Animal farm: A fairy story.* London: Secker & Warburg.

Owens, J., Anker, M., Duncan, B., & Sparks, J. (2009). *Therapist variability, the alliance, and therapist experience in couple therapy.* Manuscript submitted for publication.

Pinsof, W. M., & Catherall, D. R. (1986). The integrative psychotherapy alliance: Family, couple, and individual therapy scales. *Journal of Marital and Family Therapy, 12,* 137–151.

Pinsof, W. M., & Wynne, L. C. (1995). The efficacy of marital and family therapy: An empirical overview, conclusions, and recommendations. *Journal of Marital and Family Therapy, 21,* 585–614.

Quinn, W. H., Dotson, D., & Jordan, K. (1997). Dimensions of therapeutic alliance and their associations with outcome in family therapy. *Psychotherapy Research, 7,* 429–438.

Raytek, H. S., McCrady, B. S., Epstein, E. E., & Hirsch, L. S. (1999). Therapeutic alliance and the retention of couples in conjoint alcoholism treatment. *Addictive Behaviors, 24,* 317–330.

Robbins, M. S., Alexander, J. F., Newell, R. M., & Turner, C. W. (1996). The immediate effect of reframing on client attitude in family therapy. *Journal of Family Psychology, 10*, 28–34.

Robbins, M. S., Alexander, J. F., Turner, C. W., & Perez, G. A. (2003). Alliance and dropout in family therapy for adolescents with behavior problems: Individual and systemic effects. *Journal of Family Psychology, 17*, 534–544.

Sexton, T. L., Alexander, J. F., & Mease, A. L. (2004). Levels of evidence for the models and mechanisms of therapeutic change in family and couple therapy. In M. J. Lambert (Ed.), *Bergin and Garfield's handbook of psychotherapy and behavior change* (5th ed., pp. 590–646). New York: Wiley.

Sexton, T. L., Ridley, C. R., & Kleiner, A. J. (2004). Beyond common factors: Multilevel-process models of therapeutic change in marriage and family therapy. *Journal of Marital and Family Therapy, 30*, 131–149.

Shadish, W. R., & Baldwin, S. A. (2002). Meta-analysis of MFT interventions. In D. H. Sprenkle (Ed.), *Effectiveness research in marriage and family therapy* (pp. 339–379). Alexandria, VA: American Association of Marriage and Family Therapy.

Shadish, W. R., & Baldwin, S. A. (2005). Effects of behavioral marital therapy: A meta-analysis of randomized controlled trials. *Journal of Consulting and Clinical Psychology, 73*, 6–14.

Shadish, W. R., Montgomery, L., Wilson, P., Wilson, M., Bright, I., & Okwumabua, T. (1993). The effects of family and marital psychotherapies: A meta-analysis. *Journal of Consulting and Clinical Psychology, 61*, 992–1002.

Shelef, K., Diamond, G. M., Diamond, G. S., and Liddle, H. A. (2005). Adolescent and parent alliance and treatment outcome in multidimensional family therapy. *Journal of Consulting and Clinical Psychology, 73*, 689–698.

Shirk, S. R., & Karver, M. (2003). Prediction of treatment outcome from relationship variables in child and adolescent therapy: A meta-analytic review. *Journal of Consulting and Clinical Psychology, 71*, 452–464.

Snyder, D. K., Mangrum, L. F., & Wills, R. M. (1993). Predicting couples' response to marital therapy: A comparison of short- and long-term predictors. *Journal of Consulting and Clinical Psychology, 61*, 61–69.

Snyder, D. K., & Wills, R. M. (1989). Behavioral versus insight-oriented marital therapy: Effect on individual and interspousal functioning. *Journal of Consulting and Clinical Psychology, 61*, 61–69.

Sparks, J. A., Duncan, B. L., & Miller, S. D. (2007). Common factors in psychotherapy. In J. Lebow (Ed.), *21st century psychotherapies* (pp. 453–497). Hoboken, NJ: Wiley.

Sprenkle, D. H. (2003). Effectiveness research in marriage and family therapy: Introduction. *Journal of Marital and Family Therapy, 29*, 85–96.

Sprenkle, D. H., Blow, A. J., & Dickey, M. H. (1999). Common factors and other nontechnique variables in marriage and family therapy. In M. A. Hubble, B. L. Duncan, & S. D. Miller (Eds.), *The heart and soul of change: What works in therapy* (pp. 329–359). Washington, DC: American Psychological Association.

Stanton, M. D., & Shadish, W. R. (1997). Outcome, attrition, and family-couple treatment for drug abuse: A meta-analysis and review of the controlled, comparative studies. *Psychological Bulletin, 122,* 170–191.

Stanton, M. D., Todd, T. C., & Associates. (1982). *The family therapy of drug abuse and addiction.* New York: Guilford Press.

Symonds, D., & Horvath, A. O. (2004). Optimizing the alliance in couples therapy. *Family Process, 43,* 443–455.

Tetzlaff, B., Hahn, J., Godley, S., Godley, M., Diamond, G., & Funk, R. (2005). Working alliance, treatment satisfaction, and post-treatment patterns of use among adolescent substance users. *Psychology of Addictive Behaviors, 19,* 199–207.

Waldron, H. B., Turner, C. W., Barton, C., Alexander, J. F., & Cline, V. B. (1997). Therapist defensiveness and marital therapy process and outcome. *American Journal of Family Therapy, 25,* 233–243.

Wampold, B. E. (2001). *The great psychotherapy debate: Models, methods, and findings.* Hillsdale, NJ: Erlbaum.

Wampold, B. E. (2002). An examination of the bases of evidence-based interventions. *School Psychology Quarterly, 17,* 500–507.

Wampold, B. E., & Brown, G. (2005). Estimating therapist variability in outcomes attributable to therapists: A naturalistic study of outcomes in managed care. *Journal of Consulting and Clinical Psychology, 73,* 914–923.

Wampold, B. E., Minami, T., Tierney, S. C., Baskin, T. W., & Bhati, K. S. (2005). The placebo is powerful: Estimating placebo effects in medicine and psychotherapy from clinical trials. *Journal of Clinical Psychology, 61,* 835–854.

Weiner-Davis, M., de Shazer, S., and Gingerich, W. J. (1987). Building on pretreatment change to construct the therapeutic solution. *Journal of Marital and Family Therapy, 13,* 359–363.

Weisz, J. R., Jensen-Doss, A., & Hawley, K. M. (2006). Evidence-based youth psychotherapies versus usual clinical care: A meta-analysis of direct comparisons. *American Psychologist, 61,* 671–689.

Zane, N., Hall, G. C. N., Sue, S., Young, K., & Nunez, J. (2004). Research on psychotherapy with culturally diverse populations. In M. J. Lambert (Ed.), *Bergin and Garfield's handbook of psychotherapy and behavior change* (5th ed., pp. 767–804). New York: Wiley.

# 13

# WHAT WORKS IN SUBSTANCE ABUSE AND DEPENDENCE TREATMENT

DAVID MEE-LEE, A. THOMAS McLELLAN, AND SCOTT D. MILLER

> Discovery consists of seeing what everybody has seen and thinking what
> nobody has thought.
> —Albert Szent-Gyorgyi

The misuse of alcohol and other drugs is a serious and widespread problem. According to the Substance Abuse and Mental Health Services Administration (SAMHSA) of the Department of Health and Human Services, an estimated 23.2 million people ages 12 and older needed treatment for illicit drug or alcohol use in 2007 (National Survey on Drug Use and Health; SAMHSA, 2008). Data from the National Institute on Alcohol Abuse and Alcoholism further show that problem drinking alone is associated with more than 100,000 deaths per year (Stinson & Proudfit, 1994). By way of comparison, this is the statistical equivalent of a plane crash killing 274 people every single day. Substance abuse and addiction cost federal, state, and local governments at least $467.7 billion in 2005 (National Center on Addiction and Substance Abuse at Columbia University, 2009), and substance abuse has been reported to be the nation's number one health problem. (Ericson, 2001; U.S. Department of Health and Human Services, 2000). Approximately 40% of traffic fatalities in the United States are alcohol related (National Highway Traffic Safety Administration, 2006).

The consequences of substance abuse and dependence for the family are well established. In the January 2000 issue of the *American Journal of Public Health*, for example, researchers found that 25% of all U.S. children are exposed to alcohol abuse or dependence in the family (Grant, 2000). This dry recitation of statistics takes on added urgency when the abuse of alcohol in the home is linked with poorer school performance, increased risk of delinquency, neglect, divorce, homelessness, and violence. Regarding the latter, available evidence indicates that as many as 80% of incidents of familial violence are associated with alcohol abuse (Collins & Messerschmidt, 1993; Eighth Special Report to the U.S. Congress on Alcohol and Health, 1993). Whether or not clinicians are interested, the prevalence of substance use problems and the impact on the user, significant others, and society makes avoiding the problem unthinkable in any clinical, health, or medical setting. By 2010, the need for addictions professionals and licensed treatment staff with graduate-level degrees is expected to increase by 35% over 2003 staffing levels (National Association of State Alcohol and Drug Abuse Directors [NASADAD], 2003). Although there is an overabundance of mental health professionals, as documented in chapter 9 of this volume, too few are skilled in alcohol and other drug use problems. Many agencies are understaffed and have difficulties recruiting and training enough qualified professionals to meet current needs (SAMHSA, 2006). It is unfortunate that less than 10% of those in need of services receive professional help, and the majority of those in most levels of care do not complete treatment (SAMHSA, 2008a, 2008b) Worse still, many of those who stay the course fare no better, with more than 50% resuming problematic alcohol or drug use within 6 months. Despite such poor results, the treatment of substance-related problems has not changed appreciably in the last 75 years. In health care, and behavioral health care in particular, addressing substance use problems and addiction treatment has encompassed at least four macro approaches to service delivery (Mee-Lee, 2001a; Mee-Lee & Shulman, 2003). Most have been, and continue to be, either *complications-driven* or *diagnosis- and program-driven* in nature.

As the name implies, in complications-driven care professional time and attention is principally devoted to treating the gastrointestinal, psychiatric, orthopedic, or trauma-related consequences of substance abuse. Typically, continuing treatment for problems (physical and otherwise) is superficial or nonexistent, as the focus is on addressing the primary presenting complaint. By contrast, in diagnosis- and program-driven therapy, the abuse of and dependence on substances take center stage. Clients are admitted to a program in which the content, structure, and length are fixed. Aftercare is common and dedicated to reinforcing program goals and objectives.

Recognizing that complications- and diagnosis-driven care fail to address the underlying substance use problem or meet the specific needs of the individual, researchers and theoreticians have proposed two additional approaches: (a) *individualized, assessment-driven treatment*; and (b) most recently, *outcome-informed treatment*. The first emphasizes the need to tailor services to the individual. It offers a broad continuum of care to accommodate the diverse needs and preferences of clients. Placement criteria for multiple levels of treatment were developed by the American Society of Addiction Medicine (ASAM), first published in 1991 and most recently updated in 2001 (Hoffmann, Halikas, Mee-Lee, & Weedman, 1991; Mee-Lee, Shulman, Fishman, Gastfriend, & Griffith, 2001).

The second approach, outcomes-driven treatment, uses feedback from clients to enhance the fit and effect of services. As such, it is an extension of, rather than an alternative to, individualized, assessment-driven care. The main difference between the two is that in outcome-informed treatment, clients' rather than the clinicians' assessments drive service planning and delivery. For all the rhetoric regarding individualized treatment and data-driven quality improvement (Institute of Medicine [IOM], 2006; National Institute on Drug Abuse, 2009; SAMHSA, 2000), the field of addiction treatment has not fully implemented either approach.

The ASAM Patient Placement Criteria have been available since 1991. Although they recommend flexible, individualized treatment stays, most addiction programs still hold to programmatic, fixed lengths of stay. The IOM, in their *Quality Chasm Series*, indicated "successful quality improvement requires that quality measurement be linked with activities at the locus of care to effect change and that understanding and use of these change (quality improvement) techniques be woven into the day-to-day operations of health care organizations and provider practices" (IOM, 2006, p. 193). The report also said that "the understanding and use of modern quality improvement methods have not yet permeated the day-to-day operations of organizations and individual clinicians" (IOM, 2006, p. 141).

Luckily, several factors are coming together, challenging how treatment is currently delivered, monitored, and evaluated. Chief among these is the rise of consumerism. Those in need of help are less and less inclined to assume the patient role. Instead they want, and even demand, to play an active part. Another significant pressure comes from payers and other stakeholders who demand accountability and transparency, including evidence of return on investment for money spent. Last, but certainly not least, a new generation of researchers and clinicians is now in charge. Familiar with the field's shortcomings and armed with 40 years of evidence about what works, this group is pushing for paradigmatic change, away from complications- and diagnosis-driven care, and toward the revolutionary model described by Orford (2006) in the following passage:

> [It] give[s] far greater weight to patient choice and far less to professional allocation rules . . . shift[ing] away from a preoccupation with the psychobiological characteristics of individual clients (e.g., substance use patterns, degree of dependence, "comorbidity," and motivation for change) [and]

towards taking a far greater interest in people's social positions and identities . . . not so much whether we could establish rules about allocating certain kinds of clients to certain kinds of therapists, but rather what was the process whereby the patient decided to trust the therapist, to communicate openly. The therapist would be seen not as a more or less faithful exponent of the technology, but as someone who adjusted continuously what she or he did in response to the client and the developing client–therapist relationship. (pp. 653–654)

We begin this chapter with a systemic review of the empirical evidence regarding what works in substance abuse and dependence treatment and the broader field of psychotherapy. We then identify key curative factors and propose a series of empirically tested strategies for remedying problems associated with high dropout and low success rates in substance-related treatment. Finally, we present and illustrate the principles, practices, and overall organizational structure of a consumer-driven, outcome-informed treatment system.

## THE SEARCH FOR WHAT WORKS IN ADDICTION TREATMENT

Efforts to identify the elements of effective care have been marked by contention and debate. Historically, the most popular view among practitioners and the public has been that people can recover from drug and alcohol abuse and dependence but can never be cured. For many years, the correct treatment involved a hospital-based detoxification followed by a stay in a 28-day residential facility, lifelong commitment to abstinence, and continuing participation in some form of mutual help group (e.g., Alcoholics Anonymous, Rational Recovery).

Concurrently, a smaller group of researchers, academics, and clinicians published data critical of virtually every aspect of the dominant perspective. For instance, research did not provide any evidence of superior outcomes for traditional long-term (and expensive) treatment over brief, targeted intervention or even a single session of advice given by a family physician (Bein, Miller, & Tonigan, 1993; W. R. Miller & Hester, 1986b; Orford & Edwards, 1977). Whereas detox was once thought an essential first step toward sobriety, later research has found that the practice actually provoked future episodes of medically supervised withdrawal that, in turn, increased the risk of impaired neurocognitive functioning (Duka, Townshend, Collier, & Stephens, 2003; W. R. Miller & Hester, 1986a).

In 1986, when the U.S. Congress was deliberating the extension of appropriations for alcohol and drug research, it received a report that treatment services for alcohol and drug problems were becoming increasingly important to the nation's health care system. Consequently, it authorized a critical review of available research knowledge. In 1990, the the results of two major IOM studies were published two landmark volumes, *Broadening the Base of Treatment for Alcohol Problems* (IOM, 1990) and *Treating Drug Problems* (Gerstein, Henrick, & Harwood, 1990). Both volumes examined existing evidence and reached similar conclusions regarding the effectiveness of treatments for alcohol and drug abuse and dependence. Namely, no single approach worked for everyone. The report further noted that the lack of differential effectiveness among competing approaches had long been cited by those advocating a move away from complications- and diagnosis-driven treatment to the individualized, assessment-driven model in which services are matched to the individual (Gotheil, McLellan, & Druley, 1981; McLellan, McKay, Forman, & Kemp, 1983; Mee-Lee, 1995; W. R. Miller & Hester, 1986a).

The idea of matching treatments to clients has common sense appeal and empirical support. The literature shows, for example, that clients vary significantly in their response to different approaches (Duncan, Miller, & Sparks, 2004). As far back as 1941, Bowman and Jellinek, in the first major review of the treatment of alcohol problems, stressed the need for matching (IOM, 1990, p. 279). Since then, numerous matching variables have been proposed and tested. Additionally, over time a variety of matching hypotheses have been studied on the basis of demographic variables, psychiatric diagnosis plus alcohol problems, personality factors, severity of alcohol problems, and antecedents to drinking (IOM, 1990). Unfortunately, few studies have been replicated. Moreover, in the few cases in which matching hypotheses were tested more than once, the data have been mixed and contradictory.

Enter Project MATCH (Matching Alcoholism Treatments to Client Heterogeneity), the largest and most statistically powerful clinical trial in the history of alcohol and drug treatment (Project MATCH Research Group, 1997). In brief, this National Institute on Alcohol Abuse and Alcoholism organized and funded study was designed to carefully examine questions regarding differential efficacy and treatment matching. Three conceptually and methodologically different approaches were included: motivational enhancement therapy, 12-step facilitation, and cognitive–behavioral therapy. A range of reliable and valid measures were used to test the effectiveness of the three treatments, as well as 21 specific, matching hypotheses. Along with the suggestions of leading researchers, the latter were derived from a review of the literature and included severity of alcohol involvement, cognitive impairment, psychiatric severity, conceptual level, gender, meaning seeking, motivational readiness to change, social support for drinking versus abstinence, sociopathy, and typology of alcoholism.

Hopes were dashed. The results of this $33 million study did not provide support for the individualized, assessment-driven model. To begin with, although participants in the study showed considerable and sustained improvement, no differences in outcome emerged among the three approaches. More telling, of 64 possible matching interactions tested, only 1 match proved significant—hardly compelling evidence that clinicians can successfully match clients to treatments. If doubts persist about the durability of the findings, the same results were observed in a follow-up study conducted 10 years later. As researchers Tonigan et al. (2003) concluded, "No support for differential treatment response was found using PDA [percent days abstinent], DDD [drinks per drinking day], and total standard drink measures in comparing CBT [cognitive–behavioral], MET [motivational enhancement], and TSF [twelve-step facilitation] therapies 10-years after treatment" (p. 1).

More recently, researchers did not find any evidence regarding the impact of other factors believed to influence success. These include the following: the age of those receiving services; the specific substance being abused; and the amount, intensity, and type of care offered. The Cannabis Youth Treatment (CYT) Study is representative. In short, the CYT examined the outcomes of 600 adolescent marijuana users. Participants were randomized into one of five different treatments of either 5 or 12 weeks duration. Every effort was made to include adolescents who were rated as clinically similar or slightly more severe than those seen in routine clinical practice in public settings. Furthermore, the treatment approaches used in the study represented the best approaches considered research supported and evidence based (Dennis et al., 2004). As with Project MATCH, no differences in outcome were found. Overall, individually delivered services fared no better than those provided in a group setting. Involving the family in the therapy did not yield an advantage over services extended to the adolescent alone. Moreover, outcome was not affected by the duration of treatment. It is surprising that 5 weeks was as effective as 12, though the smaller dose had actually been designed as a minimal treatment control group.

The Combined Pharmacotherapies and Behavioral Interventions (Project COMBINE; Anton et al., 2006), as the acronym suggests, studied the effects of medication either alone or in combination with counseling in the treatment of alcohol dependence. The 3-year investigation included 1,383 participants randomly assigned to 16 weeks of naltrexone (100 milligrams/day), acamprosate (3 grams/day), placebos, or both, either alone or in combination with behavioral intervention. One group received counseling and no pills. In addition to these primary treatments, some groups received medication management and support aimed at ensuring medication compliance and abstinence from alcohol. Echoing prior studies, all of the therapies, delivered alone or in combination, succeeded in reducing drinking rates and promoting short-term abstinence. Only the drug acamprosate (Campral) showed poorer than expected results on the drinking measures. Regardless of the treatment, half of the participants in the study still had their drinking under control at 1 year follow-up.

In 2003, Berglund, Thelander, and Jonsson published an evidence-based review of all published randomized controlled trials of psychological treatments for alcohol abuse. Using a variety of methodologies, including meta-analysis, tallying of significance tests, and scholarly review, the researchers came to several determinations. First, treatment was more effective than no treatment or being placed on a waiting list. Second, specific treatments (e.g., treatments with a theoretical base, trained therapists, manuals) were more effective than standard or nonspecific treatments (e.g., supportive counseling, social work intervention). Third, no specific treatment approach was superior. Last, little supporting evidence existed for matching the type, level, or intensity of treatment to the individual client.

Most recently, Imel, Wampold, and Miller (2008) published the results of a meta-analysis specifically designed to test whether differences in efficacy exist among treatment approaches for alcoholism. The results of this state-of-the art analysis leave little room for doubt. There was no difference in outcome obtained among competing treatment approaches. Berglund et al. (2003) concluded as much, but their results were based in part on studies that included treatment conditions not intended to be therapeutic. The superiority of one approach over another is properly tested when two or more therapies intended to be therapeutic are compared within the same study (S. D. Miller, Wampold, & Varhely, 2008; Shadish and Sweeney, 1991; Wampold et al., 1997). In addition, because a wide variety of approaches were compared (e.g., 12-step facilitation, motivational enhancement therapy, behavioral self-control training, Alcoholics Anonymous, aversion therapy, relapse prevention, psychodynamic treatment) the finding of equivalent effects cannot be attributed to any similarity of treatments.

## Bringing Psychotherapy and Addiction Treatment Outcomes Research Together

As disconcerting as the results discussed to this point may be to some in the addiction industry, they are entirely consistent with findings from psychotherapy. Wampold (2001) concluded in his review of the data, "decades of research" conducted by different researchers using different methods on a variety of treatment populations provide clear evidence that the type of treatment is irrelevant, and adherence to a protocol is misguided (p. 202). Simply put, the method does not matter. In fact, available data indicate that the particular approach used accounts for 1% or less of the outcome variance (Wampold et al., 1997).

The same evidence, showing the broad equivalence of treatment approaches, provides important clues about the predictors of successful intervention (Hubble, Duncan, & Miller, 1999). No matter the type or intensity of approach, research makes clear that client engagement is the single best predictor of outcome. Orlinsky, Grawe, and Parks (1994) concluded:

> The quality of the patient's [sic] participation stands out as the most important determinant of outcome ... these consistent process–process outcome relations, based on literally hundreds of empirical findings, can be considered *facts* established by 40-plus years of research. (p. 361)

High on the list of factors mediating the critical link between participation and outcome is the quality of the therapeutic relationship, in particular, the consumer's experience early in treatment (Bachelor & Horvath, 1999; Luborsky, Barber, Siqueland, McLellan, & Woody, 1997; Orlinsky et al., 1994). Meta-analytic studies indicate "a little over half of the beneficial effects of psychotherapy . . . are linked to the quality of the alliance" (Horvath, 2001, p. 366).

Similar findings have been reported in the alcohol treatment literature, in which between 50% and 66% of the variance in outcome is attributable to qualities of the alliance between client and therapist (W. R. Miller, Wilbourne, & Hettema, 2002; Luborsky et al., 1997). In other words, the therapeutic relationship contributes 5 to 10 times more to outcome than the model or approach used (Bachelor & Horvath, 1999; Duncan et al., 2004; Wampold, 2001). Given such findings, it is not surprising that a post hoc analysis of the Project MATCH data found that client ratings of the therapeutic relationship, regardless of the treatment used, was a significant predictor of participation, drinking behavior during treatment, and drinking at 12-month follow-up (Connors, Carroll, DiClemente, Longabaugh, & Donovan, 1997). Similarly, in the CYT Study, the client's ratings of the helping alliance predicted premature dropout, substance abuse and dependence symptoms posttreatment, and cannabis use at 3- and 6-month follow-up (Godley, Jones, Funk, Ives, & Passetti, 2004; Shelef, Diamond, Diamond, & Liddle, 2005).

Another significant predictor of outcome first identified in research on psychotherapy is the client's subjective experience of improvement early in treatment (Duncan et al., 2004). In a study of more than 2,000 therapists and thousands of clients, Brown, Dreis, and Nace (1999) found that treatments for mental health problems in which no improvement occurred by the third visit did not, on average, result in improvement over the entire course. Moreover, this study also showed that clients who worsened by the third visit were twice as likely to drop out as those reporting progress. Contrary to what is usually thought to be predictive of outcome, variables such as diagnosis, severity, family support, and type of therapy were "not . . . as important [in predicting outcome] as knowing whether or not the treatment being provided [was] actually working" (Brown, Dreis, & Nace, 1999, p. 404). Once again, similar results have been reported in studies of alcohol treatment. In Project MATCH, for example, all the change on the dependent measures occurred within the first 4 weeks (Stout et al., 2003).

Such research demonstrates that the best way to improve retention and outcome is to attend to clients' experience of progress and the therapeutic relationship early in treatment. In use in psychotherapy research for over a decade, real-time monitoring of results allows for rapid and responsive modifications in the treatment plan and content (Howard, Moras, Brill, Martinovich, & Lutz, 1996; Johnson, 1995). In an exemplary study, clients whose therapists had access to outcome and alliance information were less likely to show deteriorated performance, apt to remain engaged longer, and twice as likely to achieve a clinically significant reduction in symptoms (Whipple et al., 2003). Perhaps of most importance, these results were obtained without any attempt to organize, systematize, or otherwise control the treatment process. Neither were the therapists in this study trained in any new modalities, techniques, or diagnostic procedures. Rather, the individual clinicians were completely free to engage their clients in the manner they saw fit. The only constant in an otherwise diverse treatment environment was the availability of formal client feedback.

Of late, much is made of client-centered treatment planning in the addictions field. Even so, little actual research has been conducted on using formal client feedback and considering the alliance and outcome to organize and improve service delivery. McLellan, McKay, Forman, Cacciola, and Kemp (2005) proposed the concurrent recovery monitoring model. In this article, the authors persuasively argued for a shift away from conventional approaches based on assessment, diagnosis, treatment selection, and post-treatment outcome evaluation and toward consumer engagement and adaptive models of continuing care management (Barry, 1999; IOM, 2001, 2006; McKay et al., 2004; Murphy, 2003; Rush et al., 2004). To date, S. D. Miller, Duncan, Sorrell, and Brown (2005) published the only study on the use of client feedback in substance abuse services. Similar to findings reported for mental health populations, feedback significantly improved retention and outcome. Such results, though preliminary in nature, represent an important opportunity for improving addiction treatment.

### Role of Evidence-Based Treatments, Specific Ingredients, and Common Factors

If alliance and outcome data generated in real time during treatment have a much greater influence on retention, symptom improvement, and longer term client functioning, what then is the role of evidence-based treatments (EBTs)? What is to be made of efforts to assure treatment or technique fidelity? Most addiction, mental health, and psychotherapy training and practice have continued to focus on technique and model. To ensure funding, policies and procedures on assessment, service planning, and treatment options all expect fidelity to placement criteria, accreditation standards, and sometimes manualized treatments. Quality audits and licensing inspections yield piles of paperwork. Compliance with regulations emphasizing technique, model, and structure are valued over measures of alliance, engagement, and real-time outcomes.

Many clinicians report spending 40% to 60% of their time documenting assessments, treatment plans, and progress notes. These activities have nothing to do with alliance and progress data, information that provides formal feedback for therapists and clients (thus reinforcing the alliance) or assists in modifying the treatment when early results are unsatisfactory. With current pressures in some states to pay only for EBTs, even more documentation is needed to verify allegiance to these practices. It makes sense to serve clients with therapies, medications, and services that have proven efficacy, notwithstanding, as has been observed by W. R. Miller, Zweben, and Johnson (2005), that "perhaps the proper attitude toward EBTs is one of respect not reverence" (p. 274).

Again, results from psychotherapy research offer some insights. In the past decade, psychotherapy research has shown that common therapeutic factors, rather than specific techniques or models, are the most robust predictors of client engagement, retention, and outcome (Luborsky, 1995; Morgenstern and McCrady, 1992; Morgenstern, Morgan, McCrady, Keller, & Carroll, 2001; Prochaska, 1995). These therapist behaviors, common across most therapies, consist primarily of relationship variables such as warmth, empathy, acceptance, and encouragement of risk-taking. In a series of monographs on *Ensuring Solutions to Alcohol Problems* from George Washington University Medical Center, Hon (2003) specified active ingredients of effective treatment for alcohol problems. His list included some of the same common factors seen in psychotherapy research, along with process and performance factors such as comprehensive assessment and individualized treatment plan, care management, individually delivered professional interventions, and contracting with clients.

So, how do EBTs, awareness of common factors, and the measuring and monitoring of alliance and outcome data fit together in the real world? Should programs and practitioners focus exclusively on the common factors, measures of alliance and engagement, and real-time outcomes? Should they abandon assessment, service planning, and detailed accreditation and licensure standards? In practice, both individual practitioners and the larger health care systems in which most work require structure and direction to operate. From a larger system's viewpoint, Bickel and McLellan (1996) suggested that simply funding systems in the current manner, on the basis of the number of clients served or a negotiated fee for an episode of care, has simply rewarded utilization. It is not an incentive to improve treatment quality or outcome.

They suggested alternative funding systems based on competition for outcomes and the use of measures of treatment retention and substance use during treatment (McLellan, Brooks, Carise, & Kemp, 2008).

Funding based on outcomes would certainly refocus priorities on engagement and outcome-informed changes in service design and delivery. At the practitioner level, too, management (and reimbursement) based on engagement and outcome is consistent with trends in disease and illness management, especially if conducted in real time during the treatment experience (as with management of hypertension or diabetes). The movement toward consumer empowerment, client self-management, transparency of clinical information and the treatment plan, and general collaborative care (IOM, 2001, 2006) will be further advanced if treatment is client directed and informed by alliance and outcome data. Technique and model do contribute to effectiveness of outcome, though far less than what most believe. And of course, client participation in care requires freedom of choice and the availability of various treatment options (Rush et al., 2004).

On balance, a better course is to view EBTs as diet and exercise regimens, as various classes of medications have been viewed in hypertension treatment (ALLHAT Research Group, 1996) or as therapies and medications have been most recently used in managing depression (Rush et al., 2004). In both instances, the provider's role is as an expert consultant, able to evaluate the complex problems presented by the client at the outset and to address the client's goals thoroughly. In this light, treatment initiation involves a comprehensive discussion between caregiver and client, delineating the available options, projected course of effectiveness, and potential side effects. From this discussion, a negotiated initial treatment plan is constructed that includes the setting, the goals, the components of treatment, and an agreement to evaluate together the outcomes.

The approach, as just described, communicates collaboration, respect for a client's interests and wishes, and the availability of multiple options. It also stresses the importance of client participation in the total effort, with the understanding that if the initial plan does not work, alternatives will be promptly considered. Working this way provides a sound basis for a true helping alliance, engagement, positive expectancy, and the prospect of continuing care, especially if early efforts fall short.

Finally, EBTs do provide valuable options for practitioners and their clients. As treatment is being planned, they can be presented as part of *informed consent*: the duty to advise clients of the available alternatives, along with the evidence supporting their use. From our perspective, their effectiveness in a therapy will be enhanced when combined with a consumer orientation. This involves using EBTs in a client-centered approach and relying on direct client feedback to inform and guide the care. In all, rather than have

EBTs imposed on the client by the therapist, as has been proposed (see SAMHSA, 2007), it is far better to see them as possibilities and strategies, not the final word. Regardless of what intervention is selected, any time spent collaborating with the client, measuring and monitoring outcome, and ensuring a goodness of fit in the therapeutic relationship will surely advance the work.

As clients and practitioners know, the real challenge in treatment is not figuring out what works for clients with alcohol or drug addictions in general but rather what will work for this client seated in this office on this day at this stage in his or her recovery. The report of the American Psychological Association Task Force on Evidence-Based Practice agreed on a definition of evidence-based practice (EBP) in psychology that represented a major move away from the overly simplistic and medicalized idea of specific treatments for specific disorders popular among proponents of EBP. Instead, the Task Force defined EBP as "the integration of the best available research with the clinical; expertise in the context of patient characteristics, culture, and preferences" (American Psychological Association, 2006, p. 273).

## EVOLUTION OR REVOLUTION IN DELIVERING WHAT WORKS IN ADDICTION TREATMENT?

From the perspective of mainstream health care, especially so for chronic illnesses, the proposals offered in this chapter are unoriginal or conventional. Nonetheless, given the methods used in many addiction treatment programs (Knudsen & Roman, 2004; Roman, 2002; McGlynn et al., 2003; McLellan, Kleber, & Carise, 2003) and the usual basis for reimbursement (IOM, 2006), these consumer-oriented, client-centered, adaptive care principles are a marked departure from business as usual. Some might say they are revolutionary.

If one were to propose a revolution that would espouse no fixed assessments, predetermination of models or techniques, rigid rules for client assignment, prescriptions, or manualized treatments, it might be more than the field can bear. As noted earlier, practitioners and health care systems require structure and direction to operate. Novel recommendations for applying the latest research in real-world clinical settings will involve innovative thinking about a combination of addiction and its treatment. An evolution in established practices, policies, and programs currently operating within treatment is also required. Three fundamental changes are necessary, possible, and supported by clinical research in and outside the addictions field:

1. a highly individualized service delivery plan for each client in care;
2. rapid, formal, and continuing feedback from clients regarding the plan, process, and outcome of treatment; and

3. the integration of both the plan and feedback into a continuum of care that is maximally responsive to the individual client (see McKay, 2005; S. D. Miller, Mee-Lee, Plum, & Hubble, 2005).

Of course, these procedures are not magic. By themselves, they do not have the power to ensure a positive outcome. Nevertheless, they do bring advantages. To wit, they are ethical to and respectful of clients. They are feasible and practical to implement in contemporary care settings. Furthermore, they already work in several other areas of health care (see ALLHAT Research Group, 1996; Rush et al., 2004). These three key changes have also been specifically adapted for addiction treatment settings (S. D. Miller, Mee-Lee, et al., 2005). A brief discussion of each now follows.

### Developing an Individualized Service Delivery Plan

The individualized service delivery plan is a prepared summary that captures a snapshot of the alliance between a client and therapist (or treatment team) at a given point in time. Although definitions vary, most agree that an effective alliance contains three essential ingredients: (a) shared goals; (b) consensus on means, methods, or tasks of treatment; and (c) an emotional bond (Bachelor & Horvath, 1999; Bordin, 1979; Horvath & Bedi, 2002). To these three, Hubble, Duncan, and Miller (1999) have added a fourth, namely, the client's frame of reference regarding the presenting problem, its causes, and potential remedies. This last component has been termed the *client's theory of change*. Data indicate that congruence between a person's beliefs about the causes of his or her problems and the treatment approach results in stronger therapeutic relationships, increased duration in treatment, and improved rates of success (Duncan et al., 2004; Hubble et al., 1999).

A client-centered and consumer-directed treatment develops individualized service plans that are driven by a partnership focused on what the client wants. If counselors and therapists take alliance, engagement, and self-change seriously, their task is to join with clients to help them get what they want, not what the counselors or therapists think they need. For instance, clients may want to stay out of jail, keep their job or partner, get their children back from Child Protective Services, find housing, or get people to leave them alone (Mee-Lee, 2001b; Mee-Lee, 2007).

If the individualized plan is considered collaborative, drafted to achieve what the client wants, both the document and the process leading to its creation represent a departure from traditional care. Instead of being a static statement of how treatment will proceed given the client's diagnosis, severity of illness, level of functioning, and available programming, the plan becomes a dynamic document. Indeed, it is a summary of goals and specifies both the type and level of interaction the client wants from the counselor or system of care.

Because any division or disagreement between the clinician and client risks disengagement and dropout, a method for monitoring the status of the alliance and progress is needed. This leads to the second recommendation: Develop feasible and reliable procedures for obtaining and incorporating client feedback during treatment.

## Formal Client Feedback

Therapy is a complex undertaking, full of nuance and uncertainty. Proponents of each specific technique or model provide examples in manuals and textbooks in which the treatment, if performed in the manner described, effortlessly flows toward the predetermined outcome. For all that, because outcome is often influenced more by what the client brings to the treatment and what happens outside the treatment, finding what works for a given client frequently proceeds by trial and error. Traditionally, clinical practice has been managed by standardized packages or treatment tracks. Clients are assigned to these programs and their progress judged on their compliance and movement from one level to the next.

In contrast, a client-directed, outcome-informed approach begins with the outcome the client desires. Then, it works backwards to create the means by which the client's goals will be achieved. All along, the client is in charge, helping to fine-tune or alter, continue or end treatment through their feedback.

Incorporating outcome and process instruments into treatment can be as simple as scoring the scales and discussing the results with clients at each session. Or, it can be as complex as an automated, computer-based data entry, scoring, and interpretation software program (see chap. 8, this volume). The approach chosen depends on the needs, aims, and resources of the user. Regardless of the method, the purpose of the measures is explained to clients, and their active participation is solicited before treatment commences. Encouraging therapists, moreover, to adopt a strengths-based or problem-solving approach over depth-oriented, confrontational, or other intensive strategies can help secure engagement but minimize the risk of regression.

In situations that include multiple participants or stakeholders (e.g., family or group therapy, court-referred clients) the same guidelines apply for interpreting alliance and outcome measures. Depending on the circumstances, the kind of information assessed by the measure and how it is used during treatment vary. As an illustration, consider mandated clients. It is common for these individuals to complete the measures in a manner that suggests that all is going well personally, interpersonally, and socially. Rather than trying to convince clients their status is actually worse than they acknowledge, therapists invite them to rate themselves from the perspective of the referral source. These outcome ratings are then plotted and used to assess change over the course of treatment

(S. D. Miller, Mee-Lee, et al., 2005). In such cases, the client and therapist are technically working together to resolve the problem the referrer (e.g., probation officer, employer, family) has with the client. The process is the same when treatment is delivered through groups. The underlying principle is to use outcome and alliance scales in a manner that increases the engagement of everyone involved.

Formal client feedback allows clinicians to check in with their clients and address any concerns about the work. Exploring options for changing the interaction before ending the session is critical. Research shows clients rarely report problems with the relationship until they have already decided to terminate (Bachelor & Horvath, 1999). Indeed, in a study of 160 participants treated in an alcohol and drug program, S. D. Miller, Duncan, et al. (2005) found that failure to seek feedback regarding the alliance at the first session was significantly higher among unsuccessful clients. Success in this instance was defined as maintaining employment, absence of positive urine screens, and compliance with treatment recommendations. Such findings suggest that clinicians would be well served by making extra efforts to collect an alliance measure with all cases.

### Integrating the Plan and Feedback Into a Flexible Continuum of Care

As observed, the overarching intent of many substance abuse programs is to make the client complete a treatment of predetermined length and a fixed number of steps. Many clients are mandated to addiction treatment and common lore says most are in denial or simply lying. For these reasons, client choice, client-centered therapy, jointly negotiated treatment plans, and other staples of contemporary mainstream health care have not been adopted. Unfortunately, the programming often takes precedence over clients' preferences and, in turn, has a negative impact on their engagement and retention. If a key to effective services exists, it is, in a word, flexibility. The third recommendation speaks to services that contain no fixed content, length of stay, or levels of care. Instead, a continuum of possibilities is made available to the client that includes everything from community resources and natural alliances with the family and significant others to formal treatment and care within health care settings. Everything is on the table from EBTs, healing rituals specific to a given culture, and spiritual practices.

A flexible continuum of care encompasses a wide variety of EBTs and multiple levels of care as delineated in the ASAM Patient Placement Criteria (American Society of Addiction Medicine [ASAM], 1996; Mee-Lee et al., 2001). In treatment systems, in which the setting and resources are by definition limited in scope (e.g., private practice, rural settings), practitioners may serve their clients by outsourcing, a standard business practice. Even under optimal conditions, no provider or system of care can be the end all to all clients.

When formal client feedback indicates that the partnership with a therapist or treatment center is not working, a therapy can still be saved. Turning to a network of informal yet organized contacts in the local community can help ensure a continuity of care. In truth, a broad continuum of possibilities (e.g., church, service and support groups, volunteer organizations, community leaders, local healers, contacts via e-mail or the internet) are now available to clients and their therapists.

## CONCLUSION

Increasingly, policymakers and payers are insisting that to be paid, therapists and the systems of care in which they provide addiction treatment must "deliver the goods." Consumers are also demanding results. In an attempt to provide effective and efficient services, the field of alcohol and drug treatment has embraced the notion of EBP. The idea behind this perspective is that specific techniques or approaches identified through research and delivered with fidelity uniformly produce good outcomes. It is understood: Techniques and models do contribute to effectiveness. Yet, most research in psychotherapy and addictions treatment indicates that client characteristics, common therapeutic factors (such as the alliance and engagement), and extra-therapeutic factors powerfully impact treatment outcomes (Connors, Carroll, DiClemente, Longabaugh, & Donovan, 1997; DiClemente, 2006; Wampold, 2001).

The addiction treatment field has begun a shift toward client-directed, outcome-informed approaches. It is measuring and monitoring data and using the information to change treatment in real time. In support, we have made three practical recommendations derived from psychotherapy research and contemporary practices in mainstream care for chronic illnesses. Instead of attempting to match clients to treatments through EBP, client-directed, outcome-informed care uses practice-based evidence. The purpose is to respond rapidly to the needs of the client and, if necessary, change the therapy on the basis of the actual outcome. Evidence, versus doctrine, is emphasized and used to modify and tailor services to the individual client.

## QUESTIONS FROM THE EDITORS

1. *Are the factors responsible for change in the treatment of substance use disorders any different from those responsible for change in psychotherapy. If yes, how so? If not, what are they?*

There has not been as extensive study on the factors for change in addiction treatment as there has been for mental health psychotherapy. However, available studies indicate that findings for substance abuse treatment are similar to the psychotherapy research and that there are common factors that account for change that are the same as in psychotherapy research. The major contribution to outcome are things outside of treatment's direct influence: what the client brings to the treatment experience in terms of temperament, theory of change, values, and so forth; and extratherapeutic factors such as cultural norms, peer group, living situation, and so forth. Within treatment, outcome is most dependent on the strength of client engagement and the therapeutic alliance, as defined by agreement on goals and methods in the context of a solid emotional bond. Next in importance is the allegiance of the counselor and clinician to the treatment method, whatever model is used. The strength of the clinician's belief in the efficacy of the treatment model provided accounts for a significant contribution to outcome, followed by the actual specific technique or treatment model, which contributes least. Indeed, in the meta-analysis by S. D. Miller, Wampold, and Varhely (2008), allegiance effects accounted for 100% of the variability in outcome among approaches.

The bottom line is for the clinician to engage the client in a collaborative agreement on goals and strategies using treatments in which the clinician has confidence and belief. Couple this with direct client feedback in real time on whether there is a good fit for the client with the treatment provided and whether it is working to improve the client's personal, interpersonal, and social function. If results on the fit and effectiveness of treatment are heading in the wrong direction, then therapists should do something differently (i.e., goals, strategies, techniques, models) until results improve.

On a related note, several chapters in this volume (see chaps. 1, 2, 8, and 9) highlighted the large differences in effectiveness found to exist among clinicians in psychotherapy outcome studies. Such differences are not unknown in research on treatments for alcohol dependence. For example, despite the use of and fidelity to treatment manuals for each of the three approaches in Project MATCH, significant differences in effectiveness were found among clinicians. It is important that therapists with poor outcomes accounted for most of the variability in results (Project MATCH Research Group, 1998). As the authors of the other chapters point out, such findings indicate that the therapist is a significant factor influencing the outcome of treatment. The implications of such research are also clear. In addition to ensuring the fit between client and treatment, obtaining client feedback via the use of standardized measures can also facilitate the identification of clinicians in need of training and supervision.

*2. In your estimation, what accounts for the continuing lack of integration between mental health and addictions treatment?*

In the United States, in part because of mental health's failure to provide direct treatment for alcoholism, current addiction treatment has its historical roots in the self-help movement of Alcoholics Anonymous in the 1930s.

Even to this day, many mental health clinicians have had minimal training in substance use problems and take on the same attitudinal stigma and discriminatory practices as the larger societal culture. The mutual mistrust between those working in the field through personal life recovery versus professional training is diminishing as certification and credentialing increase. However, funding, licensure, and other systems obstacles and inequities also compromise integration. Even though mental health problems still carry their own stigma, addiction problems are shunned even more, keeping both systems fragmented.

Outside the United States, some of these same issues work against integration. But some differences bring mental health and addiction treatment closer together. Harm reduction or harm minimization are much more embraced in Europe, Canada, Australia, and other countries where addiction treatment is more developed. This is more consistent with mental health treatment, which does not require clients to commit to mental health wellness and to be symptom free as a condition for treatment. Traditional addiction treatment in the United States has usually required a commitment to abstinence as a condition for treatment and has often discharged clients for recurrence of substance use while in treatment.

With recognition that the prevalence of substance use problems in mental health populations is so great that mental health problems in substance use populations are significant, clinicians and systems of care are now increasingly focused on integrating services, systems, policies, and funding for people with co-occurring mental health and addictions problems. Changes in attitudes, discriminatory practices, training and skill building will need to be coupled with systems changes for integration to be fully realized.

3. *What are the implications of your chapter for future training and certification of practitioners?*

Given that all treatments designed to be therapeutic are equally effective and that what contributes most to the outcome in treatment are alliance and allegiance factors, practitioners require training that places the appropriate weight on the most important priorities. The current preoccupation with EBTs shifts attention from what research indicates actually requires the greater focus in work with clients. Disproportionate training, certification, and credentialing resources are centered on techniques, models, and manuals as well as audits to verify fidelity to the model and other process standards. Future training and certification, to be consistent with outcomes research findings and a more balanced emphasis, would encompass the following priorities:

- To train practitioners how to determine what will work for this client in this office or program on this day at this stage in his or her recovery. If the outcomes are good, the practitioner and client keep doing what works. If the outcomes are poor, practitioners are ready and able to change quickly what they are doing together.

- To develop skills, services, and quality and certification systems that promote a client-directed approach that engages the client in a self change, uses empowered collaboration on goals and strategies (alliance), and changes treatment strategies on the basis of outcome results measured in real time in clinical practice.
- To train practitioners how to negotiate with a patient to develop a mutually agreeable initial treatment plan.
- To reorient training, certification, and quality audits to track fidelity to client-directed, outcome-informed practices and systems rather than fidelity only to assessment and treatment models, techniques, documentation, and compliance standards.
- To train practitioners in EBTs to become proficient enough to confidently include a greater variety of methods and techniques in their clinical toolkits but to not be so self-conscious over fidelity to a model that it dilutes any natural and effective style that engages clients in an effective working alliance.
- To train practitioners to collect and use patient status and function measures at each meeting with the patient to determine whether the patient likes the progress to date and whether there is an indication of favorable response.
- To train practitioners to increase therapeutic attention on what is working or not and to be willing and able to change therapeutic approaches if there is not a suitable indication of a favorable response (i.e., practice-based evidence).

## REFERENCES

ALLHAT Research Group. (1996). Rationale and design for the Antihypertensive and Lipid Lowering Treatment to Prevent Heart Attack Trial (ALLHAT). *American Journal of Hypertension, 9*, 342–360

American Psychological Association. (2006). Evidence-based practice in psychology. *American Psychologist, 61*, 271–285.

American Society of Addiction Medicine. (1996). Patient placement criteria for the treatment of substance-related disorders (2nd ed.). Chevy Chase, MD: Author.

Anton, R. F., O'Malley, S. S., Ciraulo, D. A., Cisler, R. A., Donovan, D. M., Gastfriend, D. R., et al (2006). Combined pharmacotherapies and behavioral interventions for alcohol dependence: The COMBINE study: A randomized controlled trial. JAMA, *295*, 2003–2017.

Bachelor, A., & Horvath, A. (1999). The therapeutic relationship. In M. A. Hubble, B. L. Duncan, & S. D. Miller (Eds.). *The heart and soul of change: What works in therapy* (pp. 133–178). Washington, DC: American Psychological Association.

Barry, M. J. (1999). Involving patients in medical decisions—How can physicians do better? *JAMA, 282,* 2356–2357.

Bein, T. H., Miller, W. R., & Tonigan, J. S. (1993). Brief interventions for alcohol problems: A review. *Addiction, 88,* 315–336.

Berglund, M., Thelander, S., & Jonsson, E. (Eds.). (2003). *Treating alcohol and drug abuse—An evidence based review.* Weinheim, Germany: Wiley-VCH.

Bickel, W. K., & McLellan, A. T. (1996). Can management by outcome invigorate substance abuse treatment? *American Journal on Addictions, 5,* 281–291.

Bordin, E. S. (1979). The generalizability of the psychoanalytic concept of the working alliance. *Psychotherapy, 16,* 252–260.

Bowman, K., & Jellinek, E. M. (1941). Alcohol addiction and its treatment. *Quarterly Journal of Studies on Alcohol, 2,* 98–176.

Brown, J., Dreis, S., & Nace, D .K. (1999). What really makes a difference in psychotherapy outcome? Why does managed care want to know? In M. A. Hubble, B. L. Duncan, and S. D. Miller (Eds.), *The heart and soul of change: What works in therapy* (pp. 389–406). Washington, DC: American Psychological Association.

Collins, J. J., & Messerschmidt, M. A. (1993). Epidemiology of alcohol-related violence. *Alcohol Health and Research World, 17,* 93–100.

Connors, G. J., Carroll, K. M., DiClemente, C. C., Longabaugh, R., & Donovan, D. M. (1997). The therapeutic alliance and its relationship to alcoholism treatment participation and outcome. *Journal of Consulting and Clinical Psychology, 65,* 588–598.

Dennis, M., Godley, S., Diamond, G., Tims, F., Babor, T., Donaldson, J., et al. (2004). The cannabis youth treatment (CYT) study: Main findings from two randomized trials. *Journal of Substance Abuse Treatment, 27,* 97–213.

DiClemente, C. C. (2006). Natural change and the troublesome use of substances: A life-course perspective. In W. R. Miller & K. M. Carroll (Eds.), *Rethinking substance abuse: What the science shows, and what we should do about it* (pp. 91–95). New York: Guilford Press.

Duka, T., Townshend, J. M., Collier, K., & Stephens, D. N. (2003). Impairment in cognitive functions after multiple detoxifications in alcoholic inpatients. *Alcoholism: Clinical & Experimental Research, 27,* 1563–1573.

Duncan, B. L., Miller. S. D., & Sparks, J. (2004). *The heroic client: Principles of client-directed, outcome-informed therapy* (Rev. ed.). San Francisco: Jossey-Bass.

Eighth Special Report to U.S. Congress on Alcohol and Health from the Secretary of Health and Human Services. (1993). Rockville, MD: U.S. Department of Health and Human Services.

Ericson, N. (2001, May). *Substance abuse: The nation's number one health problem* (OJDP Fact Sheet 17). Washington, DC: U.S. Department of Justice, Office of Justice Programs, Office of Juvenile Justice and Delinquency Prevention.

Gerstein, D. R., Henrick, J., & Harwood, H. J. (1990). *Treating drug problems* (Vol. 1). Washington, DC: The National Academies Press.

Godley, S. H., Jones, N., Funk, R., Ives, M., & Passetti, L. (2004). Comparing outcomes of best-practice and research-based outpatient treatment protocols for adolescents. *Journal of Psychoactive Drugs, 36*(1), 35–48.

Gotheil, E., McLellan, A. T., & Druley, K. A. (Eds.). (1981). *Matching patient need and treatment methods in alcoholism and drug abuse*. Springfield, IL: Charles C Thomas.

Grant, B. F. (2000). Estimates of U.S. children exposed to alcohol abuse and dependence in the family. *American Journal of Public Health, 90*(1), 112–115.

Hoffmann, N. G., Halikas, J. A., Mee-Lee, D., & Weedman, R. D. (1991). *Patient placement criteria for the treatment of psychoactive substance use disorders*. Washington, DC: American Society of Addiction Medicine.

Hon, J. (2003). *The active ingredients of alcohol treatment: Primer 4. Ensuring solutions to alcohol problems*. Washington, DC: The George Washington University Medical Center.

Horvath, A. O. (2001). The alliance. *Psychotherapy, 38*, 365–372.

Horvath, A. O., & Bedi, R. P. (2002). The alliance. In J. C. Norcross (Ed.), *Psychotherapy relationships that work* (pp. 37–69). New York: Oxford University Press.

Howard, K. I., Moras, K., Brill, P. L., Martinovich, Z., & Lutz, W. (1996). Evaluation of psychotherapy. Efficacy, effectiveness, and patient progress. *American Psychologist, 51*, 1059–1065.

Hubble, M. A., Duncan, B. L., & Miller, S. D. (1999). Directing attention to what works. In M. A. Hubble, B. L. Duncan, & S. D. Miller (Eds.), *The heart and soul of change: What works in therapy* (407–448). Washington, DC: American Psychological Association.

Imel, Z. E., Wampold, B. E., & Miller, S. D. (2008) Distinctions without a difference: Direct comparisons of psychotherapies for alcohol use disorders. *Psychology of Addictive Behaviors, 22*(4), 533–543.

Institute of Medicine. (1990). *Broadening the base of treatment for alcohol problems*. Washington, DC: National Academies Press.

Institute of Medicine. (2001). *Crossing the quality chasm: A new health system for the 21st century*. Washington, DC: National Academies Press.

Institute of Medicine. (2006). *Improving the quality of health care for mental and substance-use conditions. Quality chasm series*. Washington, DC: National Academies Press.

Johnson, L. D. (1995). *Psychotherapy in the age of accountability*. New York: Norton.

Knudsen, H. K., & Roman, P. M. (2004). Modeling the use of innovations in private treatment organizations: The role of absorptive capacity. *Journal of Substance Abuse Treatment, 26*(1), 51–59.

Luborsky, L. (1995). Are common factors across different psychotherapies the main explanation for the dodo bird verdict that "Everyone has won so all shall have prizes"? *Clinical Psychology: Science and Practice, 2,* 106–109.

Luborsky, L., Barber, J. P., Siqueland, L., McLellan, A. T., & Woody, G. E. (1997). Establishing a therapeutic alliance with substance abusers. In L. S. Onken, J. D. Blaine, & J. J. Boren (Eds.), *Beyond the therapeutic alliance: Keeping the drug-dependent individual in treatment* (NIDA Research Monograph 165, pp. 233–244). Rockville, MD: National Institute on Drug Abuse.

McGlynn, E. A., Asch, S. M., Adams, J., Keesey, J., Hicks, J., DeCristofaro, A., Kerr, E. A. (2003, June 26). The quality of health care delivered to adults in the United States. *New England Journal of Medicine, 348,* 2635–2645.

McKay, J. R. (2005). Is there a case for extended interventions for alcohol and drug use disorders? *Addiction, 100,* 1594–1610.

McKay, J. R., Lynch, K. G., Shepard, D. D., Ratichek, S., Morrison, R., Koppenhaver, J. & Pettinati, H. M. (2004). The effectiveness of telephone-based continuing care in the clinical management of alcohol and cocaine use disorders: 12 month outcomes. *Journal of Consulting and Clinical Psychology, 72,* 969–979.

McLellan A. T., Brooks, A., Carise, D., & Kemp, J. (2008). Improving public addiction treatment through performance contracting: The Delaware experiment. *Health Policy, 87,* 296–308.

McLellan, A. T., Kleber, H. D., & Carise, D. (2003). The national addiction treatment infrastructure: Can it support the public's demand for quality care? *Journal of Substance Abuse Treatment, 25,* 117–121.

McLellan, A. T., McKay, J. R., Forman, R., Cacciola, J., & Kemp, J. (2005). Reconsidering the evaluation of addiction treatment—From retrospective follow-up to concurrent recovery monitoring. *Addiction, 100,* 447–458.

McLellan, A. T., Woody, G. E., Luborsky, L., & O'Brien, C. P. (1983). Increased effectiveness of substance abuse treatment: A prospective study of patient–treatment "matching." *Journal of Nervous and Mental Disease, 171,* 597–605.

Mee-Lee, D. (1995). Matching in addictions treatment: How do we get there from here? *Alcoholism Treatment Quarterly, 12*113–127.

Mee-Lee, D. (2001a). Persons with addictive disorders, System failures, and managed care. In E. C. Ross (Ed.), *Managed behavioral health care handbook* (pp. 225–266). Gaithersburg, MD: Aspen.

Mee-Lee, D. (2001b). Treatment planning for dual disorders. *Psychiatric Rehabilitation Skills, 5*(1), 52–79.

Mee-Lee, D. (2007). Engaging resistant and difficult-to-treat patients in collaborative treatment. *Current Psychiatry, 6*(1), 47–61.

Mee-Lee, D., & Shulman, G. D. (2003). The ASAM Patient Placement Criteria and matching patients to treatment. In A. W. Graham, T. K. Schultz, M. F. Mayo-Smith, R. K. Ries, & B. B. Wilford (Eds.), *Principles of addiction medicine* (3rd ed., pp. 453–465). Chevy Chase, MD: American Society of Addiction Medicine.

Mee-Lee, D., Shulman, G. D., Fishman, M., Gastfriend, D. R., & Griffith J. H. (Eds.). (2001). ASAM *Patient Placement Criteria for the treatment of substance-related disorders* (2nd ed. rev.). Chevy Chase, MD: American Society of Addiction Medicine.

Miller, S. D., Duncan, B. L., Sorrell, R., & Brown, G. S. (2005). The partners for change outcome management system. *Journal of Clinical Psychology, 61,* 199–208.

Miller, S. D., Mee-Lee, D., Plum, B., & Hubble, M. (2005). Making treatment count: Client-directed, outcome informed clinical work with problem drinkers. In J. Lebow (Ed.), *Handbook of clinical family therapy* (pp. 281–308). New York: Wiley.

Miller, S. D., Wampold, B. & Varhely, K. (2008). Direct comparisons of treatment modalities for youth disorders: A meta-analysis. *Psychotherapy Research, 18,* 5–14.

Miller, W. R., & Hester, R. (1986a). The effectiveness of alcoholism treatment: What research reveals. In W. R. Miller & R. K. Hester (Eds.), *Treating addictive behaviors: Processes of change* (pp. 121–174). New York: Plenum Press.

Miller, W. R., & Hester, R. (1986b). Inpatient alcoholism treatment: Who benefits? *American Psychologist, 41,* 794–805.

Miller, W. R., Wilbourne, P. L., & Hettema, J. E. (2002). What works? A summary of alcohol treatment outcome research. In R. K. Hester & W. R. Miller (Eds.), *Handbook of alcoholism treatment approaches: Effective alternatives* (pp. 13–63). New York: Allyn & Bacon.

Miller, W. R., Zweben, J., & Johnson, W. R. (2005). Evidence-based treatment: Why, what, where, when, and how? *Journal of Substance Abuse Treatment, 29,* 267–276.

Morgenstern, J., & McCrady, B. S (1992). Curative factors in alcohol and drug treatment: behavioral and disease model perspectives. *Addiction, 87,* 901–912.

Morgenstern, J., Morgan, T. J., McCrady, B. S., Keller, D. S., & Carroll, K. M. (2001). Manual-guided cognitive–behavioral therapy training: A promising method for disseminating empirically supported substance abuse treatments to the practice community. *Psychology of Addictive Behaviors, 15,* 83–88.

Murphy, S. A. (2003). Optimal dynamic treatment regimes. *Journal of the Royal Statistical Society, Series B, 65,* 331–366.

National Association of State Alcohol and Drug Abuse Directors. (2003). *NASADAD Policy Position Paper: Recommendations related to closing the treatment gap.* Retrieved June 17, 2009, from http://www.nasadad.org/resource.php?base_id=37

National Center on Addiction and Substance Abuse at Columbia University. (2009). *Shoveling up II: the impact of substance abuse on federal, state and local budgets.* Retrieved June 21, 2009, from http://www.casacolumbia.org/absolutenm/templates/PressReleases.aspx?articleid=556&zoneid=66

National Highway Traffic Safety Administration. (2006). *Motor vehicle traffic crash fatalities and injuries: 2005 Projections.* Retrieved June 21, 2009, from http://www-nrd.nhtsa.dot.gov/Pubs/810583.PDF

National Institute on Drug Abuse. (2009). *Principles of drug addiction treatment: A research-based guide* (2nd ed.; NIH Publication No. 09-4180). Rockville, MD: Author.

Orford, J. (2006). Is treatment matching dead? Comments on Buhringer (2006). *Addiction, 101*, 653–654.

Orford, J. & Edwards, G. (1977). *Alcoholism: A comparison of treatment and advice, with a study of the influence of marriage.* Oxford, England: Oxford University Press.

Orlinsky, D. E., Grawe, K., & Parks, B. K. (1994). Process and outcome in psychotherapy—Noch einmal. In A. E. Bergin & S. L. Garfield (Eds.), *Handbook of psychotherapy and behavior change* (4th ed., pp. 270–378). New York: Wiley.

Prochaska, J. (1995). Common problems: Common solutions. *Clinical Psychology: Science and Practice, 2*, 101–105.

Project MATCH Research Group. (1997). Matching alcoholism treatments to client heterogeneity: Project MATCH posttreatment drinking outcomes. *Journal of Studies on Alcohol, 58*, 7–29.

Project MATCH Research Group. (1998). Therapist effects in three treatments for alcohol problems. *Psychotherapy Research, 8*, 455–474.

Roman, P. (2002). Adoption and implementation of new technologies in substance abuse treatment. *Journal of Substance Abuse Treatment, 22*, 211–218.

Rush, A. J., Fava, M., Wisniewski, S. R., Lavori, P. W., Trivedi, M. H., Sackeim, H. A., et al. (2004). Sequenced treatment alternatives to relieve depression (STAR*D): Rationale and design. *Controlled Clinical Trials, 25*, 119–142.

Shadish, W. R., & Sweeney, R. (1991). Mediators and moderators in meta-analysis: There's a reason we don't let dodo birds tell us which psychotherapies should have prizes. *Journal of Consulting and Clinical Psychology, 59*, 883–893.

Shelef, K., Diamond, G., Diamond, G., & Liddle. H. (2005). Adolescent and parent alliance and treatment outcome in MDFT. *Journal of Consulting and Clinical Psychology, 73*, 689–698.

Stinson, F. S., & Proudfit, A. H. (1994, July). *County alcohol problem indicators. U.S. Alcohol epidemiologic data reference manual* (Vol. 3, 4th ed.). Rockville, MD: National Institute on Alcohol Abuse and Alcoholism.

Stout, R., Del Boca, F., Carbonari, J., Rychtarik, R., Litt, M. D., & Cooney, N. L. (2003). Primary treatment outcomes and matching effects: Outpatient arm. In T. F. Babor & F. K. Del Boca (Eds.), *Treatment matching in alcoholism* (pp. 105–134). Cambridge, England: Cambridge University Press.

Substance Abuse and Mental Health Services Administration. (2000, November). *Improving substance abuse treatment: The National Treatment Plan Initiative—Changing the conversation* (DHHS Publication No. SMA 00-3479. Rockville, MD: Author.

Substance Abuse and Mental Health Services Administration. (2004). *National Survey of Substance Abuse Treatment Service (N-SSATS)*. Rockville, MD: Author.

Substance Abuse and Mental Health Services Administration. (2006, October). *Report to Congress: Addiction treatment workforce development*. Rockville, MD: Author.

Substance Abuse and Mental Health Services Administration. (2007). *The National Registry of Evidence-Based Programs and Practices: A decision–support tool to advance the use of evidence-based services*. Rockville, MD: Author. Retrieved June 21, 2009, from http://www.nrepp.samhsa.gov

Substance Abuse and Mental Health Services Administration, Office of Applied Studies. (2008a). *Results from the 2007 National Survey on Drug Use and Health: National findings* (NSDUH Series H-34, DHHS Publication No. SMA 08-4343). Rockville, MD: Author.

Substance Abuse and Mental Health Services Administration, Office of Applied Studies. (2008b). *Treatment episode data set (TEDS): 2005. Discharges from substance abuse treatment services* (DASIS Series: S-41, DHHS Publication No. SMA 08-4314). Rockville, MD: Author.

Tonigan, J. S., Miller, W. R., Chavez, R., Porter, N., Worth, L., Westphal, V., et al. (2003). *Project MATCH 10-year treatment outcome: Preliminary findings based on the Albuquerque Clinical Research Unit*. Retrieved June 21, 2009, from http://casaa.unm.edu/posters/project%20match%2010-year%20treatment%20outcome.pdf

U.S. Department of Health and Human Services. (2000). *Tenth Special Report to U.S. Congress on Alcohol and Health from the Secretary of Health and Human Services*. Rockville, MD: Author.

Wampold, B. E. (2001). *The great psychotherapy debate: Models, methods, and findings*. Hillsdale, NJ: Erlbaum.

Wampold, B. E., Mondin, G. W., Moody, M., Stich, F., Benson, K., & Ahn, H. (1997). A meta-analysis of outcome studies comparing bona fide psychotherapies: Empirically, "all must have prizes." *Psychological Bulletin, 122*, 203–215.

Whipple, J. L., Lambert, M. J., Vermeersch, D. A., Smart, D. W., Nielsen, S. L., & Hawkins, E. J. (2003). Improving the effects of psychotherapy: The use of early identification of treatment and problem-solving strategies in routine practice. *Journal of Counseling Psychology, 50*, 59–68.

# IV

## CONCLUSIONS

# 14

## DELIVERING WHAT WORKS

SCOTT D. MILLER, MARK A. HUBBLE, BARRY L. DUNCAN,
AND BRUCE E. WAMPOLD

It is not the strongest of the species that survives, nor the most intelligent, but the one most responsive to change.

—Charles Darwin

Ten years ago, the first edition of *The Heart and Soul of Change* was published. Then, as now, the practice environment was undergoing rapid and dramatic change, much of it decidedly hostile to the interests of therapists and equally inimical to clients. The profession, we recognized, was at a crossroads. The direction chosen would determine its standing and future as a healing practice (Hubble & Miller, 2001). With so much at stake, the science of the common factors not only provided the best conceptual framework for meeting the challenges at hand but also the strongest empirical basis for advancing the field.

The response to the book was gratifying and in no small way surprising. In addition to receiving highly positive reviews from both clinicians and researchers, it became a bestseller for the American Psychological Association Press (APA Books), and went on to win Menninger's 15th Annual Writing Awards Competition in the scientific books category. Though it is tempting to attribute the success to the power and persuasion of our writing and that of the contributors, another explanation readily presents itself. Readers welcomed the clear, empirically based delineation of what works in a field so accustomed to ambiguity and contentious and competing claims.

In time, most—actually all—of the conclusions drawn in the first edition were upheld. On this score, research by Wampold and others provided overwhelming support for the common factors. This same body of research undermined the belief in specificity. To be frank, any assertion for the superiority of special treatments for specific disorders should be regarded, at best, as misplaced enthusiasm, far removed from the best interests of consumers. In the past decade, moreover, concerns over the unfortunate predilection for narrowly sanctioning some treatments as official or privileged (e.g., by designating them as empirically supported treatments) has sponsored more sensible policies. These broaden the concept of evidence-based practice to include research on the process and outcomes of psychotherapy and recognize the importance of clinical expertise, client characteristics, and cultural context (American Psychological Association Presidential Task Force on Evidence-Based Practice, 2006).

*The Heart and Soul of Change, Second Edition,* continues to highlight the common factors and honors the pivotal role of clients in successful psychotherapy. As seen, this volume also documents a major innovation in psychotherapy: the development and use of monitoring and feedback systems. When used routinely, outcome measurement and management mobilize the common factors and facilitate real gains in clinical improvement, including accountability for clients, payers, and therapists. This final chapter offers a summary reflection on state of the field, with particular attention directed to "what works"; considers the implications of therapy informed by ongoing monitoring and feedback; and takes up the next frontier for clinical research.

## SPECIFIC, COMMON, AND THERAPEUTIC FACTORS: WHAT'S IN A WORD?

Following the first edition, ample opportunity existed for evidence to emerge refuting the common factors thesis. It did not happen and, to use the popular idiom, "not to put too a fine point on it," not for any lack of effort. And so it can be affirmatively stated: Theoretical schools and the impassioned rivalry they nurtured for many years at the center of professional discourse have outlived whatever meaning or function they once provided. For the sake of our clients and our own progress, it is better to regard them as subjects for historians. As Heine (1953; see Prologue, this volume) said so long ago and Frank (1973) later elaborated, psychotherapy is a single, unitary phenomenon, the effectiveness of which depends on factors common to all approaches.

As doctrinaire declarations endorsing specificity have wilted under reasoned scrutiny and now are not at issue, invoking the word *common* suggests little about common factors other than they are there across different therapies.

More, even saying "common factors" inadvertently presupposes or implies the existence of "uncommon factors"—that is, specific curative factors—that research has repeatedly failed to establish. Despite the precedent for their use, the words *specific* and *common* keep the profession bogged down in false distinctions and needless polemics. In the end, without doubt, it is not a matter of what therapies have in common. Instead, it is all about the factors that make therapy work, regardless of theory or orientation. The profession is and will be better served by attending to what are termed *therapeutic factors*, introduced by Lambert (1986), which gives emphasis to all the elements that promote and sustain change. We debated whether to substitute *therapeutic factors* for *common factors* in this edition and decided not to buck the convention. In truth, it can be confusing to change words midstream. Using terms that accord priority to what works versus what is common holds considerable merit, pointing as they do to what is most important in therapy: a good outcome.

## MEASUREMENT, FEEDBACK, AND OUTCOME MANAGEMENT: ENLISTING THE CLIENT'S PARTICIPATION

Knowing what works in therapy represents a major step forward. Notwithstanding, without a reliable and feasible way to deliver what works, the advance in science will have little value to practitioners, consumers, and anyone who pays for the work. In facing this dilemma, psychotherapy is not alone. It is the same in any discipline involved in providing health and human services. Basic research, the kind that acquires knowledge for knowledge's sake and firmly establishes our understanding of the curative factors, then depends on applied research: investigations designed to solve real problems in the field. In short, one without the other is but a half measure, a weak or imperfect line of action.

The research reported in the first edition put across the critical role common factors exert on outcome. As unquestionably material as that contribution was, once completed, we and others struggled with how to help therapists mobilize therapeutic factors (to mix the language). Additionally, all were left without a way to know whether therapists, regardless of their good intentions in heeding the factors, actually improved their effectiveness. In short, missing was a means to assess or measure results on the ground: how effective a particular practitioner is with a particular client in real time. From a broader perspective, knowledge about outcomes, the applied end of the science of psychotherapy, was sorely needed.

Over time, owing in large part to Michael J. Lambert's groundbreaking research, the technology and tools for monitoring and measuring improvement have been developed, distributed, and widely used. Information generated from these systems and then provided or returned to therapists and clients in the form of feedback on progress greatly improves the benefits of therapy. As detailed many times in this volume, both retention rates and outcomes soar when the client's ongoing experience of the alliance and improvement in treatment is continually assessed and integrated into care. Regular and purposeful collection of outcome data has the potential for becoming a core feature of therapeutic change. Therapists do not need to know ahead of time what approach to use for a given diagnosis. It is far more fruitful to know whether the current relationship is a good fit and, if not, be able to adjust the treatment and accommodate the client's experience and goals (Duncan, Miller, & Sparks, 2004). An additional bonus, given the current practice environment, is that the process addresses accountability. Monitoring and feedback provide proof of value and evidence of return on investment to both payers and policymakers. The structured use of standardized measurements at every session and the conscientious application of the findings to the work at hand are, without exaggeration, revolutionizing our ability to affect outcomes. Using formal client feedback to inform, guide, and evaluate treatment is the strongest recommendation coming from this volume.

Assessing progress and providing feedback also affirmatively connect with the most enduring result of more than 40 years of psychotherapy research: The quality of the client's participation is the major determinant of outcome (Orlinsky, Rønnestad, & Willutzki, 2004). When clients are asked to reflect and report on the relationship and their improvement, it is as though they are being told,

> Your input is crucial; your participation matters. We invite you to be a partner in your care. We respect what you have to say, so much so that we will modify the treatment to see that you get what you want.

## THE NEXT FRONTIER: THERAPIST FACTORS

This edition has added the clinician to the mix of what is critical to effective therapy. In 1974, researcher D. F. Ricks coined the term *supershrinks* to describe a group of exceptional therapists. His study examined the long-term outcomes of "highly disturbed" adolescents. When the research participants were later examined as adults, he found that a select group, treated by one particular provider, fared notably better. In the same study, boys treated by the "pseudoshrink" demonstrated alarmingly poor adjustment as adults. It is unfortunate that following Rick's first examination, and despite accumulating evidence that therapists make a difference, little effort has been expended on studying the characteristics or actions of effective therapists. One only has to consult Larry Beutler's latest chapter on therapist variables in *Bergin and Garfield's Handbook of Psychotherapy and Behavior Change* (Beutler et al., 2004) to realize how little we know about successful therapists; it is somewhat distressing how little research has been devoted to this subject. Instead, the field became preoccupied with identifying effective "therapies."

With the therapeutic factors now firmly established and feedback acknowledged as a viable approach for realizing appreciable gains in effectiveness, a new finding is directing us to the next frontier in psychotherapy research. Studies tracking the outcomes of thousands of therapists and clients have confirmed the significant role clinicians play in the outcome of therapy. As just noted, a cadre of clinicians consistently achieves superior results. The existence of large-scale databases now opens the door for researchers to isolate the best from the rest and identify patterns associated with excellence. In what amounts to a form of reverse engineering, mining of the data allows hypotheses to be generated and tested to establish the links among particular actions, processes, or events and superior outcomes. To illustrate, our own research shows that superior practitioners are much more likely to ask for and receive negative feedback about the quality of their work and their contribution to the alliance. This finding has been confirmed in several large, independent samples of practitioners working in diverse settings with a wide range of presenting problems. The best clinicians— those falling in the top 25th percentile—often have initial low alliance scores and then work to engage clients in therapy and address potential problems in the relationship. Median therapists, by contrast, commonly receive negative feedback later in treatment, at a time when clients have already disengaged and are at heightened risk for dropping out (Miller, Hubble, & Duncan, 2007).

Such research pushes the field beyond the limits imposed by randomized clinical trials. Instead of repeatedly testing the overall efficacy of whole treatment packages (i.e., models), attention is turned to the moment-by-moment, encounter-to-encounter processes associated with effective psychotherapy. Once identified, tested, and confirmed, the field is set to empower the next generation of therapists to emulate empirically derived patterns of excellence. The same approach is already being implemented in professions far removed from therapy. The behaviors of world-class musicians, athletes, mathematicians, chess players, pilots, medical diagnosticians, and air traffic controllers has been and continues to be studied. Because of this work, the performance of these professionals has consistently improved. In contrast, despite 30 years of feverish effort, the overall outcomes of therapy have remained unchanged (Smith & Glass, 1977; Wampold, 2001).

# THE FUTURE

At the conclusion of the first edition of *The Heart and Soul of Change*, when formal monitoring and feedback were still very recent developments, we proposed systematic data collection both as an alternative to the policies then guiding service delivery and an answer to the call for accountability. Although only one managed-care company (and no public behavioral health system) was systematically collecting outcome data at that time, now many—including the two largest providers of private and public behavioral health care—have either implemented or are in the process of instituting outcome management systems. Further, many state behavioral health systems are mandating that outcomes be measured, and some are even specifying the instruments to be used. With national rollout of data collection a growing possibility, professional psychological services are entering a new era.

Beyond increasing the overall effectiveness of therapy and expediting research into the behavior of the most successful clinicians, several advantages could be realized with the large-scale introduction of outcome measurement and management. First, systematic data collection and the use of feedback could give consumers a real voice in their own care. As suggested earlier, this would align mental health and substance abuse professionals with their clientele, as partners, focused together on the client's recovery and the best way to get there. Consumers have grown weary of services that treat mental illness and substance abuse as lifelong conditions, precluding full recovery (Bassman, 2007). Recovery proponents argue instead that human struggles are temporary and that each individual should be expected to pull through, given appropriate supports. A recovery-focused service requires a shift from professional interventions based on diagnostic labels and prescriptive treatments to individually tailored, consumer-directed planning (National Consensus Conference on Mental Health Recovery and Mental Health Systems Transformation, 2004). In all, collaborative measurement and monitoring of progress provides a tangible way to support and include the consumer voice.

Second, a national database could supply the impetus for reevaluating funding models and the conventions used to justify services. As more and more evidence accrues (and becomes public) showing the lack of relationship among diagnoses, so-called empirically based treatments, length of stay, and improvement, interest may turn to investigating the real predictors of progress. Once identified, practices improving outcomes could be implemented systemwide, and those that are irrelevant could be eliminated. It is already known that historical questionnaires, biopsychosocial assessments, manuals, and other methods currently in favor exert no impact on outcome.

Finally, databased outcome management allows clinicians, agencies, professional organizations, and the field at large to become players at the reimbursement table. For too long, clinicians and the guilds representing them have deferred to the whims of payers. The numbers speak for themselves, offering as they do an alternative to entreaties of "it's not fair and we deserve it," ineffective marketing strategies (e.g., specialization, boutique practices), and parroting professions that have the ear of those with the money (i.e., psychiatry). Proof is persuasive.

For all that, institutionalized data collection may have its downside. The jury is still out regarding how third-party payers will use the information. Some may use the data to improve outcomes, whereas others may use it for other purposes. For example, many clinicians worry the data might be used to do profiling, resulting in removing therapists from provider panels or limiting referrals. If an organization takes up outcome management to provide real-time (or relatively close in time) feedback to clients and therapists about progress, thus allowing for modification of services for a better outcome, that suggests the intent is positive. Monitoring without feedback will have little worth to consumers.

As with any good idea, measuring outcomes can be used for unintended purposes. As we have described, it can be used clinically to improve the quality of the services provided. However, these data (i.e., the outcomes) could be used for other purposes, such as reducing costs and limiting access to therapy. Used appropriately, outcome data can improve outcomes, reduce health disparities, and improve access. Recently, APA passed a policy on quality improvement programs (QIP; APA Performance Improvement Advisory Group, 2008). This document provides well-grounded principles that are relevant to using practice-based evidence. The first criterion of a good QIP, according to this policy, is that "QIPs are designed to ensure and promote quality of care. Cost containment is never the sole purpose of a well-designed QIP" (APA Performance Improvement Advisory Group, 2008, p. 4).

## CONCLUSIONS

Research and the clinical recommendations summarized in this volume, in each of the subject areas, provide guidance in creating a culture of accountability and clinical excellence. These recommendations, if put into action in their entirety, also have the potential for revolutionizing every aspect of professional life, including training, licensure and certification, continuing education, supervision and quality assurance, the funding and conduct of clinical research, reimbursement policy, marketing, management of customer and client relationships, and the very bedrock of our identity as helpers. We are encouraged by practitioners, agencies, and payers that are already implementing ideas and practices consistent with those reported here. Despite significant obstacles, they are progressing. Of course, not everyone is doing it. Though growing, the number of practitioners and institutions using outcomes remains few. Once more, using formal monitoring and feedback to inform, guide, and evaluate treatment is the strongest proposal tendered in this edition. We believe, and the evidence supports, that the profession has the means to deliver more effective services. This could transform the nature of mental health and substance abuse services. The question is, will we?

We concede that the pull toward the old paradigm is strong. The medical model for psychotherapy remains robust, and its reach into every aspect of clinical work is deep. To move beyond it, to accept and then put to use the latest science, will require nothing short of a paradigmatic shift. Such a change will naturally take time, in combination with strong and consistent leadership. If the material in the present volume in any way serves to inspire and support this cultural transformation, the editors and contributors will have accomplished their purpose.

## REFERENCES

American Psychological Association Presidential Task Force on Evidence-Based Practice. (2006). Evidence-based practice in psychology. *American Psychologist*, *61*, 271–285.

APA Performance Improvement Advisory Group. (2008). *Criteria for the evaluation of quality improvement programs and the use of quality improvement data*. Retrieved July 7, 2009, from http://www.apa.org/practice/Criteria-for-Eval-2008.pdf

Bassman, R. (2007). Building alliances with the recovery movement. In B. L. Duncan & J. A. Sparks (Eds.), *Heroic clients, heroic agencies: Partners for change* (Rev. ed., pp. 155–162). Ft. Lauderdale, FL: Author.

Beutler, L. E., Malik, M., Alimohamed, S., Harwood, T. M., Talebi, H., Noble, S., et al. (2004). Therapist variables. In M. J. Lambert (Ed.), *Bergin and Garfield's handbook of psychotherapy and behavior change* (5th ed., pp. 227–306). New York: Wiley.

Duncan, B. L., Miller, S. D., & Sparks, J. A. (2004). *The heroic client: A revolutionary way to improve effectiveness through client-directed, outcome-informed therapy* (Rev. ed.). San Francisco: Jossey-Bass.

Frank, J. D. (1973). *Persuasion and healing* (2nd ed.) Baltimore: Johns Hopkins University Press.

Heine, R. W. (1953). A comparison of patients' reports on psychotherapeutic experience with psychoanalytic, nondirective and Adlerian therapists. *American Journal of Psychotherapy*, *7*, 16–23.

Hubble, M. A., & Miller, S. D. (2001). In pursuit of folly. *Academy of Clinical Psychology Bulletin*, *7*, 2–7.

Lambert, M. J. (1986). Implications of psychotherapy outcome research for eclectic psychotherapy. In J. C. Norcross (Ed.), *Handbook of eclectic psychotherapy* (pp. 436–462). New York: Brunner/Mazel.

Miller, S. D., Hubble, M. A., & Duncan, B. L. (2007). Supershrinks. *Psychotherapy Networker, 31*(6), 26–35, 56.

National Consensus Conference on Mental Health Recovery and Mental Health Systems Transformation. (2004). *National consensus statement on mental health recovery.* Retrieved September 22, 2007, from http://mentalhealth.samhsa.gov/publications/allpubs/sma05-4129/

Orlinsky, D. E., Rønnestad, M. H., & Willutzki, U. (2004). Fifty years of psychotherapy process–outcome research: Continuity and change. In M. J. Lambert (Ed.), *Bergin and Garfield's handbook of psychotherapy and behavior change* (5th ed., pp. 307–390). New York: Wiley.

Ricks, D. F. (1974). Supershrink: Methods of a therapist judged successful on the basis of adult outcomes of adolescent patients. In D. F. Ricks, M. Roff, & A. Thomas (Eds.), *Life history research in psychopathology* (Vol. 3, pp. 275–297). Minneapolis: University of Minnesota Press.

Smith, M., & Glass, G. (1977). Meta-analysis of psychotherapy outcome studies. *American Psychologist, 32,* 752–761.

Wampold, B. E. (2001). *The great psychotherapy debate: Models, methods, and findings.* Mahwah, NJ: Erlbaum.

# INDEX

Abilify. *See* Aripiprazole
Absolute efficacy, 358
Acamprosate (Campral), 398
Accountability
    and EBTs, 186
    and outcomes management,
        241–243, 424
    in psychotherapy, 31, 39–40
    in substance abuse and dependence
        treatments, 408
    of therapists, 72
ACORN (A Collaborative Outcomes
    Resource Network), 287–288
Action stage, of change, 128, 129
Active collaborators, clients as, 97
Activity, of clients, 89
Adderall, 206
Addictions field. *See also* Substance
    abuse and dependence treatment
    client-centered treatment in,
        401, 408
    integration of mental health field
        with, 409–410
Adequacy, of therapy, 12
ADHD. *See* Attention-deficit/
    hyperactivity disorder
Adherence, to treatment protocol,
    65–66, 370
Administrators, support for CDOI by, 312
Adolescents, 325. *See also* Youth
    psychotherapy
Agency, of clients, 89
Agreement(s)
    about goals of therapy, 70
    interrater, 175
Ahn, H., 62
Akathisia, 213
AKQUASI system, 251–253
Alcohol dependence and abuse,
    398–401. *See also* Substance
    abuse and dependence
Alcoholics Anonymous, 396, 399, 409
Alexander, J. F., 365, 372
Allegiance
    in couple and family therapy,
        361–363, 366, 373

in EBT efficacy studies, 328
as model or technique factor, 36, 37,
    57–58, 73
and psychiatric drug efficacy, 221
in substance abuse and dependence
    treatment, 409
and treatment as myth, 157–158
in youth psychotherapy, 361
Allgood, S. M., 367
Alliance. *See also* Therapeutic
    alliance (TA)
    assessments of, 134
    and collaboration, 122
    in couple and family therapy, 368,
        370–372
    family, 372
    feedback on, 375
    gender differences in, 372
    parent–counselor, 371
    positive, 37
    and psychiatric drug efficacy, 219
    and recovery, 304, 306
    repairing ruptures of, 124–125, 131
    split vs. intact, 372
    in substance abuse and dependence
        treatment, 405, 407
    in therapeutic relationship, 120–121
    as therapist effect, 425
    working, 68–69, 120
Alternative treatments, 154. *See also*
    Supportive counseling
Aman, M. G., 215
American Psychological Association
    Task Forces
    on Evidence-Based Practice, 29–30,
        118, 242, 317, 326, 404
    on Identification and Dissemination of
        Psychological Procedures, 242
    on Promotion and Dissemination of
        Psychological Procedures,
        52–53, 99
American Psychological Association
    Working Group, 225
American Society of Addiction Medicine
    Patient Placement Criteria,
        395, 407

Amphetamine, 206
Analysis of results, in research
     syntheses, 176
Anaphora, 23
Anker, M., 249, 256, 368, 372, 375,
     376, 378
Annapolis Coalition on the Behavioral
     Health Workforce, 301–303
Antidepressants
     and children, 204–206, 212, 217
     clinical trials of, 199–202
     placebo effects for, 212–213, 220
Antipsychotics, 199, 203–204, 208–210,
     213, 217
Antisocial behavior, 85
Antonuccio, D. O., 210
Anxiety disorders
     and contextual model of
          psychotherapy, 146
     self-help for, 94
     treatments for, 58–60
     in youth, 329, 338
Aparsu, R., 203
Applicability, of models and techniques,
     144–145
Aripiprazole (Abilify), 213, 214
Arizona, CDOI care in, 300, 307–317,
     319
Arkowitz, H. S., 94
Arndt, I., 363
Asay, T. P., 84
Assessment-driven treatment, for
     substance abuse and dependence,
     394–395, 397–398
Assumptions, and therapeutic
     relationship, 130–131
Atkinson, D. R., 148
Atomoxetine (Strattera), 206
Attachment style, and therapeutic
     relationship, 129
Attendance rates, CDOI care and,
     308–311
Attention-deficit/hyperactivity disorder
     (ADHD), 206–209, 217–218, 329
Attunement, of psychotherapy,
     126–127
Authority, prescriptive, 224–225
Authorization process, for PBH, 300–301
Autism, 216
Azocar, F., 286

Bachelor, A., 96–97
Baekeland, F., 304
Baldwin, S. A., 38–39, 69, 358, 360, 361
Bandura, A., 70
Bangor, Maine, CDOI care in, 310–311
Barkham, M., 253
Barlow, D. H., 53, 56, 58, 66, 151
Baskin, T. W., 62
Bateman, M., 85
Beck, A. T., 279
Behavioral approaches, for ADHD, 207
Behavioral health services, as commodity,
     275–278
Behavioral marital therapy (BMT),
     358–360, 368
Behavioral treatment (BT), for
     depression, 62
Behaviorism and behaviorists, 51, 52,
     144
Benedetti, F., 153
"The Benefits to the Clinician of
     Psychotherapy Research"
     (L. Luborsky), xx
Bergin, A. E., xx, 36, 84, 86
Berglund, M., 399
Berking, M., 249
Best, K. M., 87
Best, S. R., 87
Best practices
     for children and adolescents, 325
     defined, 307
     and outcomes management, 242–243
Beutler, L. E., 93, 357, 368, 425
Beyebach, M., 367
Bhati, K. S., 149
Bias
     confirmation, 181, 184, 189
     experimental, 19
     and pharmaceutical industry-
          sponsored research, 210–211
     in psychiatric drug trials, 214–215
     publication, 174, 189, 201, 206
     in research syntheses, 173–174,
          186, 189
     selection, 215
Bibliotherapy, 93–94, 331
Bickel, W. K., 402
Bickman, L., 333, 337
Bipolar disorder
     and alliance, 120–121

in children, 208, 209
differential efficacy of treatments for, 364–365
psychiatric drugs for, 204, 213, 220
Bischoff, R. J., 368
Blackburn, I., 57
Blaschke, T., 306
BMT. *See* Behavioral marital therapy
Bohanske, R., 341
Bohart, A. C., 89
Bona fide treatments, 329
Bonds, relational, 121
Bordeleau, V., 96–97
Borderline personality disorder, 85
Boston, P., 358
Boston School of Psychopathology, 50, 270
Bowman, K., 397
Boyd, G., 89
Bristol-Myers Squibb, 214
*Broadening the Base of Treatment for Alcohol Problems* (Institute of Medicine), 397
Brondino, M. J., 370
Brotman, M. A., 68–69
Brown, G. S., 32, 255, 258, 283, 401
Brunk, M., 183–185
BT (behavioral treatment), for depression, 62
Burke, B. L., 94
Business, psychotherapy as, 267, 270

Cacciola, J., 401
CADT (Center for Alcohol and Drug Treatment), 311, 312
Calabrese, J. R., 214
Calhoun, L. G., 87
California Psychotherapy Alliance Scales, 120
Campaign for Mental Health Reform (CMHR), 302
Campbell, D. T., 187
Campbell Collaboration, 176, 188
Campral (acamprosate), 398
Cannabis Youth Treatment (CYT) Study, 329–330, 360, 371, 373, 398, 400
Cantor, N., 96
Caplan, E., 280
Caregivers, in youth psychotherapy, 333–334, 341–343

Caregiver strain, 333–334
Carlton, P. L., 173
Carr, A., 358
Carroll, Lewis, 8, 9
CATIE. *See* Clinical Antipsychotic Trials of Intervention
CBMT. *See* Cognitive–behavioral marital therapy
CBT. *See* Cognitive–behavioral therapy
C'de Baca, J., 86
CDOI care. *See* Client-directed outcome-informed care
Center for Alcohol and Drug Treatment (CADT), 311, 312
Center for Family Services (CFS), 308
Centers for Disease Control and Prevention, 171
Centers for Medicare and Medicaid Services (CMS), 302
Centricity, therapist, 131
CFIT. *See* Contextual feedback intervention and training
CFS (Center for Family Services), 308
Chalmers, I., 177, 186
Chambless, D. L., 52, 169, 170, 181
Change
  client's theory of, 405
  early, 91–92
  human potential for, 85–88
  pretreatment, 367
  quantum, 86
  self-generated, 85–86
  stages of, 128–129
Child and Adolescent Functional Assessment Scale, 341
Childhood disorders, 59–60
Child Outcome Rating Scale (CORS), 341–342, 376, 383, 384
Children. *See also* Youth psychotherapy
  and antidepressants, 204–206, 212, 217
  best practices for, 325
  bipolar disorder in, 208, 209
  cognitive–behavioral therapy for, 329, 338
  and dodo verdict, 58
  exposure to alcohol abuse, 393–394
  psychiatric drugs for, 208–210
  psychosocial interventions for, 218
Chorpita, B. F., 338

Chrismer, S. S., 185
Christensen, A., 358–360, 362, 368
Christian Science, 50, 270
Churchill, R., 184
Churchill, Winston, 149, 239
Clarkin, J. F., 368
Claud, D., 341
Claud, David, 308, 309
Clemmer, Jim, 325
Client-based feedback, 39, 40
Client-centered theory, 144. *See also*
    Person-centered care
Client-centered treatment, in addictions
    field, 401, 405, 408
Client-directed outcome-informed
    (CDOI) care
  defined, 308
  ESTs vs., 318
  implications of, 317–320
  in public behavioral health care,
    307–316
  in substance abuse and dependence
    treatment, 408
Client expertise, 102
Client factors (client effects), xxii,
    xxviii, 35–36, 83–104
  and clients as self-healers, 94–95
  clinical practice implications of,
    95–98
  in couple and family therapy,
    366–368, 379–380
  and efficacy of psychotherapy, 88–92
  and human potential for change,
    85–88
  and psychiatric drug efficacy, 219
  in psychotherapy field, 99–101
  in traditional model of psychother-
    apy, 92–94
  training implications of, 98–99
  and variance in therapeutic out-
    come, 83–85
  in youth psychotherapy, 332–334
Clients
  in evidence-based practice, 29
  functional impairments of, 128
  mandated, 406–407
  in paradigms for psychotherapy, xxi
  as participants, 395–396
  reactance of, 127–128
  reality of, xxiii

as self-healers, 103
stages of change for, 128–129
therapeutic relationship and prefer-
    ences of, 129
view of therapeutic relationship by,
    115–118
Client's theory of change, 405
Client–therapist relationship, 114. *See
    also* Therapeutic alliance (TA)
Client variability, 70
Clinical Antipsychotic Trials of
    Intervention (CATIE), 203–204,
    213, 217
Clinical expertise, 242
Clinical implications
  of CDOI care, 317–318
  of client factors, 95–98
  of evidence-based practice, 188–189
  for future of psychotherapy, 427–428
  of treatment with psychiatric drugs,
    221–223
Clinical Outcomes in Routine Evalua-
    tion (CORE) system, 253
Clinical Support Tool (CST), 244,
    247–248
Clinical support tools, for outcomes
    management, 247–250
Clinical trials, 154, 157. *See also*
    Randomized clinical trials
  of antidepressants, 199–202
  for psychiatric drugs, 210–217
  standards for reporting, 186–187
  of treatments, 57, 71
Clinician-rated scales, for clinical trials,
    212
Clinicians, roles of, 222. *See also*
    Therapists
CMHR (Campaign for Mental Health
    Reform), 302
CMS (Centers for Medicare and
    Medicaid Services), 302
Cochrane Collaboration, 176, 188
Coffey, R. M., 275
Cognitive–affective processes, 129
Cognitive–behavioral marital therapy
    (CBMT), 359, 360
Cognitive–behavioral therapy (CBT)
  for children, 60, 329, 338
  for depression in adolescents, 205,
    220–221

efficacy of, 57–59, 62
for PTSD, 150
and response prevention/exposure, 65
Cognitive dissonance, 343
Cohen, O., 100
Cohesion, in therapeutic relationship,
    121–122
Collaboration, 96–97, 122
Collaborative Cocaine Treatment
    Study, 86
A Collaborative Outcomes Resource
    Network (ACORN), 287–288
Combined Pharmacotherapies and
    Behavioral Interventions (Project
    COMBINE), 398
Common factor(s)
    client and extratherapeutic factors,
        35–36
    and dodo verdict, 8–9
    feedback as, 377–378
    integrated models of, 67
    interdependence of, 34–35
    model and technique factors, 36–37
    origin of, 4–8
    in psychotherapy, 9–13, 28–29,
        33–39, 422–423
    Saul Rosenzweig as founder of, 3–9,
        13–20
    specific factors vs., 143
    therapeutic relationship/alliance,
        37–38
    therapist factors as, 38–39
    and treatment outcome, 33
Common factor controls, 61, 154–155
Community Health and Counseling
    Services, 310–311
Community Mental Health Centers
    Act, 271
Comparisons, unequal, 363–365
COMPASS system, 250–251
Competence, adherence of therapist
    and, 65–66
Complementarity, of psychotherapies,
    17, 18
Complications-driven care, for substance
    abuse and dependence, 394
Component studies, 62, 338
Computer-assisted therapy, 93–94
Computers, in outcomes management,
    240, 339, 425

Concerta (methylphenidate), 206
Concurrent recovery monitoring
    model, 401
Confirmation bias, 181, 184, 189
Conflicts of interest, in psychiatric drug
    trials, 214
Confounding variables, in meta-analyses,
    57, 58
Confrontation, and therapeutic
    relationship, 130
Congruence, in therapeutic relation-
    ship, 123–124
Consent, informed, 403
Consistency, in psychotherapy, 7, 11
Constantino, M. J., 154
Consumer-centered services, 302–303
Consumer-oriented, client-centered,
    adaptive care, 404–408
Contemplation stage, of change,
    128, 129
Contextual feedback intervention and
    training (CFIT), 342–344,
    346–347
Contextual model of psychotherapy,
    143–160
    and definitions of models, 144–145
    emotionally charged, confiding rela-
        tionship in, 151–152
    healing setting or culture in, 148
    myth or rationale in, 148–149
    and placebos, 152–154
    practice implications of, 156–157
    research implications of, 154–156
    ritual or technique in, 149–151
Continuums of care, 314–315, 407–408
Controls and control groups
    common factor, 61, 154–155
    for EBT efficacy studies, 327–328
    placebo-controlled research, 61–63,
        211–212
    usual care, 382
Converging Themes in Psychotherapy
    (M. R. Goldfried), 8
Coping style, and therapeutic relation-
    ship, 129
CORE.net (Web system), 253
CORE-OM. See CORE Outcome
    Measure
CORE Outcome Measure (CORE-OM),
    253, 254

CORE-PC software, 253
CORE (Clinical Outcomes in Routine
    Evaluation) system, 253
CORS. *See* Child Outcome Rating
    Scale
Cosgrove, L., 210
Cottraux, J., 57
Cottrell, D., 358
Counseling, supportive, 57–58, 61, 150,
    154–155
*Counseling and Psychotherapy*
    (Carl Rogers), 5
Countertransference, in therapeutic
    relationship, 125
Couple and family therapy, 357–384
    allegiance factors in, 361–363
    alliance factors in, 370–372
    and common factors, 365–378
    efficacy of, 358–360
    feedback in, 374–378
    model and technique factors in,
        373–374
    practice implications of common
        factors for, 379–382
    therapist factors in, 368–370
    unequal comparisons in, 363–365
Creativity, of clients, 90
Credibility, of therapists, 155
Creed, T. A., 122
Crits-Christoph, P., 58
Croonenberghs, J., 216
CST. *See* Clinical Support Tool
Cucherat, M., 57
Culture
    in contextual model of psycho-
        therapy, 148, 156–157
    in person-centered care, 101
    and placebo effect, 153
    psychotherapy as epiphenomenon of,
        158–159
    and therapeutic relationship, 129
Cummings, Nicholas, 291
Customization, of therapeutic relation-
    ship, 126–130
CYT Study. *See* Cannabis Youth
    Treatment Study

Daleiden, E. L., 338
Danton, W. G., 210
Darwin, Charles, 421

DAS (Dyadic Adjustment Scale), 362
Data collection, for outcomes manage-
    ment, 425–427
Data extraction, in research syntheses,
    175
Dauber, S., 374
Davies, P., 169
DeGeorge, J., 154
Demographic factors, in couple and
    family therapy, 367
Dependence treatment. *See* Substance
    abuse and dependence treatment
Depression
    and alliance, 120
    and contextual model of psycho-
        therapy, 146
    dodo verdict for, 64
    EBT for, 327–328
    effectiveness of treatments for, 55,
        58–59
    self-help for, 94
    specific factors for, 279
    specificity of treatments for, 62
    and therapeutic relationship, 116
    and therapist effects, 281
    treatment resistant, 201
    in youth, 329, 338
DeRubeis, R. J., 68–69
Desensitization, systematic, 63
De Shazer, S., 367
DeSmedt, G., 216
Deterioration. *See also* Dropout rates
    as client outcome, 239–240
    and feedback from PCOMS system,
        256–257
    and outcomes management, 245,
        252
Detoxification, 396
Dew, S. E., 337
DHHS (U.S. Department of Health and
    Human Services), 171
Diagnosis-driven care, for substance
    abuse and dependence, 394
*Diagnostic and Statistical Manual of
    Mental Disorders* (DSM), 52, 225
Diamond, G., 358
Diamond, G. M., 371
Diamond, G. S., 371
Dickens, Charles, 23
DiClemente, C. C., 86

Differential efficacy, 359
Dimidjian, S., 59
Directiveness, reactance and, 127–128
Disability, mental illness as, 299
Disclosure, as client factor, 87–88
Disruptive behaviors, in children, 216
Dissonance, cognitive, 343
Distress levels, as predictors of change,
        91, 102–103
Diversification, in psychotherapy, 27
Dixon, L. B., 184
Dodo verdict, 4, 14–15
    and children, 58
    and common factors, 8–9
    in couple and family therapy,
        365, 382
    and treatment of depression, 64
    in youth psychotherapy, 330
Dose–effect relationship, 91
Dotson, D., 371
Dreier, O., 90
Dries, S., 258
Drinking, problem, 393
Dropout rates. See also Deterioration
    in public behavioral health care,
        301, 304, 306
    and socioeconomic status, 367
    and therapeutic alliance, 336, 372
    and treatment rationale, 155–156
    for youth, 331
Drug abuse, 359, 363, 364. See also
        Substance abuse
Drugs, psychiatric. See Psychiatric drugs
DSM (Diagnostic and Statistical Manual
        of Mental Disorders), 52
Duluth, Minnesota, CDOI care in,
        311, 312
Duncan, B. L., xx, xxvii, 13–20, 31, 67,
        95, 103, 146, 149, 249, 255, 258,
        290, 308, 312, 315, 341, 366,
        401, 405, 407
Dunn, R. L., 360
Durability, of interventions, 362
Dyadic Adjustment Scale (DAS), 362
"A Dynamic Interpretation of Psycho-
        therapy Oriented Towards
        Research" (Saul Rosenzweig), 18

Early change, client factors and, 91–92
Early responders, 91

EBM (evidence-based medicine), 168
EBP. See Evidence-based practice
EBPP. See Evidence-based practice in
        psychology
EBTs. See Evidence-based treatments
Eclecticism, technical, 64
Economic factors, reimbursement and,
        270–274
Economics of psychotherapy, 277–278
Effect size, 176
Efficacy, 358, 359
EFT. See Emotionally focused therapy
Eliot, George, 130
Elliott, Robert, 104
Ellwood, Paul, 272
Emery, G., 279
Emmanuel Movement, 50
Emotionally charged, confiding
        relationships, 7, 151–152
Emotionally focused therapy (EFT),
        359–362, 371, 376
Empathy, in therapeutic relationship,
        118–119
Empirically supported therapies, 301
Empirically supported treatments
        (ESTs), 169. See also Evidence-
        based treatments (EBTs)
    CDOI care vs., 318
    and EBPP, 326
    and outcomes management, 241–242
    and specificity of therapy, 52, 59
Empirically validated treatments
        (EVTs), 169. See also Evidence-
        based treatments (EBTs)
Empowerment, 305, 334
Emslie, G. J., 204, 207, 212
End of Therapy Form, for CORE system,
        253
Epstein, E. E., 370
Equivalence, structural, 62
Error variability, 70
ESTs. See Empirically supported
        treatments
Ethnicity, as therapist effect, 368
Etiology, of mental health disorders, 64
Etrafon (perphenazine), 203
Evans, Mary Ann, 130
Evidence-based medicine (EBM), 168
Evidence-based practice (EBP), 99–100,
        167–190, 404

Evidence-based practice (EBP), *continued*
  clinical implications of, 188–189
  defined, 29–30, 100
  history of, 168–169
  limitations of, 171–172
  and policymakers, 189
  politics and power in, 357
  practice-based evidence vs., 39
  psychiatric drugs in, 222
  research on process and outcomes of
      psychotherapy in, 422
  and research syntheses, 172–177
  and reviews of Multisystemic
      Therapy, 177–186
  for substance abuse and dependence,
      408
  treatments in, 169–171
  weaknesses of, 186–188
Evidence-based practice in psychology
    (EBPP), 242, 326, 344
Evidence-based treatments (EBTs)
  and common factors, 380–381
  in couple and family therapy, 382
  in evidence-based practice, 169–171
  for substance abuse and dependence,
      401–404
  for youth, 325–331, 344–346
EVTs (empirically validated treatments),
    169
Exclusion criteria, for research
    syntheses, 175
Expectancy and expectations, 70
  in couple and family therapy, 366,
      373–374
  and model or technique factors, 36
  and placebos, 152–155
  and psychiatric drug efficacy, 220, 221
  in youth psychotherapy, 337, 338
Expected treatment response (ETR),
    243, 244, 250
Experience, of therapist, 370
Experience of treatment, monitoring,
    125, 130–131, 400–401
Experiences of clients, privileging,
    117, 131
Experimental bias, 19
Expertise
  client, 102
  clinical, 242
  of therapists, 92–93

Externalizing disorders, 336
Extrapyramidal symptoms, 209
Extratherapeutic factors, 33
  as common factors, 35–36
  in couple and family therapy,
      366–368
  and psychiatric drug efficacy,
      218–219
  for youth, 332
Eysenck, Hans, 54, 56, 57

*Facets of Psychotherapy*
    (Saul Rosenzweig), 18
Family Adaptability and Cohesion
    Evaluation Scales, 180
Family alliance, 372
Family drug education (FDE), 364
Family therapy. *See also* Couple and
    family therapy
  efficacy of, 358–359
  in youth psychotherapy, 333–334,
      336
Family violence, 394
Fancher, Robert, 143
FDA. *See* Food and Drug Administration
FDE (family drug education), 364
Feedback, 156, 423–424. *See also*
    Measurement feedback systems
    (MFSs)
  about therapist's listening skills, 99
  on alliance, 375
  and CDOI care, 316–318
  client-based, 39, 40
  as common factor, 377–378
  in couple and family therapy, 366,
      374–378, 380
  and empathy, 119
  in evidence-based practice, 30
  feasibility of, 384
  improving quality of service with, 71
  and outcomes management,
      240–250
  and PCOMS system, 256–257
  retrospective vs. real-time, 341
  in substance abuse and dependence
      treatment, 395, 405–407, 409
  and therapeutic relationship, 124
  and therapist prediction of outcome,
      261
  and training, 262

and treatment success, 117
  for youth psychotherapy, 339–344
Fee-for-service indemnity plans, 270
FFT (functional family therapy), 363
Fidelity, treatment, 190
Findling, R. L., 216
Fischer, A. R., 148
Five-component model, of behaviorism,
  52
Flexibility, for substance abuse and
  dependence treatment, 407–408
Fluoxetine (Prozac), 204–205, 211, 212,
  220–221
Foa, E. B., 57–59
Follette, W. C., 64
Fonagy, P., 85
Food and Drug Administration (FDA),
  52, 210, 211
Formal consistency, in psychotherapy,
  7, 11
Forman, R., 401
Foundation of Idiodynamics, Personality
  Theory, and Literary Creativity, 16
Frank, J. B., 67, 69, 70, 147–149, 151–153
Frank, J. D., 6–8, 19, 23–24, 53, 61, 63,
  67, 69, 70, 147–149, 151–153,
  331, 422
Frankenburg, F. R., 85
Franklin, Benjamin, 221
Freud, Sigmund, 50, 51, 144, 270
Friedlander, M. L., 374
Functional family therapy (FFT), 363
Functional impairments, of clients, 128
Funding. *See also* Reimbursement
  and EBTs, 185–186
  for substance abuse and dependence
  treatment, 402–403

GAF scores. *See* Global Assessment of
  Functioning scores
Gamache, D., 96–97
Gandhi, A. G., 185
Garfield, S. L., xx, 6, 8, 19, 36, 53, 84
Garfinkel, H., 89
Garmazy, N., 87
GAS (Goal Attainment Scale), 362
Gassman, D., 95
Gender differences, in alliance, 372
Generic model of psychotherapy,
  146, 147

Generic psychotherapy, 53
Genuineness, in therapeutic relation-
  ship, 123–124
Gerstein, D. R., 397
Gibbons, C. J., 68–69
Gibbs, L. E., 169
Gide, Andre, 167
Gingerich, W. J., 367
Glass, G. V., 54, 56–57
Gloaguen, V. A., 57
Global Assessment of Functioning
  (GAF) scores, 128, 250
Goal Attainment Scale (GAS), 362
Goal consensus, in therapeutic
  relationship, 122
Goldfried, M. R., 8
Goldman, A., 362
Goldman, H. H., 184
Goldstein, M. J., 365
Gollan, J. K., 358–359
Gorman, D. M., 185
Gorman, J. M., 66
Grawe, K., 95, 144, 400
Gray, J. S., 329
Gray literature, 175
Greaves, A. L., 89
Greenberg, L., 362
Greenberg, R. P., 218, 221
Greenwood, P. W., 186
Gregory, R. J., 93
Grencavage, L. M., 67
Grissom, R. J., 86
Group therapy, 121–122, 407
Growth, posttraumatic, 87

Hakuda, Ken, 267
Hall, G. Stanley, 50, 270
Hamilton Depression Rating Scale,
  200, 212
*Handbook of Psychotherapy and Behavior
  Change* (S. L. Garfield & A. E.
  Bergen), xx
Hannan, C., 240, 261
Hannöver, W., 251
Harm reduction (minimization), in
  addiction treatment, 410
Harwood, H. J., 397
Hawkins, E. J., 243
Hawley, K. M., 328, 337, 382
Healers, native, 158–159

Healing setting, 7, 148, 156
Health care, public behavioral. *See* Public behavioral health care
Health Maintenance Organization Act, 272
Health maintenance organizations (HMOs), 271–273
Heavey, C. L., 360, 362
Heine, R. W., 5, 8, 422
Henggeler, S. W., 364, 370
Hennen, J., 85
Henrick, J., 397
Heres, S., 210
Heroic Agency ListServ, 289
Hirsch, L. S., 370
HMOs (health maintenance organizations), 271–273
Hoch, Paul, 5, 19, 149
Hodges, K., 341
Hoerner, C., 89
Hogan, Michael F., 300
Hogue, A., 374
Holistic approach, in NCSMHR, 305
Hollon, S. D., 52
Hon, J., 402
Honors for Outcomes initiative, 283–284
Honos-Webb, L., 86
Hope, 36, 152, 306, 337–338
Horan, F. P., 253
Horvath, A. O., 372
Houts, A. C., 64
Howard, K. I., 25, 91, 146, 250
Hubble, M. A., xx, xxvii, 31, 34–35, 103, 146, 290, 312, 405
Huey, S. J., 370
Human Affairs International Outcomes Clinical Information System Project, 282
Humanistic interaction, of therapist and client, 53
Human potential for change, 85–88
Huppert, J. D., 66

Imel, Z. E., 149, 281, 399
Implementation
    of CDOI, 319–320
    of outcomes management, 259–260
Implicit common factors, 66–67
Incarceration, 179

Inclusion criteria, for research syntheses, 174–175
Income, of psychologists, 30–31
Individualized, assessment-driven treatment, for substance abuse and dependence, 394–395, 397, 405–406
Individualized care, in NCSMHR, 305
Information technology, client care and, 240
Informed consent, 403
Inpatient care, 251–253, 273, 275
Insight, in common factors model, 69
Insight-oriented marital therapy (IOMT), 359, 360, 368
Intact alliance, 372
Integrated models of common factors, 67
Integrated systemic therapy, 362
Integrative couple therapy, 359
Integrity in Science (website), 214
Interdependence, of common factors, 34–35
Interpersonal skills, of therapists, 368
Interpretations
    of psychological events, 11
    relational, 125–126
Interrater agreements, 175
Interviewing, motivational, 119
*Introductory Clinical Psychology* (Sol Garfield), 6
Ioannidis, J. P., 186
IOMT. *See* Insight-oriented marital therapy
Iowa, EBTs in mental health centers of, 171
Item torture test, 287

Jacobs, M. K., 93
Jacobson, N. S., 62, 251, 358–359, 368
James, William, 50, 270
Janssen (company), 216
Jellinek E. M., 397
Jensen, P. S., 331
Jensen-Doss, A., 328, 382
Joanning, H., 364
Johansson, L., 97
Johnson, Ann, 300
Johnson, S. M., 361, 362, 367, 368
Johnson, W. R., 402
Johnson-Jennings, M. D., 149

Johnson & Johnson (company), 216
Jome, L. M., 148
Jonsson, E., 399
Jordan, J. V., 151
Jordan, K., 371
Jordan, Michael, 291
Jospehson, A., 358
Jureidini, J. N., 206

Karver, M. S., 333–335, 337, 371
Kasanin, Jacob, 16
Keck, P. E., 214
Keller, M. B., 202
Kemp, J., 401
Kendall, P. C., 122
Kennedy, Edward, 271
Kirsch, I., 86, 200, 201
Klein, D. N., 132
Kleiner, A. J., 359
Knobloch-Fedders, L. M., 372
Kopp, Sheldon, 315
Kordy, H., 251, 252
Kraus, D. R., 253
Krimsky, S., 210
Kuhn, Thomas, 25
Kühnlein, I., 91

Lam, A. G., 157
Lambert, M. J., 33, 34, 36, 84, 86, 156,
    243, 345, 378, 423
Lambert, W., 333
Laverdière, O., 96–97
Legitimacy, of treatments, 159–160
Lehman, A. F., 184
Length of treatment, in outcomes
    management, 245, 247
Levant, R. F., 29, 357
Levitt, H. M., 88, 93
Levy, K. N., 368
Liddle, H. A., 371, 374
Lieberman, J. A., 204
Lipsey, T. L., 87
Listening skills, of therapists,
    97–99, 116
Literature, gray, 175
Literature reviews, 215
Luborsky, L., xx, 8, 9, 361
Lueger, R. J., 250
Lundwall, L., 304
Lutz, W., 249

Mackrill, T., 89–91
Magellan (company), 286
Mainstream media, pharmaceutical
    industry and, 223–224
Maintenance, withdrawal from
    psychiatric drugs vs., 211–212
Maintenance stage, of change, 128, 129
Major depressive disorder (MDD),
    205, 220
Managed behavioral health care organi-
    zations (MBHOs)
    evaluations of therapists by, 281–282
    in history of psychotherapy, 273–274
    outcomes management by, 285–286,
        289
    and reimbursement of therapists,
        277–278
Managed care
    and field of psychotherapy, 31
    and HMOs, 271–273
    and outcome assessment, 239–240
    and public behavioral health care,
        300
    and reimbursement rates, 269, 278
Mandated clients, 406–407
Marc Center (MC), 307, 309, 311,
    315, 319
Marital therapy, 358–359. See also
    Couple and family therapy
Mark, T. L., 275
Marmor, Judd, 53
Marriage and family therapy (MFT),
    357–358. See also Couple and
    family therapy
Masten, A. S., 87
Matching Alcoholism Treatments to
    Client Heterogeneity (Project
    MATCH), 397, 400–401, 409
MBHOs. See Managed behavioral
    health care organizations
MC. See Marc Center
McCarty, C. A., 327, 328
McClanahan, T. M., 210
McCrady, B. S., 370
McFall, J. P., 60
McFarlane, W. R., 365
McKay, J. R., 401
McKay, K. M., 219, 281
McLellan, A. T., 363, 401, 402
MDD. See Major depressive disorder

MDFT. *See* Multidimensional family therapy

Mease, A. L., 365

Measurement feedback systems (MFSs), 339–345

Media, pharmaceutical industry and, 223–224

Medicaid, 271

Medical influence on psychotherapy, 49–73
    and common factors model, 53–54, 66–71
    and comparative effectiveness of treatments, 56–60
    and effectiveness of treatment, 54–56
    and future of psychotherapy, 428
    historical, 50–54
    measurement feedback systems vs., 339
    and reimbursement, 270, 279
    research and practice implications of, 71–72
    and specificity, 60–66

Medical model of psychotherapy, xxvii–xxix, 50–53

Medicare, 271, 272

Medicine
    evidence-based, 168
    placebo effect in, 152

Mee-Lee, D., 312, 405

Melton, G. B., 364

Menchola, M., 94

Mental health disorders, etiology of, 64

Mental health field
    growth and diversification in, 27
    integration of addictions field with, 409–410

Mental Health Outcomes and Assessment Tools, 340

Mental Health Parity and Addiction Equity Act, 285

Mesmer, Franz Anton, 51–52

Meta-analysis, xx, 33, 176

Methadone, 363

Methylphenidate (Concerta, Ritalin), 206, 207

Metzer, D., 363

MFSs (measurement feedback systems), 339–345

MFT (marriage and family therapy), 357–358. *See also* Couple and family therapy

Mihalic, S., 184

Miklowitz, D. J., 365

Miller, S. D., xx, xxvii, 31, 60, 67, 103, 146, 148, 149, 255, 290, 307, 308, 312, 325, 329, 341, 361, 399, 401, 405, 407, 409

Miller, W. R., 86, 119, 402

Minami, T., 27

Minnesota Multiphasic Personality Inventory Paranoid, Defensive, and Hostility scales, 127

Mitchell, John K., 50

Model and technique factors
    as common factors, 35–37
    in couple and family therapy, 366, 373–374
    as specific factors, 143
    and treatment outcome, 33
    for youth psychotherapy, 332, 336–338

Models
    definitions of, 144–145
    in psychotherapy, 24–26

Moertl, K., 90

Moher, D., 176

Mondin, G. W., 329

Monitoring
    of experience of treatment, 125, 130–131, 400–401
    probation, 364

Moore, T. J., 200

Morejon, A. R., 367

Morgan, Christiana, 13, 14

Motivation, 96, 334, 342

Motivational interviewing, 119

MST. *See* Multisystemic Therapy

MST Adherence Measure, 370

MTA. *See* Multimodal Treatment Study of Children with ADHD

Mullen, R., 364

Multidimensional family therapy (MDFT), 360, 374

Multimodal Treatment Study of Children with ADHD (MTA), 207, 212, 213

Multisystemic Therapy (MST), 177–186, 364, 370

Munsey, C., 224–225
Muran, J. C., 248
Murdock, T. B., 57–58
Murphy-Graham, E., 185
Murray, E. J., 88
Murray, Henry, 13
Mutual collaborators, clients as, 97
Myth, as common factor, 7, 69,
    148–149, 157

Nace, D., 258
Naltrexone, 398
Narrative reviews, 172–173
National Consensus Statement on
    Mental Health Recovery
    (NCSMHR), 303–306
National Institute of Mental Health
    (NIMH), 224
National Institute of Mental Health
    Treatment of Depression Collab-
    orative Research Program, 116
National Registry of Evidence-Based
    Programs and Practices, 259
Native healers, 158–159
NCSMHR (National Consensus
    Statement on Mental Health
    Recovery), 303–306
"The Necessary and Sufficient Condi-
    tions of Therapeutic Personality
    Change" (Carl Rogers), 6
Negative communication patterns, 117
Negative processes, and therapeutic
    relationship, 130
Negative results, in research syntheses,
    173, 181
Nervous exhaustion, 270
Neurasthenia, 270
New Thought movement, 50, 270
Nicholls, S. N., 200
Nielsen, S. L., 243
NIH. See U.S. National Institutes of
    Health
NIMH (National Institute of Mental
    Health), 224
Nixon, Richard, 272
NNT (number needed to treat), 55
Nonlinearity, in NCSMHR, 305
Nonspecific treatments, 61
Norcross, J. C., 30, 67, 86, 93, 357
Normal science, 25

Norsworthy, L., 257
Norway Couple Feedback Project, 368
Null results, in research syntheses,
    173, 181
Number needed to treat (NNT), 55

O'Brien, C., 363
Obsessive–compulsive disorder, 65
Office of the Surgeon General, 184
Ohio Youth Problems, Functioning, and
    Satisfaction Scales (Ohio Scales),
    342, 375
Okiishi, J., 32
Olanzapine (Zyprexa), 203, 204, 210
Olfson, M., 275
Ollendick, T. H., 170
OQ-45. See Outcome Questionnaire
OQ-Analyst (program), 244–246,
    259–261
OQ Measures Web site, 260
Oregon
    EBTs in, 171
    outcomes-informed care in, 287
Orford, J., 395–396
Orlinsky, D. E., 25, 83–84, 88, 96, 144,
    146, 374, 400
ORS. See Outcome Rating Scale
Orth, U., 249
Osterberg, L., 306
Ostrich behavior, 131
Outcome-informed treatment, 395, 403
Outcome Questionnaire (OQ-45), 243,
    244, 251, 257
Outcome Rating Scale (ORS), 249,
    318, 341–342, 375, 383
Outcomes-informed practice, 286–287,
    289
Outcomes management, 30, 239–262.
    See also Feedback
    and accountability, 241–243
    AKQUASI system, 251–253
    clinical support tools for, 247–250
    COMPASS system, 250–251
    CORE system, 253
    and future of psychotherapy,
        423–424, 426–427
    history of, 239–241
    implementation of, 257–259
    with OQ measures, 251
    PCOMS system, 255–257

Outcomes management, *continued*
  rationale for implementation, 259–260
  and reimbursement, 269–270,
      282–290
  research on, 243–247
  software for, 289
  in substance abuse and addiction
      treatment, 406–407
  systems for, 250–260
  TOP system, 253–255
  training about, 291–293
  in youth psychotherapy, 339–345
Outpatient services, 273, 275
Outsourcing, of substance abuse and
      dependence treatment, 407–408
Owen, J., 369, 372
Ozer, E. J., 87

PacifiCare Behavioral Health (PBH)
      ALERT project, 282–283
Palenzuela, D. L., 367
Palm Beach County, Florida, CDOI in,
      308–309
Panic disorder, 64, 66
Parent–counselor alliance, 371
Parent Management Training, Oregon
      Model (PMTO), 382–383
Parents
  in therapeutic relationship, 331, 336
  in youth psychotherapy, 333–334,
      341–343, 364
Parham, K. B., 367
Park, C. L., 87
Parkinson's disease, 152
Parks, B. K., 144, 400
Participation, of clients, 334, 400
Partners for Change Outcome Manage-
      ment System (PCOMS) system,
      255–257, 286, 341–342
Partnerships, between clients and thera-
      pists, 37
Pasek, L. F., 60
Passive resistance, 340
Pathway thinking, 338
Patient–therapist relationship, xxi. *See
      also* Therapeutic relationship
Paul Wellstone and Pete Domenici
      Mental Health Parity and Addic-
      tion Equity Act, 285
PBE. *See* Practice-based evidence

PBH (PacifiCare Behavioral Health)
      ALERT project, 282–283
PCOMS. *See* Partners for Change Out-
      come Management System
PCT (present-centered therapy), 150
Peabody Treatment Progress Battery,
      342–343
Peer review system, 189–190
Peer support, in NCSMHR, 305
Pekarik, G., 301, 304
Perez, G. A., 372
Perphenazine (Etrafon), 203
Personality, 12
Personality disorders, 85
Person-centered care, 100–101, 305. *See
      also related topics, e.g.:* Client-
      centered theory
*Persuasion and Healing* (Jerome Frank),
      7, 8
Petrosino, A., 185
Pharmaceutical industry
  and mainstream media, 223–224
  research funded by, 210–211, 214
Pharmacology-based paradigm, for
      psychotherapy, xxi–xxiii
Pickrel, S. G., 370
Picture-Frustration Study, 14
Pinsof, W. M., 359
Placebo-controlled research, 61–63,
      211–212
Placebo factors (placebo effects)
  in antidepressant trials, 201
  as client effects, 86–87
  as common factors, 218–220
  in couple and family therapy, 373
  as model and technique factors, 36–37
  and time of trial, 212–213
Placebos, 33, 70, 150, 152–154
Placebo washout, 214–215
Plum, B., 312
PMTO (Parent Management Training,
      Oregon Model), 382–383
PNFCMH. *See* President's New Free-
      dom Commission on Mental
      Health
Policymakers, EBP and, 189
Political correctness, 157
Politics
  and EBP, 189, 357
  in reimbursement, 270–274

Positive alliances, 37
Positive regard, in therapeutic relationship, 123
Positive results, in research syntheses, 173–174, 181, 187
Posttraumatic growth, 87
Posttraumatic stress disorder (PTSD), 58–60, 150
Power, in EBP, 357
Practice-based evidence (PBE)
    evidence-based practice vs., 39
    in youth psychotherapy, 339–345
Practice implications
    of common factors for couple and family therapy, 379–382
    of contextual model of psychotherapy, 156–157
    of EBT in youth psychotherapy, 344–345
    of medical influence on psychotherapy, 71–72
    of therapeutic relationship, 132–134
Precontemplation stage, of change, 128, 129
"Pre-paradigmatic stage," of science, 25
Preparation stage, of change, 128, 129
Preschool ADHD Treatment Study, 207
Prescription drugs, 199. See also Psychiatric drugs
Prescriptive authority, 224–225
Present-centered therapy (PCT), 150
President's New Freedom Commission on Mental Health (PNFCMH), 299–300, 302, 303
Pretreatment change (PTC), 367
Prince, Morton, 280
Privileged data, events in therapy as, xxiii
Probation monitoring, as treatment, 364
Problem drinking, 393
Problem-solving treatments, in couple and family therapy, 362
Process–experiential treatment, 59
Process–outcome research, xxii–xxiii, 374
Prochaska, J. O., 85, 86
Procrustean bed, and therapeutic relationship, 131
Productivity rates, CDOI care and, 310
Project COMBINE (Combined Pharmacotherapies and Behavioral Interventions), 398

Project MATCH. See Matching Alcoholism Treatments to Client Heterogeneity
Prozac. See Fluoxetine
Psychiatric drugs, 199–226
    antidepressants, 200–202, 204–206
    antipsychotics, 203–204, 209–210
    for children, 204–210
    clinical implications of treatment with, 221–223
    and common factors, 218–221
    efficacy of psychotherapy vs., 55
    expenditures for, 275
    flaws of treatment with, 210–217
    pyschotropics, 208–210
    risk–benefit profiles of, 217–218
    stimulants, 206–207
    and therapist effects, 281, 283
Psychoanalysis, 50, 51
Psychodynamic therapy, 115
Psychoeducation, 364–365
Psychological treatments, 53
Psychologists
    incomes of, 30–31
    prescriptive authority for, 224–225
Psychology, evidence-based practice in, 326, 344
Psychopathology, 270
Psychosocial interventions, for children, 218
Psychotherapy, 23–40, 421–428
    accountability in, 39–40
    areas of concern in, 30–33
    clients' participation in, 423–424
    and common factors, 28–29
    common factors in, 9–13, 28–29, 33–39, 422–423
    effectiveness of, 27–28
    efficacy of psychiatric drugs vs., 55
    encouraging developments in, 24–30
    evidence-based practice in, 29–30
    formal consistency in, 7, 11
    growth and diversification in, 27
    history of, 50–54
    history of research and practice in, xx–xxi
    medical model of, 50–53
    model development in, 24–26
    perceived value of, 267–269

Psychotherapy, *continued*
  research- vs. pharmacology-based
    paradigm for, xxi–xxiii
  scientific foundation for, xix–xx
  state of field of, 421–428
  stigma in, 26–27
  therapist competency in, 32–33
  underutilization of, 32
  as viable profession, 30–31
*Psychotherapy Research and Practice*
  (L. Luborsky), xx
PTC (pretreatment change), 367
PTSD. *See* Posttraumatic stress disorder
Publication bias, 174, 189, 201, 206
Public behavioral health care, 299–320
  CDOI in, 307–316
  common factors in, 304–306
  consumer-centered services in,
    302–303
  current state of, 299–301
  and implications of CDOI, 317–318
  and recovery, 303–306
  reformation of, 301–307
Pyschotropics, 208–210

QIPs (quality improvement programs),
  427
Quality Chasm Series, 395
Quality improvement programs
  (QIPs), 427
Quality of Life Scale, 204
Quality of Reporting of Meta-analyses
  (QUOROM) statement, 176, 188
Quantitative analysis, clients' narratives
  vs., 116
Quantum change, 86
Quetiapine (Seroquel), 203
Quinn, W. H., 364, 371, 372
QUOROM statement. *See* Quality of
  Reporting of Meta-analyses
  statement

Radical behaviorism, 144
Randomized clinical trials (RCTs). *See
  also* Clinical trials
  and efficacy of treatments, 381
  of psychiatric drugs, 214–215
  and specificity of treatments, 52, 72
Rational Recovery, 396
Rationale, as common factor, 7,
  148–149, 366, 373

Raytek, H. S., 370
RCTs. *See* Randomized clinical trials
Reactance, of clients, 127–128
Reality, of clients, xxiii
Real-time feedback, 341
Reattribution, 374
Recovery
  in couple and family therapy, 362
  and public behavioral health care,
    303–306
  spontaneous, 86
Recovery-focused services, 426
Reese, R. J., 257
Reflexivity, of clients, 89–90
Reframing, 374
Regence (company), 287, 288
Reich, D. B., 85
Reimbursement, 267–290. *See also*
  Funding
  and behavioral health services as
    commodity, 275–278
  current trends in, 274–275
  increasing levels of, 288–290
  and outcomes management,
    269–270, 282–290
  and perceived value of treatment,
    267–269
  political and economic factors affect-
    ing, 270–274
  and psychotherapists as commodity,
    278–281
  training about, 291–293
Relational bonds, 121
Relational elements, treatment outcomes
  and, 118–126, 132
Relational interpretations, in therapeu-
  tic relationship, 125–126
Relationship, therapeutic. *See* Thera-
  peutic relationship
Relationship factors, as common
  factors, 33
Relative efficacy, 359
Religious commitment, and therapeutic
  relationship, 129
Religious ministers, as healers, 158–159
Remen, Rachel, 113
Remission, spontaneous, 219
Remoralization, 304
Rennie, D. L., 88
Report cards, for clients, 252

Research
    and contextual model of psycho-
        therapy, 154–156
    funded by pharmaceutical industry,
        210–211, 214
    in future of psychotherapy, 427–428
    and medical influence on psycho-
        therapy, 71–72
    on outcomes management, 243–247
    and practice in psychotherapy, xx–xxi
    process–outcome, xxii–xxiii
    on therapeutic relationship, 132–134
    translational, 171
"Research-Based Knowledge as the
    Emergent Foundation for Clinical
    Practice" (D. E. Orlinsky), xx
Research-based paradigm, for
    psychotherapy, xxi–xxiii
"Research Cannot Yet Influence Clini-
    cal Practice" (L. Luborsky), xx
Research syntheses, 172–177, 186
Resilience, 87, 103, 333
Resistance, passive, 340
Resources for Living®, 316
Resources for Living SIGNAL
    system, 282
Respect, in NCSMHR, 305
Responders, early, 91
Response prevention/exposure (RPE), 65
Responsibility, in NCSMHR, 305
Responsiveness, of psychotherapy,
    126–127, 135
Results, in research syntheses, 173–174,
    176, 181, 187
Retrospective feedback, 341
Reviews
    literature, 215
    narrative, 172–173
    in research syntheses, 184
    systematic, 174–176, 188
    utilization, 272–273
Reyes, M., 215, 216
Richard, M., 251
Ricks, D. F., 424
Ridley, C. R., 359
Riggs, D. S., 57–58
Rigidity, and therapeutic relationship,
    131
Risk–benefit profiles, of psychiatric
    drugs, 217–218

Risks, in psychiatric drug studies,
    213–214
Risperdal. See Risperidone
Risperidone (Risperdal), 203, 208–209,
    211, 215, 216
Ritalin (methylphenidate), 206, 207
Ritual, as common factor, 7, 69,
    149–151, 157, 366, 373
Robbins, M. S., 372
Robinson, L. A., 57
Robinson, Maria, 299
Rodriguez-Arias, J. L., 367
Rogers, C., 5, 6, 8, 17–19, 37, 118,
    124, 144
Rønnestad, M. H., 83–84, 374
Rosenthal, D., 61, 63
Rosenthal, R., 28
Rosenzweig, Saul, 3–9, 13–20, 53, 54,
    56, 66, 280, 365
Ross, R. G., 210
Rothbaum, B. O., 57–58
Rowlands, S., 257
RPE (response prevention/exposure), 65
Ruptures in alliance, repairing,
    124–125, 131
Rush, A. J., 279
Rusk, G., 95

Sackett, D. L., 168, 170, 185
Sackettisation, 185
Safran, J. D., 248
Salts, C. J., 367
Samuolis, J., 374
Sapirstein, G., 200
SBHS. See Southwest Behavioral
    Health Services
Schizophrenia, 100
    differential efficacy of treatments for,
        364–365
    MFT for, 359
    psychiatric drugs for, 208–210, 219
Schneider, L., 210
Schoolism, 25
"Schools of Psychotherapy" (Saul
    Rosenzweig), 16–17
Schwebel, A. I., 360
Science
    in foundation of psychotherapy,
        xix–xx
    stages of, 25

Scoboria, A., 200
Search strategies, for research syntheses, 175
Segal, D. L., 88
Selby, C. E., 90
Selection bias, 215
Selective serotonin reuptake inhibitors (SSRIs), 86, 201, 202, 205–206, 216, 217
Self-defeating behavior, 96
Self-direction, in NCSMHR, 305
Self-disclosure, in therapeutic relationship, 125
Self-expression, as client factor, 87–88
Self-generated change, 85–86
Self-healers, clients as, 94–95, 103
Self-help programs, 93–94, 409–410
Sequenced Treatment Alternatives to Relieve Depression (STAR*D), 201, 213, 217, 224
Serious mental illness (SMI), 319
Seroquel (quetiapine), 203
SES (socioeconomic status), drop-out rates and, 367
Session Rating Scale (SRS), 249, 375, 383
Setting, healing, 7, 148, 156
Sexton, T. L., 359, 365
Shadish, W. R., 358–361, 363, 364
Shapiro, D. A., 86
Shaw, B. F., 65, 279
Shear, M. K., 66
Shelef, K., 371
Shirk, S. R., 371
Short-term therapy, 268
Side effects, of psychiatric drugs, 211, 213–214, 216
Signal-alarm cases, 243, 248, 252
Silence, 99
Silk, K., 85
Skinner, B. F., 144
Smart, D. W., 243
SMI (serious mental illness), 319
Smith, L. A., 364
Smith, M. L., 54, 56–57
Smith, Richard, 214
Smith, T. A., 367
Snyder, C. R., 338
Social support, outcomes management and, 247–248

Socioeconomic status (SES), drop-out rates and, 367
Software, for outcomes management, 289
Solovey, A., 95
Somatic discontinuation syndrome, 211
"Some Implicit Common Factors in Diverse Forms of Psychotherapy" (Saul Rosenzweig), 9–13, 16
Sorrell, R., 255, 401
Southwest Behavioral Health Services (SBHS), 307, 308, 310–313, 315, 319
Sparks, J. A., 67, 249, 308, 312, 341, 372
Specialization, by therapists, 278–279
Specific factors (specific effects), xxii, 423
   for depression, 279
   model and technique factors as, 143
   in youth psychotherapy, 326–327
Specificity, of psychotherapy, 51, 52, 60–66
Spending, on mental health treatment services, 274–275
Spielmans, G. I., 60, 329
Split alliance, 372
Spontaneous recovery, 86
Spontaneous remission, 219
Sprenkle, D. H., 365, 368
SRS. See Session Rating Scale
SSRIs. See Selective serotonin reuptake inhibitors
Standardized mean difference, 176
Stanton, M. D., 359, 363, 364
STAR*D. See Sequenced Treatment Alternatives to Relieve Depression
STEP-BD. See Systemic Treatment Enhancement Program for Bipolar Disorder
Stevenson, Robert Louis, 83
Stigma, in psychotherapy, 26–27
Stimulants, 206–207, 217–218
Strain, caregiver, 333–334
Strategic therapy, 359
Strawderman, W. E., 173
Strength-based approaches, in NCSMHR, 305
Strength-based approaches, in psychotherapy, 95–96
Structural equivalence, 62

Strupp, H. H., 25, 133
Study quality, for research syntheses, 175
Substance abuse and dependence
        treatment, 393–411
    assessment-driven and outcome-
        informed, 394–395
    CDOI in, 408
    consumer-oriented, client-centered,
        adaptive care in, 404–408
    EBT for, 401–404
    effectiveness of, 396–404
    family therapy for, 360
    feedback in, 406–407
    flexible continuum of care for,
        407–408
    individualized service delivery plans
        for, 405–406
    outcomes management for, 247
    and self-generated change, 85–86
    for youths, 334, 360
Substance abuse disorder, 329–330
Success of therapy, validity of theory
        and, 9–10
Sue, S., 157
Suicidality, 202, 205, 206, 210
Supershrinks, 424
"Supershrinks" (S. D. Miller, M. Hubble,
        & B. L. Duncan), 290–291
Supervision and supervisors
    and CFIT, 343, 346–347
    in PBH, 314
Supportive counseling, 57–58, 61, 150,
        154–155
Symonds, D., 372
Symptom Checklist-90, 252
Symptoms, extrapyramidal, 209
Systematic desensitization, 63
Systematic reviews, in research syntheses,
        174–176, 188
Systemic Treatment Enhancement
        Program for Bipolar Disorder
        (STEP-BD), 204, 217
System-specific sequence, in psycho-
        therapy, 63–66
Szent-Gyorgyi, Albert, 393

TA. See Therapeutic alliance
TADS. See Treatment for Adolescents
        With Depression Study
Talent, of therapists, 290

Talitman, E., 367, 368
Talking cure, 279
Talmon, M., 90
Target Complaints (TC) Scale, 362
TAT (Thematic Apperception Test), 13
TAU (treatment as usual) controls,
        327–328
Taylor, C. A., 119
TBCT. See Traditional behavioral
        couple therapy
TC (Target Complaints) Scale, 362
TDCRP. See Treatment of Depression
        Collaborative Research Project
Technical eclecticism, 64
Technique
    in contextual model of psychotherapy,
        149–151
    defined, 144
Tedeschi, R. G., 87
TEOSS (Treatment of Early Onset
        Schizophrenia Spectrum
        Disorders), 209–210
Thase, M. E., 202
Thelander, S., 399
Thematic Apperception Test (TAT), 13
Therapeutic alliance (TA), 120
    as common factor, 37–38
    in couple and family therapy, 366,
        368–369
    and placebo-controlled research, 62
    in youth psychotherapy, 335–336,
        339, 371, 372
Therapeutic factors, xxii, 423
Therapeutic relationship, 113–135
    clients' view of, 88–89, 115–118
    as common factor, 10–11, 37–38
    customization of, 126–130
    elements of effective, 118–126
    integrating research and practice for,
        132–134
    parents in, 331
    strategies to avoid in, 130–132
    in substance abuse and dependence
        treatment, 400
Therapist centricity, 131
Therapist factors (therapist effects),
        6, 11, 68
    as common factors, 38–39
    in couple and family therapy, 366,
        368–370

Therapist factors (therapist effects),
    *continued*
    in evidence-based practice, 29
    and feedback, 375–376
    and outcomes management, 280–281
    and psychiatric drug efficacy, 219, 283
    in psychotherapy, 424–425
    in substance abuse and dependence
        treatment, 402
    in youth psychotherapy, 332–335,
        338–339, 346
Therapists
    adherence to treatment protocol by,
        65–66
    cognitive dissonance in, 343
    as commodity, 278–281
    competency of, 32–33
    effectiveness of, 290–291
    expertise of, 92–93
    as key determinants of outcome,
        xxviii
    listening skills of, 97–99
    in measurement feedback systems,
        340–341
    prediction of outcomes by, 261
    resistance to outcomes monitoring
        by, 258
    specialization by, 278–279
Therapy
    short-term, 268
    as single entity, 7
    tool kit approach to, 338
Therapy Assessment Form, for CORE
    system, 253
"Therapy in America" Harris Poll, 26
Thomas, F., 364
Thomas, K. B., 153
Threats-to-validity approach, 175
Time of measurement, for psychiatric
    drug trials, 212–213
Todd, T. C., 363
TOGs (transition oversight groups),
    313–314
Tonigan, J. S., 398
Tool kit approach to therapy, 338
TOP (Treatment Outcome Package)
    system, 253–255
Traditional behavioral couple therapy
    (TBCT), 359, 360
Traditional model of psychotherapy,
    92–94

Training
    about client factors, 98–99
    about outcomes management,
        291–293
    about reimbursement, 291–293
    about therapeutic relationship,
        134–135
    and allegiance, 361
    in CDOI care, 313–314
    client's voice in, 383
    contextual feedback intervention
        and, 342–344, 346–347
    in couple and family therapy, 380
    EBTs in, 170–171
    and feedback, 262
    psychiatric drugs in, 225–226
    in substance abuse and dependence
        treatment, 394, 410–411
Training Institute, 319
Transition oversight groups (TOGs),
    313–314
Translational research, 171
*Treating Drug Problems* (D. R. Gerstein,
    J. Henrick, and H. J. Harwood),
    397
Treatment as usual (TAU) controls,
    327–328
Treatment fidelity, 190
Treatment for Adolescents With
    Depression Study (TADS), 205,
    212, 220
Treatment of Depression Collaborative
    Research Project (TDCRP), 86,
    212–213, 219, 220
Treatment of Early Onset Schizophrenia
    Spectrum Disorders (TEOSS),
    209–210
Treatment Outcome Package (TOP)
    system, 253–255
Treatment resistant depression, 201
Tricyclic antidepressants, 204, 212
Truax, P., 251
Tuason, M. T., 374
Turgay, L., 216
Turner, C. W., 372
Turnover, in PBH system, 318–319
Twain, Mark, 9

UBH. *See* United Behavioral Health
UC controls. *See* Usual care controls

Understanding, communication of, 119
Underutilization, of psychotherapy, 32
Unequal comparisons, in couple and
    family therapy, 363–365
Uniform efficacy, 359
United Behavioral Health (UBH), 285,
    286, 288
Universal applicability, of models and
    techniques, 144–145
University of Rhode Island, 383
Updating, in research syntheses, 176
U.S. Department of Health and Human
    Services (DHHS), 171
U.S. National Institutes of Health
    (NIH), 171, 184–185, 210
Usual care (UC) controls, 327–328, 382
Utilization reviews, 272–273

Vaillant, G. E., 87
Valeri, S. M., 327, 328
Validity of theory, success of therapy
    and, 9–10
Value index, 284
ValueOptions, 288
Vandecreek, Leon, 30
Varhely, K., 60, 325, 409
Variability, client and error, 70
Vermeersch, D. A., 243
Vijayaraghavan, M., 210
Violence
    family, 394
    youth, 170
Vote counting, 173

Wachtel, P. L., 146
Wampold, B. E., 32–34, 37, 38, 58–60,
    62, 63, 67, 84, 92, 93, 149, 218,
    279, 281, 308, 325, 329, 333,
    381, 399, 409, 422
Wang, P. S., 32
Washington State
    EBTs in mental health centers, 171
    outcomes-informed care initiatives
        in, 287
Watson, G., 4–5, 17
Weiner-Davis, M., 367
Weiss, C. H., 185
Weiss, D. S., 87
Weisz, J. R., 327–329, 337, 338, 382
Werbart, A., 97

West, J. C., 119
Western culture, psychotherapy in,
    158–159
Whipple, J. L., 243, 247
Wierzbicki, M., 301
Wilberforce, William, 199
Willman, D., 210
Willutzki, U., 83–84, 374
Withdrawal, maintenance of psychiatric
    drugs vs., 211–212
Wolpe, J., 63
Woods, S. W., 66
Woody, G., 363
Woody, S. R., 170
Work and Social Adjustment Scale, 204
Working alliance, 68–69, 120. See also
    Therapeutic alliance
World Health Organization, 252
World War II, 270–271
Wotring, J., 341
Wynne, L. C., 359

Youth Outcome Questionnaire (YOQ),
    341
Youth psychotherapy, 325–347
    allegiance in, 361
    and alliance, 372
    and antidepressants, 202
    client factors in, 333–334
    common factors in, 331–339
    effectiveness of, 326–331
    future of, 338–339
    measurement feedback system for,
        339–344
    multisystemic therapy in, 364
    practice implications of EBT in,
        344–345
    specific vs. general aspects of
        techniques for, 336–338
    substance abuse and dependence
        treatment for, 398
    therapeutic alliance in, 335–336,
        371
    therapist effects in, 334–335,
        424–425
Youth violence, 170

Zanarini, M. C., 85
Zweben, J., 402
Zyprexa. See Olanzapine

# ABOUT THE EDITORS

**Barry L. Duncan, PsyD,** is a therapist, trainer, and researcher with more than 17,000 hours of clinical experience. He is director of the Heart and Soul of Change Project (http://www.heartandsoulofchange.com), a practice-driven training and research initiative that focuses on what works in therapy and, more importantly, how to deliver it on the front lines via client-based outcome feedback. Dr. Duncan received the Wright State University School of Professional Psychology's first annual Outstanding Alumnus Award for his contributions to the field, and the *Psychotherapy Networker* 20th Anniversary All Time Top Ten Award for the article "Exposing the Mythmakers." He has more than 100 publications, including 15 books, most recently *Brief Intervention for School Problems* (with John Murphy); *What's Right With You; The Heroic Client* (with Scott Miller and Jacqueline Sparks); and the forthcoming volume, *On Becoming A Better Therapist.* He is the codeveloper of the Outcome Rating Scale (ORS), Session Rating Scale (SRS), Child ORS, and Child SRS, measures designed to give clients the voice they deserve as well as to provide clients, clinicians, administrators, and payers with feedback about the client's response to services, thus enabling more effective care tailored to client preferences.

**Scott D. Miller, PhD,** is a cofounder of the Center for Clinical Excellence, an international consortium of clinicians, researchers, and educators dedicated to promoting excellence in behavior health. Dr. Miller conducts workshops and training in the United States and abroad, helping hundreds of agencies and organizations, both public and private, to achieve superior results. He is one of a handful of "invited faculty" whose work, thinking, and research are featured at the prestigious Evolution of Psychotherapy Conference. Over the past 20 years, his presentation style and command of the research literature have inspired practitioners, administrators, and policymakers to make effective changes in service delivery. He is the author of numerous articles and a co-author of *Working With the Problem Drinker: A Solution-Focused Approach* (with Insoo Berg); The *"Miracle" Method: A Radically New Approach to Problem Drinking* (with Insoo Kim Berg), *Finding the Adult Within: A Solution-Focused Self-Help Guide* (with Barbara McFarland); *Handbook of Solution-Focused Brief Therapy: Foundations, Applications, and Research* (with Mark Hubble and Barry Duncan); *Escape From Babel: Toward a Unifying Language for Psychotherapy Practice* (with Barry Duncan and Mark Hubble); *Psychotherapy With Impossible Cases: Efficient Treatment of Therapy Veterans* (with Barry Duncan and Mark Hubble); *The Heart and Soul of Change: What Works in Therapy* (with Mark Hubble and Barry Duncan); *The Heroic Client: A Revolutionary Way to Improve Effectiveness Through Client-Directed, Outcome-Informed Therapy* (with Barry Duncan and Jacqueline Sparks); and the forthcoming *Achieving Clinical Excellence: Lessons From the Field's Most Effective Practitioners*.

**Bruce E. Wampold, PhD, ABPP,** who was trained in mathematics (BA from the University of Washington) before earning his doctorate in counseling psychology (PhD from the University of California, Santa Barbara) is professor and chair of the Department of Counseling Psychology at the University of Wisconsin–Madison. He is a fellow of the American Psychological Association (APA) Divisions 12 (Society of Clinical Psychology), 17 (Society of Counseling Psychology), and 29 (Psychotherapy); a diplomate in Counseling Psychology of the American Board of Professional Psychology; and a recipient of the APA Distinguished Professional Contributions to Applied Research Award. Currently, his work involves understanding counseling and psychotherapy from empirical, historical, methodological, and anthropological perspectives. His analysis of empirical evidence, which led to the development of a contextual model from which to understand the benefits of counseling and psychotherapy, is found in *The Great Psychotherapy Debate: Models, Methods, and Findings*. He is the author of more than 100 books, chapters, and articles related to counseling, psychotherapy, statistics, and research methods and has given lectures on these subjects nationally and internationally.

**Mark A. Hubble, PhD,** a national consultant, has coauthored and coedited several books, including *The Handbook of Solution-Focused Brief Therapy*, *Escape From Babel: Toward a Unifying Language for Psychotherapy Practice*, and *Staying on Top and Keeping the Sand Out of Your Pants: A Surfer's Guide to the Good Life*, and was the lead editor for the award-winning first edition of *The Heart and Soul of Change: What Works in Therapy*. Dr. Hubble is a graduate of the postdoctoral fellowship in clinical psychology at Menninger and formerly served on the editorial review board for the *Journal of Systemic Therapies*. In years past, he founded and directed the Brief Therapy Clinic at the University of Missouri, Kansas City, and was a contributing editor for *The Family Therapy Networker*. Beyond his consulting work with individuals and companies, he is a senior advisor and founding member of the International Center for Clinical Excellence, Chicago, Illinois.